Learning Disabilities in Older Adolescents and Adults

CRITICAL ISSUES IN NEUROPSYCHOLOGY

Series Editors

Antonio E. Puente
University of North Carolina at Wilmington

Cecil R. Reynolds
*Texas A&M University
and Bastrop Mental Health
Associates*

Current Volumes in this Series

HANDBOOK OF CROSS-CULTURAL NEUROPSYCHOLOGY
Edited by Elaine Fletcher-Janzen, Tony L. Strickland, and Cecil R. Reynolds

INTERNATIONAL HANDBOOK OF NEUROPSYCHOLOGICAL
REHABILITATION
Edited by Anne-Lise Christensen and B. P. Uzzell

LEARNING DISABILITIES IN OLDER ADOLESCENTS AND ADULTS
Clinical Utility of the Neuropsychological Perspective
Lynda J. Katz, Gerald Goldstein, and Sue R. Beers

MEDICAL NEUROPSYCHOLOGY, Second Edition
Edited by Ralph E. Tarter, Meryl Butters, and Sue R. Beers

NEUROPSYCHOLOGICAL INTERPRETATION OF OBJECTIVE
PSYCHOLOGICAL TESTS
Charles J. Golden, Patricia Espe-Pfeifer, and Jana Wachsler-Felder

NEUROPSYCHOTHERAPY AND COMMUNITY INTEGRATION
Brain Illness, Emotions, and Behavior
Tedd Judd

PRACTITIONER'S GUIDE TO EVALUATING CHANGE WITH INTELLECTUAL
ASSESSMENT INSTRUMENTS
Edited by Robert J. McCaffrey, Kevin Duff, and Holly J. Westervelt

PRACTITIONER'S GUIDE TO EVALUATING CHANGE WITH
NEUROPSYCHOLOGICAL ASSESSMENT INSTRUMENTS
Edited by Robert J. McCaffrey, Kevin Duff, and Holly J. Westervelt

RELIABILITY AND VALIDITY IN NEUROPSYCHOLOGICAL ASSESSMENT,
Second Edition
Michael D. Franzen

A Continuation Order Plan is available for this series. A continuation order will bring delivery of each
new volume immediately upon publication. Volumes are billed only upon actual shipment. For further
information please contact the publisher.

Learning Disabilities in Older Adolescents and Adults

Clinical Utility of the Neuropsychological Perspective

Lynda J. Katz
Landmark College
Putney, Vermont

Gerald Goldstein
VA Pittsburgh Healthcare System and
University of Pittsburgh
Pittsburgh, Pennsylvania

and

Sue R. Beers
University of Pittsburgh
Pittsburgh, Pennsylvania

Kluwer Academic / Plenum Publishers
New York, Boston, Dordrecht, London, Moscow

Library of Congress Cataloging-in-Publication Data

Katz, Lynda J.
  Learning disabilities in late adolescence and early adulthood: clinical utility of the neuropsychological perspective/Lynda J. Katz, Gerald Goldstein, and Sue R. Beers.
      p. ; cm. — (Critical issues in neuropsychology)
  Includes bibliographical references and index.
  ISBN 0-306-46633-3
    1. Learning disabilities—Diagnosis. 2. Attention-deficit hyperactivity disorder—Diagnosis. 3. Autism—Diagnosis. 4. Neuropsychological tests. I. Goldstein, Gerald, 1931– II. Beers, Sue R.. IV. Title. V. Series.
    [DNLM: 1. Learning Disorders—Adolescence. 2. Learning Disorders—Adult. 3. Attention Deficit Disorder with Hyperactivity. 4. Autistic Disorder. 5. Nervous System Diseases—psychology—Adolescence. 6. Nervous System Diseases—psychology—Adult. 7. Neuropsychology—methods. WS 110 K19L 2001]
  RC394.L37 K38 2001
  616.85′889075—dc21
                                                                                        2001029888

ISBN 0-306-46633-3

©2001 Kluwer Academic / Plenum Publishers, New York
233 Spring Street, New York, N.Y. 10013

http://www.wkap.nl/

10 9 8 7 6 5 4 3 2 1

A C.I.P. record for this book is available from the Library of Congress.

Printed in the United States of America

PREFACE

While numerous books have been written on diagnostic practices and intervention strategies for school-age children, much less information is available for the clinician and educator who works primarily with older adolescents and young adults who meet criteria for a diagnosis of a specific learning disorder and/or attention deficit disorder (ADHD). Many psychologists, including the authors of this book, specialize in the area of neuropsychology. In particular, we have worked with adolescents and young adults who seek evaluations to determine the presence a learning disorder more typically diagnosed in childhood because of the significant negative impact they have begun to experience in their later academic or vocational career. Because they had not been previously diagnosed despite, often times, ongoing concerns of parents and significant others, they come to the attention of clinicians as diagnostic dilemmas in many instances. Comorbidity issues emerge as these individuals enter the young adult years, some of which have necessitated treatment at one point or another. Clinicians who will be sought out to conduct assessments, document the presence of a disability, and offer recommendations regarding treatment/interventions and reasonable accommodations will be required to have a comprehensive knowledge of the various aspects of language based learning disorders, what constitutes nonverbal learning disorders and high functioning autism, and how attention deficit disorders are typically manifest in adults in order to competently address the complex diagnostic and treatment issues raised.

This book is an effort to provide a comprehensive review of what we know about certain of these disorders, specifically, disorders of reading and written expression, mathematics, nonverbal learning disorders (NVLD), high functioning autism, and ADHD, as they manifest in the lives of young adults. It will readily become apparent to the reader that hotly contested controversies surround the diagnostic methodologies employed across the learning disorders (one of which is not even categorized in the DSM-IV) and ADHD. In addition, how to intervene and the effectiveness of any given intervention in the later years of development and maturity are open for investigation. Much of what we know is descriptive in nature as research involving adults has only recently begun to emerge in the literature. As more work clarifies diagnostic issues in childhood and the public at large grows increasingly concerned with academic failures in the high school years and beyond, researchers will be asked to deal with these concerns as well. In addition, just as many students with diagnosed learning disorders and/or ADHD have begun to benefit from special education laws or 504 Plans in their elementary and secondary school years, recognition of the need for ongoing services or accommodations in postsecondary settings and in the work place have been challenged in the courts. The *Boston University* decision as well as several other court cases sent a message to those professionals involved in the diagnostic process, defining to some degree the nature of documentation required for disability status under the law.

It was with these concerns in mind that we set out to write this book. Not only did we want to bring a historical perspective to the subject matter, but we also wanted to document relevant research including that from areas outside of the strict domain of neuropsychology (psychopharmacology, educational psychology, neurology) in order to give as holistic a picture as possible. Our own neuropsychological training and work experiences color our review to be sure, but because we attempted to remain true to underlying values concerning the need for comprehensiveness and ecological validity, we do not apologize for our bias.

The book is divided into five chapters, each one addressing one of the disorders of learning mentioned above. If particular studies pertained to more than one topical area, we made efforts to refer the reader to the more complete discussion of that area. Each chapter is divided into sections dealing with historical perspectives, definitions and diagnostic criteria, incidence and prevalence data, comorbidity studies, pertinent research from neurophysiology, neuropsychology, neuroimaging, and psychopharmacology where appropriate, educational psychology and special education studies, reasonable accommodations in academics as well as the workplace, and outcome data. Obviously, some of the disorders have been less well researched in the adult literature (e.g., math disorders, NVLD, autism), but we attempted to provide as thorough a perspective for the practicing clinician as was possible. We have made efforts also to refer the reader to more comprehensive reviews on particular aspects of the various disorders when appropriate. Finally, the reference list at the end of the book provides an excellent resource in its own right. We learned from each other as we wrote this book; we hope that our readers will have that same experience.

Lynda J. Katz
Gerald Goldstein
Sue R. Beers

ACKNOWLEDGEMENTS

We wish to extend our special thanks to Gladyce Coval, Executive Assistant to the President of Landmark College (one of the authors, Lynda J. Katz) who worked tirelessly throughout the production of this book and who assured the production of our final manuscript. We would also like to acknowledge the contribution of Dr. Michael McCue, who was an early collaborator on much of our own research and teaching in the area of adults with learning disability. We also want to thank our respective organizations, Landmark College, the Department of Veterans Affairs, and Western Psychiatric Institute and Clinic for their support of this work.

CONTENTS

1

READING AND WRITING DISORDERS

INTRODUCTION

In order to address the disorders of reading and writing as they manifest themselves in the lives of young adults, it is first necessary to define the population involved. Defining the population means that we must define the disorders. However, defining learning disabilities has been one of the most controversial subjects in the professional literature and remains so today. We will examine the nature of the controversy and then attempt to establish some consensus as we approach these two disorders from a clinical (neuropsychological) perspective. Incidence and prevalence data will be reviewed in our effort to support the occurrence of these two language based disorders in young adults. Data will be extrapolated from those found in follow up studies of individuals diagnosed with a learning disorder in childhood and survey results from major studies of literacy, transitioning of youth from special education classes, and college freshmen. A review of neurobiological correlates and the results from salient neuroanatomical and neuroimaging studies will be presented as well as issues regarding the use of various diagnostic tools and the utility of neurospsychological assessment in the evaluation of these disorders. We shall also look at co-morbidity, psychosocial issues related to adjustment, appropriate interventions, and the nature of reasonable accommodations both in academic and workplace settings with these individuals. Finally, we briefly review outcome studies and what they may tell us in regard to these salient issues.

DEFINING LEARNING DISORDERS

Educational Definitions

According to Lyon (1996), while only recognized as a federally designated handicapping condition in 1968, learning disabilities represent approximately one half of all children receiving special education services nationally. Ironically, learning disabilities remain "one of the least understood and most debated of the disabling conditions that affect children" (p. 3). Arguments over definition have been continuous from the time that the term learning disabilities was popularized in the early 1960s, with the dominant definition incorporated into federal legislation born out of compromise (Adelman and Taylor, 1986). The Education for all Handicapped Children Act of 1975 (PL-142) provides a definition based primarily on that proposed by the National Advisory Committee on Handicapped Children in 1968 and subsequently incorporated into the Individuals with Disabilities Education Act of 1990 (IDEA) as follows:

> The term specific learning disability means a disorder in one or more of the basic psychological processes involved in understanding or in using language, spoken or written, which may manifest itself in an imperfect ability to listen, speak, read, write, spell, or do mathematical calculations. The term includes such conditions as perceptual handicaps, brain injury, minimal brain dysfunction, dyslexia, and developmental aphasia. Such terms do not include children who have learning difficulties which are primarily the result of visual, hearing, or motor handicaps, of mental retardation, of emotional disturbance, or of environmental, cultural, or economic disadvantage (U.S. Office of Special Education, 1977, p. 6).

Torgeson (1991) wrote that the 1968 definition has at least four major problems. First, the definition does not indicate that learning disabilities are a heterogeneous group of disorders; second, the definition fails to recognize the persistence of learning disabilities into adulthood; third, it does not clearly specify that the final common path involves inherent alterations in the way information is processed regardless of the cause. Finally, the definition does not recognize that individuals with other disabilities or environmental limitations may have a learning disability (LD) concurrently with these conditions.

In summary, Lyon (1996) stated that the federal definition is "virtually useless with respect to providing clinicians and researchers with objective guidelines and criteria for distinguishing individuals with LD from those with other primary disabilities or generalized learning difficulties" (p. 6). In accord with Lyon's earlier statement, Stanovich (1999) has written that the umbrella term learning disabilities does nothing but confuse. "The domain specific disabilities should be treated separately and labeled separately....Comorbidity becomes an issue 'after' the initial domain-specific classification has been carried out" (p. 350). "The logic underlying the development of such a classification system is that identification, diagnosis, intervention, and prognosis...cannot be addressed effectively until the heterogeneity across and within domain-specific learning disabilities and subgroups and subtypes are delineated that are theoretically meaningful, reliable, and valid" (p. 8).

One such domain specific definition aimed at a particular subgroup has been adopted by the International Dyslexia Association (formerly the Orton Dyslexia Society). According to Lyon (1996) the new definition reduces the exclusionary language in previous definitions of LD and dyslexia and defines dyslexia using current and valid research data.

> Dyslexia is one of several distinct learning disabilities. It is a specific language-based disorder of constitutional origin characterized by difficulties in single word decoding, usually reflecting insufficient phonological processing abilities. These difficulties in single word decoding are often unexpected in relation to age and other cognitive and academic abilities; they are not the result of generalized developmental disability or sensory impairment. Dyslexia is manifest by variable difficulty with different forms of language, often including, in addition to problems reading, a conspicuous problem with acquiring proficiency in writing and spelling (Lyon, 1995b, p.10).

On the other hand, it has been observed that there are no clear operational definitions of a written language expression disorder that address all components of the written language domain (Berninger, 1994). According to Hooper *et al.* (1994) writing has been conceptualized as a complex problem-solving process which involves (1) the writer's declarative knowledge, (2) procedural knowledge, and (3) conditional knowledge, all of which interact with the instructional paradigm and the instructor's knowledge of the writing process. Declarative knowledge refers to specific writing and spelling subskills and procedural knowledge refers to the individual's competence in using such knowledge in writing (Lyon, 1996).

Research studies conducted by Poteet (1978) and Houck and Billingsley (1989) suggests that composing problems of students with learning disabilities go beyond the mechanics such as spelling, punctuation, and grammar. Wong, Wong, and Blenkinsop (1989), Newcomer and Barenbaum (1991), and Graham, Schwartz, and MacArthur (1993) report higher-order cognitive and metacognitive problems in this subgroup. The closest statement suggestive of a definition proposes that members of this subgroup are characterized by problems in basic text production skills, knowledge about writing, and lack of ability to engage in writing as a process requiring planning and revision (Graham, Harris, MacArthur, and Schwartz, 1991).

Subtyping as an identification approach

Since the early 1970s there have been numerous studies conducted whose aim has been the identification of subtypes among individuals diagnosed with learning disorders (Boder, 1973; Rourke and Finlayson, 1978; Lyon, Stewart, and Freeman, 1982; Rourke and Strang, 1983; McCue, Goldstein, Shelly, and Katz, 1986; Siegel and Heaven, 1986; Goldstein, Shelly, McCue, and Kane, 1987; Rourke, 1991; Newby and Lyon, 1991; Fletcher *et al.*, 1993; Goldstein, Katz, Slomka, and Kelly, 1993). Subtyping models have ranged from the simple dichotomy proposed by Johnson and Myklebust (1967) between language and nonverbal subtypes to one involving three subtypes as exemplified in the work of Rourke and his associates (Rourke and Finlayson, 1978; Rourke and Strang, 1983; Rourke, 1985). Further, specific subtypes with respect to reading disabilities in children have been identified by numerous researchers (Boder, 1970; 1973; Doehring and Hoshko, 1977; Lyon, Rietta, Watson, Porch, and Rhodes, 1981; Lyon, 1983; Lovett, 1984; Lyon 1985; Lovett, 1987)). For a comprehensive review of the history of the subtyping issue the reader is referred to the work of Feagans and McKinney (1991).

One example of domain specific subtyping research carried out by educational researchers is that of Siegel and her associates (Siegel and Heaven, 1986; Siegel and Ryan, 1988, 1989a, 1989b; Shafrir, Siegel, and Chee, 1990; and Morrison and Siegel, 1991). While initially proposing a classification scheme based upon a reading disability, an arithmetic/written work disability, and an attention deficit disorder, Siegel and colleagues revised their classification system based on patterns of academic achievement such as that used by Fletcher (1985); Brandys and Rourke (1991), and Russell and Rourke (1991) with children.

In subsequent work with adults, (Shafrir and Siegel, 1994) similar subtypes were identified based upon academic deficits (reading only, reading and arithmetic, arithmetic only). The question of an attention deficit disorder was not addressed because of the difficulties in establishing reliable diagnoses with the particular age group in the study. The authors apparently limited themselves to diagnosis solely based upon parent and teacher ratings as are common in the assessment of children. We will discuss the Shafrir and Siegel (1994) study in detail for a number of salient reasons. First, it is one of the few studies with adults spanning such a wide age range while taking into account educational levels (non-postsecondary and postsecondary). Previous outcome studies have differentiated groups based upon educational level, particularly groups serviced through the vocational rehabilitation system and those who are college students and/or graduates. Second, the study is methodologically sound and grounded in empirical research findings. Third, the relevance to clinical diagnostic work is readily apparent.

The study population reported by Shafrir and Siegel (1994) consisted of 130 members in a normal achieving control group, 88 persons in the Arithmetic Disorder (AD) group, 32 individuals in the Reading Disorder (RD) group, and 81 individuals in the Reading and Arithmetic Disorder (RAD) group. The age range of the population was from 16 to 72 years, with all subjects meeting the basic criterion of an estimated IQ score of 80 or more. Subjects in the AD group performed at or below the 25th percentile on the Arithmetic subtest of the Wide Range Achievement Test-R (WRAT-R) and at or above the 30th percentile on the Reading subtest of the WRAT-R. Parallel percentiles were established for the RD group with subjects in the RAD group performing at or below the level of the 25th percentile on both the Reading and Arithmetic subtests of the WRAT-R. A discrepancy criterion was not used as Siegel among others has consistently advocated its irrelevance to the definition of learning disabilities in general and reading disabilities in particular (Siegel, 1988, 1989; Stanovich, 1991).

With both the RD and RAD groups results indicated a deficit in phonological processing, in reading and spelling, and in short-term memory. However, for the RD group the phonological deficit was present independent of educational level, while a visual deficit in reading appeared only in the non-postsecondary group. The authors took this finding to support the view that a phonological deficit lies at the core of reading disability, a view previously reported by researchers such as Wagner and Torgesen (19887) and Stanovich (1988a, 1988b) among others. They go on to speculate that a " higher level of print exposure at the postsecondary level may result in better visual recognition skills for words, and may be a partial explanation for this finding" (Shafrir and Siegel, 1994, p. 131).

In contrast, the AD group did not have a deficit in reading, spelling, or phonological processing and their performance was similar to the NA group on pseudoword reading and phonological processing. In addition, at the postsecondary level a greater distinction could be drawn between the AD and NA groups. Specifically, a deficit in visual-spatial functioning was found in the AD group at the postsecondary level but not at the non-postsecondary level. The RAD group (but not the RD group) showed a generalized deficit in visual-spatial processing across both educational levels. The researchers took this finding to mean that a reading disability alone is not associated with a spatial-visual deficit. And finally, the addition of an education level criterion to the classification scheme resulted in an increase in homogeneity of the subtype groups on Block Design, visual and phonological reading tasks, and the Space Relation Task. "It appears that print exposure may play an important part in acquiring sensitivity to orthographic cues (visual aspects of reading) that are related to visual-spatial tasks" (p. 132).

One of the earlier theory based subtyping studies conducted on reading disabilities exclusively which appears to have current validity was that conducted by Lovett (1984; 1987). Lyon (1996) wrote that one of the greatest strengths of the Lovett subtyping research program has been its extensive external validation (Newby and Lyon, 1991). Lovett proposed two subtypes of reading disability, those identified as accuracy disabled and those identified as rate disabled. The accuracy disabled group were those children who failed to achieve age-appropriate word recognition skills while the rate disabled were those whose deficient performance was related to contextual reading and spelling vs. phonemic analysis. In other words, Lovett's rate-disabled group demonstrated that naming-speed deficits can exist in poor readers without the typical phonological deficits described in most dyslexia research (Wolf and Bowers, 1999). Her work coincides with the view of researchers primarily in the cognitive neurosciences (Rack, Snowling, and Olson, 1992; Wolf, 1997; Meyer, Wood, Hart, and Felton, 1998a; 1998b) who tend to view phonological processes as separate, specific sources of disability vs. the current practice among most reading researchers "to subsume naming speed under phonological processes" (Wolf and Bowers, 1999).

While restricted to the study of pre-adolescents, more recent studies have documented the presence of numerous subtypes among the dyslexic (reading disorders) subgroup. These include studies by Stanovich, Siegel, and Gottardo (1997) and Morris, Fletcher, Shaywitz, et al. (1998) among others. In the case of the work of Morris and his colleagues, seven reading-disabled subtypes were identified. Two were globally deficient in language skills and 4 of the other 5 subtypes displayed a relative weakness in phonological awareness, variations in rapid serial naming, and verbal short-term memory.

This study (Morris et al., 1998) did not yield a subtype in which spatial cognitive deficits were the predominant characteristic. The authors go on to suggest that the failure of previous studies to include measures of phonological awareness accounts for this difference and pointed out that the phonology vs. verbal short-term memory-spatial subtype would easily have resembled the nonverbal/spatial subtypes observed by numerous studies previously. They then suggest that this result "highlights the importance of approaching classification issues in children with reading disabilities from well-developed hypotheses guiding the selection of the classification attributes" (Morris et al., p. 370). Their apparent blatant disregard for the validity of previous research in this regard, including recent work by Wolf, Pfeil, Lotz, and Biddle (1994) and Wolf (1996), and their adherence to the "primacy of the decoding problem, which, with deficits in phonological awareness, appears to be the most salient characteristic of people with reading disabilities" (Shaywitz, 1996, p. 370), reminds one of the statement attributed to Gerald Coles. "If you trace the history of dyslexia research, you always find the same pattern. First, there's a paper or two claiming a new explanation for the disorder. Then replication research ultimately repudiates the initial claim" (Scientific American, 1995, p. 14).

Definitions from a Rehabilitation Perspective: Eligibility vs. Entitlement

A major system dealing with adults with disabling conditions once they leave the aegis of the education system in this country, the Rehabilitation Services Administration (RSA), only began to offer services to individuals with learning disabilities in 1981. At that time a policy directive was issued to state agencies making specific learning disabilities a medically recognized disability (Rehabilitation Services Administration, 1981). The definition then officially adopted by the RSA in 1985 stated:

> A specific learning disability is a disorder in one or more of the central nervous system processes involved in perceiving, understanding, and/or using concepts through verbal (spoken or written) language or nonverbal means. This disorder manifests itself with a deficit in one or more of the following areas: attention, reasoning, processing memory, communication, reading, writing, spelling, calculation, coordination, social competence, and emotional maturity (Rehabilitation Services Administration, 1985, p.2).

In discussing the differences between the two definitions Dowdy, Smith, and Nowell (1992) point out that the RSA definition reflects the position that a learning disability is a lifelong (permanent) disability resulting from a central nervous system dysfunction. In addition, the RSA definition exclusively lists a series of deficits (attention, reasoning, processing memory, communication, etc.) that are then used by vocational rehabilitation agencies as criteria for eligibility. The RSA definition does not include an exclusionary clause for other primary handicapping condition, and it does not reference specific discrepancy criteria as found in the special education identification criteria issued in the Federal Register (1977).

Adherence to DSM-IV Criteria

While the RSA provides a definition for a specific learning disability, diagnoses are the province of a licensed physician or psychologist. As such diagnoses are established using the *Diagnostic and Statistical Manual of Mental Disorders Fourth Edition* (DSM-IV) of the American Psychiatric Association (1994). However, as most clinicians are aware, the DSM-IV separates the category Learning Disorders from Motor Skills Disorder and Communication Disorders (oral language disorders) and uses instead specific domains of deficit that include: Reading Disorder, Mathematics Disorder, Disorder of Written Expression, and Learning Disorder Not Otherwise Specified. Similarly, the *ICD-10 Classification of Mental and Behavioral Disorders* (ICD-10) utilizes specific domains of deficit when defining, classifying, and coding learning disorders and specific developmental disorders of scholastic skills. While diagnostic labels and criteria for establishing a reading disorder or mathematics disorder are similar between ICD-10 and DSM-IV, disorders involving written language skills are classified dissimilarly, as a disorder of written language in DSM-IV and a specific spelling disorder in ICD-10.

According to the DSM-IV guidelines, learning disorders are diagnosed when the individual's achievement on individually administered, standardized tests in reading, mathematics, or written expression is substantially below that expected for age, schooling, and level of intelligence, and learning problems are judged to significantly interfere with academic achievement in these areas.   The requirement for performance that is "substantially below" that expected is "usually defined as a discrepancy of more than 2 standard deviations between achievement and IQ" (p. 46).   Exceptions to the 2 standard deviation rule of thumb may occur when "an individual's performance on an IQ test may have been compromised by an associated disorder in cognitive processing, a comorbid mental disorder or general medical condition, or the individual's ethnic or cultural background" (p. 46).

Thus, while the RSA definition of a specific learning disability does not include specific discrepancy criteria, use of such discrepancy criteria is implicit in establishing a medical diagnosis (required in order to establish eligibility for services) if one is to adhere to DSM-IV diagnostic criteria. Further, since vocational rehabilitation programs are not entitlement programs, "a diagnosis of learning disabilities by a licensed professional does not automatically entitle one to vocational rehabilitation services (Abbott, 1987)" (Dowdy, Smith, and Nowell, 1992).   Additional eligibility criteria require, among other things, that a given disability constitutes or results in a substantial handicap to employment, and there must be a reasonable expectation that vocational rehabilitation services may benefit the individual in terms of employability.   These criteria make it clear that having an academic disability does not necessarily result in a vocational handicap and highlight the importance attached to the special manifestations included in the RSA definition.

Finally, under the Americans with Disabilities Act (ADA) of 1990 and Section 504 of the Rehabilitation Act of 1973, individuals with learning disabilities are guaranteed certain protections and rights to equal access to programs and services.   However, in order to access these rights, the individual must present documentation indicating that his or her disability substantially limits some major life activity, including learning.   The term "substantially limits" means that an individual is either (1) unable to perform a major life activity that the average person in the general population can perform or (2) significantly restricted as to the condition, manner or duration of the major life activity in question, when measured against the abilities of the average person in the general population (29 C.F.R. Section 1630).

The principal purpose of documentation is the establishment of an individual's entitlement to special education and reasonable accommodations in education, testing, and employment.   The documentation must include diagnosis, evaluation of impact, and recommendations. Together they establish the existence of the disability, the areas of affected functioning, and specific strategies and/or accommodations that are made necessary by that disability in school, testing, the workplace, and personal living (Latham and Latham, 1997).

The *Policy Statement for Documentation of a Learning Disability in Adolescents and Adults*, the guidelines for test accommodations provided by the National Board of Medical Examiners for the U.S. Medical License Examination, and the LSAC Guidelines for Documentation of Cognitive Disabilities for individuals seeking accommodations on the LSAT, make clear the requirements for a "specific diagnosis." In the case of the LSAC guidelines, for example, the statement is made: "individual "learning styles," "learning differences," and "academic problems" are not by themselves cognitive disabilities for which accommodations will be granted." With the U.S. Medical Licensing Examination guidelines, the criterion establishing the requirement for a statement of a specific diagnosis of the disability is amplified: "A professionally recognized diagnosis for the particular category of disability is expected e.g., the DSM-IV diagnostic *categories* for learning disabilities" (p.2).

IQ/Achievement Discrepancy Controversy

Although federal law in the U.S. defines learning disabilities in terms of an achievement-ability discrepancy not explicable in terms of sociocultural causes or other medical problems, since the late 1980s and early 1990s studies published on reading disorders in children have cast doubt on the utility and validity of the notion of discrepancy (Siegel, 1988; Siegel, 1989; Stanovich, 1991; Fletcher, Francis, Rourke, *et al.*, 1992; Siegel, 1993). It is the IQ component of the discrepancy model to which the majority of these researchers have objected. Their objections (fully discussed in the work of Siegel [1993], Stanovich [1991], and the Connecticut Longitudinal Study group [Shaywitz *et al*, 1997]) hinge on four basic arguments: (1) The acquisition of literacy fosters the very cognitive skills that are assessed on aptitude measures, thus low scores on the IQ test are a consequence not a cause of the reading disability, commonly referred to as the "Matthew effect" (Stanovich, 1986; Walberg and Tsai, 1983); (2) Findings have demonstrated that the information processing operations that underlie the word recognition deficits of poor readers are the same for poor readers with low IQ and high IQ (Fletcher *et al*, 1994; Stanovich and Siegel, 1994; Fletcher, Foorman, Shaywitz, and Shaywitz, in press); (3) The concept of intelligence does not provide the specific model that explains poor reading but a phonological deficit model does (Share and Stanovich, 1995; Shaywitz *et al.*, 1997; Siegel, 1999); (4) There is an overidentification of children with high IQs and the underidentification of individuals with low IQs by the standard score discrepancy method (Reynolds, 1985; Fletcher *et al.*, 1994; Kavale and Forness, 1995) since it does not take account of appropriate regression calculations.

In line with these arguments, as early as 1992, Shaywitz, Escobar, Shaywitz, et al., reported that reading disability is distributed along a continuum that blends imperceptibly with normal reading ability. They went on to suggest that "the most reasonable approach" (Shaywitz, Fletcher, Holahan, and Shaywitz, 1992, p. 646) to determining eligibility for special education services may be to consider both groups of children with reading disability, discrepancy based and low achievers, as eligible for special education services. However, their suggestion did not take into account any socio-political or federal policy level implications of such an action.

As has been pointed out by Kelman and Lester (1997), the recipient of federal funds must label and categorize students as learning disabled or not; the statute does not allow for judgments that learning disabilities are invariably on a continuum. Kelman and Lester provide an extensive discussion of the conceptual and sociopolitical complexities surrounding the matter of accommodations to university level students, which is a matter of eligibility vs. entitlement based upon a diagnosis of a learning disability. However, theirs is an idealized analysis vs. "the best politically feasible alternative" (p.9). While they are quite critical of Individuals with Disabilities Education Act (IDEA) as an ideal statute with respect to children with disabilities, they "offer no real insight into the question of whether a system that would in fact be likely to replace it if it eroded would be preferable to the current system" (p.9). So much for the pundits!

Wood, Felton, Flowers and Naylor (1991) presented a set of "simple" propositions dealing with the definition of reading disability that remain instructive today. They analogize that the case definition of reading disability is often confounded, at least in childhood, by attention deficit disorder—whose separate cognitive correlates should be removed from consideration. In a way that is conceptually similar to the ADHD confound, IQ or other general ability measures, including vocabulary, can be separated from reading disability itself. While discrepancy formulae are neither the only way to accomplish this nor perhaps even the most rigorous statistical way, it would appear that the isolation of reading alone, and the separate accounting for IQ effects, can both be accomplished by statistical multivariate approaches that assess the separate variance accounted for by each variable. In any case, "Whatever definition is proposed for dyslexia should be demonstrably persistent over time—even from first grade through adulthood" (p. 21).

Finally, a relatively recent survey of departments of special education, vocational rehabilitation, adult education, and various other literacy and job training programs across all 50 states and the District of Columbia was conducted by Gregg, Scott, McPeek, and Ferri (1999). As part of the survey, the issue of discrepancy as a variable and how it was defined by the various state agencies was addressed. Results indicated that 67% of the special education programs surveyed used the term discrepancy within their definitions and 100

% applied the term to their eligibility criteria. Sixty-seven percent of the special education programs used an ability-achievement approach and those agencies relying on DSM-IV categories of disorders (all VR agencies) reported use of discrepancy within their definitions and eligibility criteria.

Following analysis of survey results, Gregg *et al.* (1999) offered suggestions regarding definitions and eligibility criteria policy across state agencies involved with adolescents and adults with learning disabilities. These included: the need to clarify the component constructs of IQ, cognitive processing, achievement, and discrepancy for adults, as those currently established for children may have limited relevance to adult needs; a clearer reflection of the identification markers for adults with learning disabilities as put forth in the DSM-IV in the definitions used by the various agencies serving adults; and support for a "clinical eligibility model" (p. 222), including psychosocial, physical, sensory, environmental, cultural, economic, and instructional variables, and the impact of an individual's strengths and weaknesses as formerly proposed by Brinckerhoff, Shaw, and McGuire (1993) and Gregg (1995).

We conclude this discussion on definitions and diagnostic criteria with the view that since ours is a clinical and neuropsychological perspective, we have adhered to the guidelines provided by the DSM-IV in the specific case materials discussed later on in this chapter. However, we do recognize the current controversies surrounding assessment particularly with respect to the IQ/achievement discrepancy issue, which has been raised most particularly in the studies of children with reading disabilities and most recently with adults.

INCIDENCE AND PREVALENCE

Learning Disabilities in General

Developmental dyslexia (specific reading disability) has prevalence rates ranging from 5% to 17.5% among children (Interagency Committee on Learning Disabilities, 1987; Shaywitz, Fletcher, and Shaywitz, 1994). In addition, learning disabilities represent approximately one half of all children receiving special education services nationally (U.S. Department of Education, 1989). In a later publication, Shaywitz and Shaywitz (1997) reported a prevalence rate for dyslexia of approximately 20% in an unselected school-aged sample comprising the Connecticut Longitudinal Study.

However, establishing the incidence and prevalence of reading and writing disorders in young adults (16-30 years of age) is complicated by the fact that most data collected on individuals within this age group are subsumed under the generic terms "learning disabilities" or "learning disabled". Further, as Zigmond (1990) pointed out, prior to the passage of Public Law 94-142 (1975), the body of literature devoted to adolescents with learning disabilities was quite limited, with even less written on adults.

Estimates of the numbers of individuals people affected by LD range from 5-20% of the population (Gerber and Reiff, 1994; Gadbow and DuBois, 1998), meaning that anywhere from 5 million to 30 million adults have a learning disability.   Of the two and a half million adults enrolled in Adult Basic Education (ABE) and General Educational Development (GED) programs, estimates of adults with learning disabilities range from 20 to 89% (Bursuck *et al.*, 1989; Minskoff *et al.*, 1989; Nightengale *et al.*, 1991).   In addition, a research and evaluation report prepared by the Urban Institute of Washington, DC (Nightengale *et al.*, 1991) states that an estimated 15 to 30% of all Job Training Partnership participants and 25 to 40 % of all adults on Aid to Families with Dependent Children have a learning disability.

Reading Disorder

Results from National Adult Literacy Survey

In our attempts to address the issues of incidence and prevalence rate among a population of young adults, several recent survey reports were reviewed in greater detail in order to determine whether they might provide some useful information.   Among the studies reviewed were the National Adult Literacy Survey (NALS) (Kirsch, Jungeblut, Jenkins, and Kilstad, 1993), the National Longitudinal Transition Study of Special Education Students (NLTS) (Wagner and Blackorby, 1996; Blackorby and Wagner, 1997), a report by the National Center for Education Statistics entitled "Students with Disabilities in Postsecondary Education: A Profile of Preparation, Participation, and Outcomes, (NPSAS) (1999), and the Connecticut Longitudinal Study (Shaywitz, Shaywitz, Fletcher, and Escobar, 1990; Shaywitz, 1998).

The National Adult Literacy Survey (NALS) was the result of efforts by the Department of Education Office of Educational Research and Improvement, National Center for Education Statistics to identify the basic educational skills needed for literacy functioning (Vogel, 1996).   This self-report survey was administered to a national representative sample of 26,000 individuals ages 16 and older drawn from a population of 191 million adults in the nation.   The target sample represented 100.6 million individuals, 48% of whom were males and 52% female.   In response to the question, "Do you currently have a learning disability?", 392 individuals in the target sample responded positively, representing 2.8 million adults (2.9% of the target population).   The age range of the self-report sample with learning disabilities (SRLD) was from 25-64 years, and there was no significant difference in the incidence rate for SRLD between African Americans and non-African Americans (3.6% and 2.7%, respectively).

Slightly more males (56%) than females (44%) were found in the SRLD category (Vogel and Reder, 1998).

Prevalence estimates were then gleaned by comparing the percentage of individuals in the SRLD category in each of the five Levels of Literacy established by the National Education Goals Panel (1993). Whereas Level 3 is regarded as meeting the national literacy goal, five times the percentage of adults with SRLD as opposed to those not reporting a learning disability scored within Level 1, the lowest literacy level. However, unlike previously reported studies where school-aged girls were found to have significantly more severe learning disabilities than boys (Levine and Fuller, 1972, Eno and Woehlke, 1980; Ryckman, 1981; Hassett and Gurian, 1984) differences by gender were not significant. Vogel's (1990) review of the literature on gender differences had found that girls identified as learning disabled were generally older, of lower intellectual ability, and functioned at a lower academic level than boys with LD. However, Vogel concluded her review with the suggestion that the system identified females with learning disabilities in the studies undertaken may not be representative of the female population with LD in general. Further, 2% of the adults in the SRLD category scored at Level 5, suggesting that they had either overcome their SRLD or "perhaps had a math disability rather than a language-based LD.... Yet, they still perceived themselves as having a learning disability" (Vogel and Reder, 1998 p. 166). While this report among many other past studies validates the persistence of learning disabilities into adulthood (Blalock, 1982; Hartzell and Compton, 1984; Bruck, 1987; Rogan and Hartman, 1990; Johnson, 1994) actual prevalence rates for reading and writing disorders have not been distinguished and depend in large part on the work of Blalock (1981, 1982), Johnson and Blalock (1987), and Zigmond and Thornton (1985) who reported that 80% or more of individuals with a learning disability in their studies had reading disabilities.

National Longitudinal Transition Study of Special Education Students

The second major survey, the National Longitudinal Transition Study of Special Education Students (NLTS, 1996), was based on a nationally representative sample of more than 8000 individuals with disabilities drawn from the rosters of special education students from more than 300 school districts across the nation (Wagner and Blackorby, 1996). Data were collected in 1987 and again in 1990 on special education students who were between the ages of 15 and 21 years in the 1985-86 school year. Approximately 55% of the population under study had been classified as learning disabled. Unlike their non-disabled peers, students with disabilities and particularly learning disabilities were more likely to be African American and male. Twenty-two percent of the students with learning disabilities were African American even though African American students constituted only 14% of the general population of students of similar age.

Again, no differentiation was made regarding the type of learning disabilities involved (reading vs. math vs. combined, etc.) in the NLTS report. However, if we are to: (1) agree with the 80% incidence of reading disorders previously established in the learning disabilities literature (Lerner, 1989); (2) take into account Lyon's (1995) statement on the incidence of reading disorders among children with learning disabilities (one in five) based on a review of the most recent scientific findings in the field; and (3) recall that a 6% prevalence rate of LD in math has been reported in children which persists through adolescence (Norman and Zigmond, 1980; Cawley and Miller, 1989), then we must assume that the majority of the students in this longitudinal study had learning disabilities related to impairments in reading.

National Postsecondary Student Aid Study

The National Postsecondary Student Aid Study (NPSAS) undertaken during the 1995-96 academic year involved a nationally representative sample of 21,000 undergraduates who were queried regarding the presence of disabilities. Of the 6% of graduates reporting a disability, 29% said they had a learning disability. These results are similar to those reported by Henderson (1999) in the triennial statistical profile of college freshmen with disabilities where 32.2% of the freshmen students surveyed reported a learning disability (double the figure reported in 1988). Of these students, 78% were Caucasian, 8-10% were African American, 4% were Asian American, and 2% were Mexican American. Caucasian males were over-represented among the group in contrast to students without disabilities (52 vs. 46%) and women were underrepresented (36 vs. 42%). Typically, students with disabilities had been out of high school longer than their nondisabled peers.

Henderson's (1999) survey results were similar to those reported through the NPSAS. Overall, those with disabilities were more likely to have taken remedial mathematics and English courses in high school, less likely to have taken advanced placement courses, had lower high school GPAs, and had lower than average SAT entrance exam scores. In summary, nearly one third of all college students with disabilities reported having learning disabilities. It is inferred that 80% of these disabilities would be related to reading given the incidence figures previously reported.

Connecticut Longitudinal Study

Finally, we turn to the longitudinal data emanating from the work of Shaywitz, Shaywitz, Fletcher, and Escobar (1990) following 414 Connecticut children identified as having a reading disability on the basis of school behavior and objective research testing. While the prevalence of reading disorders was two to four times more common in boys than girls when made on the basis of school identification, there were no significant differences in the prevalence of a reading disability between the genders when the diagnosis was made on the basis of research identification. (Shaywitz, Holford, and Holahan, *et al.*, 1995). These findings persisted well into adolescence, with delayed reading levels between disabled and nondisabled readers remaining relatively constant. There was no evidence that children identified in the "persistently poor reader" group caught up in their reading skills over time (Shaywitz, Fletcher, Holahan, *et al.*, 1999).

Disorder of Written Expression

Few epidemiological studies of disorders of written expression are available in the literature (Hooper, 1994; DSM-IV, 1994) and relatively little is known about the etiology, developmental course, prognosis, and intervention for disorders of written expression according to Lyon (1996). In an early study involving acquired disorders of written expression, Basso, Taborelli, and Vignolo (1978) reported that acquired disorders of written expression occurred infrequently, with a frequency rate of approximately 1 in every 250 subjects. According to Lyon (1996), however, given the high rate of developmental language disorders in the general population (8 to 15%) and the significantly higher rate of reading disorders in particular (15 to 20%), written language disorders could be predicted to affect at least 10% of the school-age population. However, as Hooper *et al.* (1994) have written, much of the research related to disorders of written expression and agraphia to that point in time, employed case study methodology and relied primarily on the study of individuals with acquired brain damage. Authors of the DSM-IV (1994) write that because prevalence studies have focused on learning disabilities in general, separating out prevalence rates for disorders of written expression is difficult at best. However, they conclude that a disorder of written expression is "rare when not associated with other Learning Disorders"(p.26).

   Results from various studies looking at incidence differences between the genders with respect to written language deficits are equivocal (Berninger and Fuller, 1992; Hooper *et al.*, 1994). In addition, Berninger and Abbott (1994) have found that children with LD in writing often present concomitantly with deficits in attention, executive functions, and motivation. On the other hand, Berninger, Mizokawa, and Bragg (1991) and Berninger and Hart (1992; 1993) have demonstrated that reading and writing systems can be dissociated. "As expected, many, but not all, individuals with writing disabilities manifest deficits in reading" (Lyon, 1996).

In contrast to this work, in a most recent publication, Siegel (1999) has concluded that while spelling difficulties can occur in the absence of severe reading disabilities (Bruck and Waters, 1988; Lennox and Siegel, 1993), and while there also may be problems with understanding or producing language, these problems have not been documented as distinct learning disabilities and are often components of dyslexia. The "existence of a separate written language disability has not been clearly established nor is there a clear definition of it especially in the adult population" (p. 306). However, it has been only since the mid-1980s that the study of disorders of written expression has "risen from its status as 'a poor relative of aphasia' (Shallice, 1988)" (Lyon, 1996, p. 35).

In summary, while there is a great deal of variability in the reporting of incidence and prevalence rates among children and adults, it is clear that 80% of individuals diagnosed with a learning disability do indeed meet criteria for a reading disorder. The reasons for the high degree of variability would appear to be related to factors such as methods of identification, assessment strategies, and measures of literacy. In addition, while there appears to be no differentiation in incidence rates by gender, the effects of race and socio economic status are positively correlated with the diagnosis of a learning disability. Finally, there is no reason to assume that the rates for adults should be any less than for children as the chronic nature of the disorder has been well established in the professional literature.

ETIOLOGY AND NEUROBIOLOGICAL CORRELATES

Early Work

It has been said that the investigator who put dyslexia "on the map" in the United States was Samuel Torrey Orton, a neurologist and neuropathologist, who recognized a distinctive syndrome that had symptoms in common with the classical condition of acquired alexia with agraphia (Geschwind, 1985, p.1). However, rather than being accepted by his colleagues in the medical profession his work was taken up by educators who then began to develop methods of remediation still in use today (Orton, 1966; Gillingham and Stillman, 1973). In his report entitled "Word-Blindness in School Children" (1925), Orton compared dyslexia to the aphasias, postulating that the problem was at the symbolic level, and that dyslexia did not imply low intelligence. Orton's findings of crossed-eye/hand preference led him to postulate that the mechanism of the behavior lay in a competition for the perception and memory of letters between the two hemisphere, thus introducing the role of hemispheric lateralization for language as a potential factor in reading disability (Orton, 1937; Geschwind, 1982; Duane, 1983). However, Denckla (1974) was to report later that crossed-eye/hand preference may occur in as high as 30% of the normal-achieving young male population.

Critchley (1928; 1964; 1970) who was conducting studies simultaneously with Orton on the problems of reading in children, subsequently adopted the notion of developmental dyslexia as a medical syndrome. The salient feature of the deficit was an inability to derive meaning from written symbols, as well as problems with directionality of letters, sequences of letters, and "uncertainty of what is right and left on one's body and in extrapersonal space" (Duane, 1983). Later, as president of the World Federation of Neurology, he then succeeded in having that organization endorse a definition of specific developmental dyslexia.

Genetic Research

For at least the past 30 years, genetic studies have attempted to define the nature of the familial contribution to dyslexia (Zerbin-Rudin, 1967). Bakwin (1973) had the largest single twin sample on which reading disabilities had been reported up to that point. And while his study, and those reviewed by Zerbin-Rudin previously, suffered from methodological limitations, a significantly greater concordance rate for reading retardation in monozygotic twins than in dizygotic twins was reported. Further, the observation that dyslexia aggregates in families is nearly as old as the description of the disorder itself, dating back to 1905 (Pennington and Gilger, 1996).

More recently, two methodologically sound twin studies of dyslexia have been conducted, one at the Institute for Behavior Genetics in Boulder, Colorado (the Twin Family Reading Study) and the other at the Institute for Psychiatry in London (Stevenson, Graham, Fredman, and McLoughlin, 1987). The Colorado study began in 1979 and in a 1991 update the investigators reported that "evidence has been obtained to indicate that the correlation between phonological coding and word recognition is largely due to heritable influences, whereas the relationship between orthographic coding and word recognition is due primarily to environmental influences" (DeFries, Olson, Pennington, and Smith, 1991, p. 83). Results obtained through linkage analysis suggested that reading disability is etiologically heterogeneous. Linkage analysis is based on the fact that genes that are close together on the same chromosome tend to be inherited together as they are passed on from parent to child. Twenty percent of the families with an apparent autosomal dominant transmission for reading disability manifested linkage to chromosome 15 but not to chromosome 6. Earlier case reports and family studies had led previous researchers to the conclusion that reading disability was inherited as an autosomal dominant condition (Hallgren, 1950). Subsequently, other studies demonstrated more than one mode of transmission including autosomal dominant, autosomal recessive, and multifactorial inheritance. (Finucci *et al.*, 1976; Lewitter, DeFries, and Elston, 1980). In like manner, linkage to chromosome 6 but not 15 was obtained from data on other families.

Contrary to earlier work that established that clinical correlates of reading disability included immune disorders (Geschwind and Behan, 1982; 1984), no association between reading disability and prevalence of immune disorders was obtained. However, the possible validity of a genetic subtype of reading disability concordant with atopic disorders (allergy/asthma) was suggested. While the cross-concordance analysis was based upon a relatively small sample, the preliminary findings were convergent with those preliminary results obtained from linkage analysis indicating a subtype of familial dyslexia closely linked to the HLA region of chromosome 6, which contains many genes that affect the immune system (DeFries, Olson, Pennington, and Smith, 1991).

Neuroanatomical and neuropathological Studies

With the seminal work of Galaburda in the early 1980s, the neuropathologic basis of dyslexia began to be more fully elucidated. Four consecutive male brains studied by Galaburda *et al.* (1985) showed developmental anomalies of the cerebral cortex, consisting of neuronal ectopias (displaced neurons) and architectonic dysplasias (distortions of the normal organized layering of the cortex) (Rumsey and Eden, 1998). The anomalies, thought to be of prenatal origin, were seen on both sides of the brain, but showed a predisposition for the left perisylvian language cortex.

As ectopias are densely and aberrantly connected with other brain regions, one result of ectopia formation is the alteration of brain organization. One such alteration in dyslexia is the lack of asymmetry in a language-related cortical region called the planum temporale, an auditory area that lies on the superior surface of the temporal lobe. In contrast, in individuals without dyslexia the planum temporale is usually larger in the left hemisphere (Sherman, 1995).

Also reported were developmental anomalies within the lateral geniculate nucleus, a thalamic nucleus through which visual information is transmitted to the cortex (Livingstone, Rosen, Drislane, and Galaburda, 1991). As described by Rumsey and Eden, this structure consists of two ventral magnocellular layers and four dorsal parvocellular layers. While the parvocellular (small-celled) layers of the lateral geniculate nucleus appeared normal in the dyslexic brains, the magnocellular layers were disorganized and the cell bodies within these layers appeared smaller in dyslexic than in the control brains (Livingstone, *et al*, 1991). These findings were consistent with the hypothesis that deficits in rapid temporal visual processing in dyslexia result from a dysfunctional magnocellular visual system. Sherman (1995) goes on to write that the visual processing disturbance could interfere with normal reading just as similar deficits in other sensory pathways such as the auditory system (Tallal, 1976; Tallal and Piercy,

1979; Hagman, Wood, Buchsbaum, *et al.*, 1992) could interfere with the acquisition of phonological skills.

In conjunction with the work of Livingstone *et al.*, (1991), more recently, Stein and Walsh (1997) have postulated a general timing hypothesis. Namely, that rather than singling out either phonological, visual or motor deficits, temporal processing in all three systems may be impaired. They go on to suggest that there is some evidence which seems to indicate that magnocellular temporal processing deficits are not confined to vision and audition, but extend to other systems such as the vestibular and motor systems. "Dyslexics are notoriously clumsy and uncoordinated, their writing is appalling, their balance is poor, and they show other soft cerebellar signs, such as reach and gaze overshot and muscle hypotonia" (p. 151). The cerebellum is a major target of m-type (magnocellular) efferents. They conclude by suggesting that selective damage *in utero* to a particular magnocellular neuronal cell line that plays a major role in temporal processing in all sensory, sensorimotor, and motor systems throughout the brain may occur, resulting from genetic impairment of cellular development or immunological attack.

Neuroimaging Work

According to Bigler, Lajiness-Oneill, and Howes (1998), the first CT (computerized tomography) studies in dyslexia began in the 1970s. But, by the mid 1980s other imaging techniques such as magnetic resonance imaging (MRI), single photon emission tomography (SPECT), and positron emission tomography (PET) became more readily available and clearly outperformed the earlier CT imaging studies in terms of resolution, clarity, and capacity for quantification. This paper and one previously done by Bigler (1992) present excellent reviews of studies involving the use of neurophysiological and neuroimaging techniques prior to the use of fMRI.

Riccio and Hynd (1996) have presented an excellent discussion of the findings of neurobiological research specific to adults with leaning disabilities and dyslexia. In terms of morphological findings, CT and MRI studies have provided evidence that ties deviations in normal patterns of asymmetry to the dyslexic syndrome, with the symmetry in the brains of individuals diagnosed with dyslexia due to a larger right hemisphere, which may be the result of reduced neuronal loss (Galaburda *et al.*, 1985). Differences in symmetry have also been reported with respect to brain regions implicated in language processing (plana temporale, angular gyrus).

Further, results of initial PET and rCBF studies of cognitive functions suggest that reading depends on neural activity in a widely distributed set of specific brain regions. Differences between dyslexics and non-dyslexic controls were found in a number of areas including the prefrontal region (Gross-Glenn, Duara, Barker *et al.*, 1991), left parietal and left middle temporal regions (Rumsey *et al*,

1992), caudate (Wood, Flowers, Buchsbaum, and Tallal, 1991), and the occipital lobe (Gross-Glenn *et al.*, 1991). (The reader is referred to the paper by Riccio and Hynd (1996) for a more detailed discussion of these findings). These results led Riccio and Hynd to conclude that the conceptualization that reading involves a widely distributed functional system, resulting in a heterogeneous group of adults who may be diagnosed with dyslexia. This conceptualization was supported and consistent with the interactive activation model of reading development proposed by Adams (1990), Chase and Tallal (1991) among others.

During the 1990s fMRI (functional magnetic resonance imaging) became available and has been used in studies similar to that reported by Shaywitz *et al.* (1997). Shaywitz et al. report that their neurobiologic investigations are "informed by an empirically supported model of both reading and reading disability....Identification of phonological processing as the core cognitive deficit in dyslexia provides a conceptual template for planning and interpreting studies seeking the neuronal underpinnings of dyslexia" (p. 24). Using fMRI techniques, activation of the left inferior frontal gyrus in male subjects engaged in phonological processing tasks, was found whereas females doing the very same task engaged both the left and right inferior frontal gyrus. Further, when reading letters in a word (orthography) a region in the back of the brain was activated. As the letters form sounds (phonology), the neuronal systems in the inferior frontal gyrus (Broca's area) were activated. As the sound structure of the words was used to get to the meaning of the word (assembled phonology), regions in the middle of the brain, the superior and middle temporal gyrus, were activated.

Here, we again have another example of the rigorous adherence to one particular theory by various researchers. As Stein and Walsh have written, "Although the evidence in favour of the phonological weakness of dyslexics has dominated the scene recently, it does not diminish the importance of the visual perceptual problems that many dyslexics report" (p. 148). In the words of Galaburda, the Harvard University neuroscientist in reference to Shaywitz: "She's wrong, and that's the end of it"...."The distinctions we make about the visual and auditory brain are somewhat arbitrary" (Scientific American, 1995, p. 14).

A chapter by Rumsey and Eden (1998) describes the first PET and fMRI studies of regional cerebral blood flow in dyslexia, investigating both language-based and visually-based abnormalities in men with clear, persisting cases of dyslexia. Their male subjects all had childhood histories of a developmental reading disorder, continued to show at least mild deficits in decoding, and had average intelligence. While their reading comprehension and verbal comprehension skills were good, they continued to perform poorly on measures of phonological processing, including tests of phonological awareness and pseudoword reading.

According to these investigators, results from both sets of studies, PET measures of regional cerebral blood flow during word recognition tasks (Rumsey *et al.*, 1997) and an fMRI study of visual motion sensitivity (Eden *et al.*, 1996) suggest bilateral reductions in task-related activation in the posterior temporal brain regions and nearby inferior parietal and occipital regions. Both sets of studies have identified significant neural correlates of the behavior deficits associated with dyslexia. PET studies of word recognition have implicated posterior language regions. An fMRI study of visual motion processing implicated dysfunction of the transient, magnocellular visual pathway with preservation of "visual association regions subserving pattern processing, thought to reflect the function of the sustained, parvocellular pathway" (p. 57).

Rumsey and Eden (1998) concluded that whether and how word recognition deficits and visual processing abnormalities, which were both accompanied by reduced activation in and near posterior temporal brain regions, are related remains a question in need of further study. "One possibility is that some common underlying deficit in the transient, or rapid processing of temporal information contributes to both categories of deficit" (p. 57). Further, when one combines neuroimaging experimental study results of reading and reading-related processing with those demonstrating a magnocellular visual system deficit, then the superior temporal/inferior parietal areas emerge "as likely candidates for the principal locus of cerebral dysfunction in dyslexia" (p. 57). This hypothesis is in keeping with that postulated by Stein and Walsh in their 1997 paper.

CONTRIBUTIONS OF NEUROPSYCHOLOGICAL ASSESSMENT

Neuropsychological Assessment in Learning Disabilities

Beginning in the mid to late 1980s a number of research studies emerged in the literature relating to the neuropsychological profiles of adults with learning disabilities and dyslexia in particular and the discriminant validity of neuropsychological measures (Finucci, Whitehouse, Isaacs, and Childs, 1984; McCue, 1984; Miles, 1986; Horn, O'Donnell, and Leicht, 1988; Badian, McAnulty, Duffy, and Als, 1990; Felton, Naylor, and Wood, 1990; O'Donnell, Romero, and Leicht, 1990; O'Donnell, 1991; Katz and Goldstein; 1993). Research published in the prior decade (Coles, 1978; 1987) had challenged the construct and discriminant validity of neuropsychological test batteries in so far as they obtained to children with learning disabilities. We will review two of these well-designed studies in some detail as they appear to exemplify what we know about the neuropsychological profiles of adults with learning disabilities in general and reading disabilities in specific and the discriminant validity of various neuropsychological measure in particular.

With respect to the general area of learning disabilities in adults, O'Donnell (1991) compared a group of students applying to an LD college support program matched for FSIQ and balanced for gender with a normal and head injured group. Their average ages were 18, 20.9, and 25.6 years, respectively, and their WAIS full-scale IQs averaged 103.4 for the LD group and the normal group and 101.1 for the head injured group. In addition to the WAIS and WRAT, the Halstead-Reitan Neuropsychological Battery (HRNB) was administered. Cluster analysis was applied to the data resulting in the emergence of five subtypes. Mean test scores for Subtype 1 were in the average range; Subtype 2 exhibited auditory processing deficits; Subtype 3 exhibited spatial processing deficits; Subtype 4 had deficient performance on 10 of the 12 measures (global deficits); and Subtype 5 had language processing deficits. However, all LD deficit subtypes experienced problems with flexibility and sequential processing. It is important to note that no screening for attention deficit disorder was included in this study, nor was it typically found as a rule out in any of the studies conducted during this time period.

Results from the O'Donnell study are summarized as follows: (1) Of the six orthogonal dimensions, three were related to academic achievement. (2) Dimensions subsuming nonverbal reasoning/visual-spatial abilities and attention-response speed were associated with computation skill. (3) The auditory processing dimension was associated with reading and spelling. Additional analysis of the abbreviated Aphasia Screening Test showed that items measuring phoneme articulation but not naming or sentence interpretation items were correlated with reading and spelling (findings consistent with the earlier work of Mann and Brady, 1988; Wagner and Torgesen, 1987). (4) In terms of discriminant function, the test battery correctly identified 93% of the LD group and 100% of the normal groups. (5) The strongest contributions to this discrimination came from measures of auditory processing, language, visual-motor ability, and attention-response speed. (6) In terms of homogeneous subtypes, the auditory and language subtypes were relatively more deficient in reading and spelling, and the global and language subtypes were relatively more deficient in computational skill. (7) Some young adults with LD, but not all, experience socio-emotional problems. O'Donnell concluded by writing that: "The present findings confirm the validity of the Halstead-Reitan Neuropsychological Test Battery in the assessment of young adults with learning disabilities" (p. 350).

Neuropsychological Assessment in Reading Disability

The second study conducted by Felton, Naylor, and Wood (1990) accessed 115 adults between the ages of 20 and 44 years who had initially been evaluated between 1957 and 1972 by June Lyday Orton and for whom childhood achievement and intelligence test scores were available. Finucci, Whitehouse, Isaacs, and Childs' (1984) method of classifying adults according to degree of reading deficit was used. In addition to the administration of intelligence and achievement tests, a battery of neuropsychological measures was utilized including the: Boston Naming Test (BNT), Verbal Fluency Test (FAS), Rapid Automatized Naming Test (RAN), Rapid Alternating Stimulus Test (RAS), the Lindamood Auditory Conceptualization Test (LAC), the Word Attack subtest from the Woodcock Psychoeducational Battery, Prose Recall, Rey Auditory Verbal Learning Test (AVLT), Rey Complex Figure Drawing (CFT), Trailmaking Test (Trails B), and Judgment of Line Orientation (JL).

Consistent with their original hypothesis regarding core deficits in the reading disabled group, the tasks which most clearly differentiated the RD and the NDR subjects were those requiring rapid, sequential retrieval of verbal labels, phonetic decoding of nonwords, and analysis and manipulation of phonemes. When controlling for IQ and socioeconomic status, no differences were found between reading ability groups on measures of memory for visual or verbal material, visual perception, visuomotor speed, mental flexibility, confrontation naming, or verbal fluency. (Felton, Naylor, and Wood, 1990). In terms of diagnosing dyslexia in individual adults, the accuracy of nonword reading is a "potent indicator of a history of reading disability even in subjects with relatively intact single word reading and comprehension skills" (p. 495). They state further that within the average range of intellectual ability, cognitive deficits involving rapid retrieval of verbal labels and the analysis and manipulation of phonemes are frequent correlates of childhood reading disability. They caution, however, that within these broad guidelines, there is evidence of considerable heterogeneity among adult subjects citing the work of Elbert and Seale (1988) among others.

In summary, research has confirmed that there are significant neuropsychological differences between adults with and without learning disabilities, with deficits tending to be somewhat nonspecific. However, when one controls for intelligence, educational background, and some socioeconomic status variables, deficits appear to be restricted to the language domain in individuals with dyslexia (Bigler, 1992).

Assessment of Language Domain Deficits in Dyslexia

Illustrations of Current Theoretical Frames of Reference

The literature dealing with the assessment of basic processes in adults with reading disabilities and most particularly that driven by phonological processing deficit theory appears more frequently in reading-related and developmental/educational psychology journals vs. more traditional neuropsychology literature in the United States. This may speak to the crossing-over and convergence of neurobiological and neuropsychological findings from the field of reading disabilities itself into the educational literature. In any case, the research literature reflects the specific definition of dyslexia used. As described by Rack (1997), in practice one can make a distinction between "broadly defined" and "narrowly defined" dyslexia (p.67). Narrowly defined dyslexia is developmental phonological dyslexia; broadly defined dyslexia is a difficulty in acquiring literacy skills which is related to any underlying specific learning difficulty, not solely phonological processing. We suggest that this rather generalized distinction captures the two current views of developmental dyslexia, which have been applied to studies with adults.

The first theory clusters around the primacy of phonological awareness deficits (phoneme awareness) among the phonological processing skills positively correlated with early reading skills (the others include phonological memory and rate of access for phonological information, i.e. rapid naming of letters, digits, colors, objects. Underlying this theory is the work in the early 1970s by the psycholinguist Liberman (Liberman, Shankweiler, Liberman, Fowler, and Fischer (1977), followed by systematic research in reading by investigators such as Bradley and Bryant (1978, 1983); Wagner and Torgesen (1987), Brady and Shankweiler (1991); Torgesen, Wagner, and Rashotte (1994), and Foorman et al. (1997), among others.

Work by Pratt and Brady (1988), Bruck (1992), and Elbro, Nielsen, and Petersen (1994) has confirmed the persistence of phoneme awareness deficits in adults previously diagnosed with dyslexia as children. However, in the study by Bruck (1992), her data suggested that the arrest in phoneme awareness skills found in children and adults was associated with the failure to use orthographic information when making phonological judgments. That is, in contrast to nondyslexic children, for those with dyslexia, word recognition skill has very little impact on the development of phoneme awareness and on the use of orthographic information. Consistent with the underlying theory, her hypothesis surrounding these results states: "...these data may be consistent with a more general model of the relationship between phonological awareness and word recognition by suggesting that initially dyslexic children encounter much difficulty in learning to read because of pervasively deficient phonological awareness skills. When they eventually acquire word recognition skills, there is little interaction between orthographic and phonological codes" (p. 885). Phoneme awareness skills develop as a function of word recognition skills in normal children. But, the development of phoneme awareness is associated with increases in the use of orthographic information when making phonological judgments (Bruck, 1992). Thus, coming from a broader view of dyslexia one may have reached another conclusion than that reached by this investigator Mattis, 1978; Ehri, 1980; Corcos and Willion, 1993; Willows, Kruk, and Corcos, 1993; Roberts and Mather, 1997). This view includes orthographic dyslexia (a problem with the acquisition of decoding or encoding skills that is caused by difficulty with rapid and accurate formation of word images in memory, Roberts and Mather, 1997). However, limited consensus exists with respect to the measurement and definitional operation of orthographic processing (Olson, Forsberg, Wise and Rack, 1994) despite the earlier work of Boder (1973) and Boder and Jarrico (1982) and the electrophysiological studies which appeared to validate the subtyping (Flynn and Deering, 1989).

The second theoretical cluster is exemplified in the work of Wolf (1982, 1991a, 1991b, 1997). As the reader may recall, Wolf (1991a) would support the notion that rapid naming-speed deficits can be validly separated from the phonological awareness variable. In addition, Wolf and Bowers (1999) propose an alternative conceptualization of the developmental dyslexias, the "double-deficit hypothesis" in which they argue that phonological deficits and processes underlying naming-speed deficits represent two separable sources of reading dysfunction. Their work thus far has been limited to children and they have in place a study testing the differential treatment effects of a more comprehensive model of fluency-based reading intervention, which is a direct outgrowth of the double-deficit hypothesis. Wolf and Bower's (1999) summary remarks prove noteworthy for clinicians involved in the diagnosis and treatment of individuals with reading disabilities.

> Whether either of our speculative hypotheses about the relationships connecting naming speed to reading will ultimately prove correct, the cumulative evidence ... challenges researchers to create an understanding of reading disabilities that is no longer restricted to dyslexic readers who are defined largely by phonological deficits.... A final cautionary note, however, is critical to restate. The history of dyslexia research, the well-known heterogeneity of dyslexic children, and the very complexity of the reading process argue against any single unifying explanation for reading breakdown (p. 432).

Applying Experimental Tasks to the Assessment of Adults

In summary, one of the few salient pieces of recent research that we were able to locate linking specific assessment strategies with adults to the most current causal relationship theories addressed in the reading disability literature was that of Gottardo, Siegel, and Stanovich (1997). While previous work by Bruck (1990) and others has primarily been concerned with establishing the continued presence of phonological awareness deficits in adults with reading disabilities, the relationships between phonological deficits and more general cognitive abilities investigated in children remain largely unexplored in the adult literature according to Gottardo and colleagues. These investigators sought to establish whether phonological awareness remains a unique predictor of reading ability when controlling for syntactic processing.

The battery used (Gottardo, Siegel, and Stanovich, 1997) required 2.5 hours of administration time and consisted of the Reading subtest from the WRAT-R (Jastak and Wilkinson, 1984), the Word Identification and Word Attack subtests from the Woodcock Reading Mastery Test (Woodcock, 1987), the Nelson-Denny Reading Test (Brown, Bennett, and Hanna, 1981), and the Block Design, Vocabulary, and Digit Span subtests from the WAIS-R (Wechsler, 1981). Listening comprehension was assessed via the listening comprehension subtest from the Wechsler Individual Achievement Test (Wechsler, 1992). Experimental tasks were utilized to assess working memory, syntactic processing, phonological processing skills, and pseudoword repetition. Phonological processing skills were measured via the Auditory Analysis Test (AAT) (Rosner and Simon, 1971). This instrument measures syllable and phoneme deletion performance, and a modified Pig Latin Test (Pennington *et al.*, 1990).

Results of this study comparing poor readers (reading at or below the 25th percentile on the WRAT-R word recognition test) and average readers (reading at or above the 30th percentile on the same test), with a mean age of 33 years and nonverbal IQ scores within the average range i.e. Scaled score > than 7 on the Block Design subtest of the WAIS-R, demonstrated that adults with reading disabilities performed significantly worse on all the standardized achievement tests (reading and listening comprehension) and on the experimental measures of syntactic processing, phonological processing, pseudoword repetition, and on the recall component of the working memory task. Using hierarchical regression analysis, both the AAT (phoneme deletion measure) and WAIS-R Vocabulary scores were found to be "strong unique statistical predictors" of raw scores on the word reading test (Gottardo, Siegel, and Stanovich, 1997, p. 50). However, the Pig Latin task appeared to be a stronger predictor of non-word reading ability than was phoneme deletion. The investigators suggested that performance on the Pig Latin task, which requires deleting a phoneme followed by blending that phoneme with a new syllable, may have more processes in common with novel word decoding than a simpler phoneme deletion task. "Given that verbal working memory ability was statistically controlled in these analyses, it is unlikely that performance differences on these tasks are solely the result of differences in memory load" (p. 52).

In terms of an assessment battery for adults, Gottardo, Siegel, and Stanovich (1997) recommended including a measure of phonological processing (phoneme deletion task or the modified Pig Latin task), even though normative scores for these tasks are not available for adults as well as a measure of explicit knowledge of vocabulary such as the WAIS-R Vocabulary score. They also conclude that an individual's level of reading performance may best determine the phonological processing measure to use in the assessment process.

The Comprehensive Test of Phonological Processing

Since the writing of the Gottardo *et al.* study (1997), Wagner, Torgesen and Rashotte (1999) have published the Comprehensive Test of Phonological Processing (CTOPP), the subtests of which "represent refined versions of experimental tasks we devised over the past decade of research..." (CTOPP Examiner's Manual, 1999, p. vii). The authors go on to define phonological processing as a kind of auditory processing that is most strongly related to mastery of written language and clearly implicated as the "most common cause of reading disabilities or dyslexia" (p.2). Three kinds of phonological processing are deemed relevant to the mastery of written language: phonological awareness, phonological memory, and rapid naming. The CTOPP was developed for individuals between the ages of 5-0 and 24-11, thus its utility in the evaluation of adolescents and adults. There are six core subtests and six supplemental subtests with composite scores derived from them. The various subtests include: Elision ("Say bold without saying /b/"); Blending Words ("What word do these sounds make?"); Sound Matching ("Which word starts with the same sound as pan? Pig, hat, or cone?"); Memory for Digits; Nonword Repetition; Rapid Color Naming; Rapid Object Naming; Rapid Digit Naming; Rapid Letter Naming; Blending Nonwords ("What made-up word do these sounds make: nim-by?"); Segmenting Words; Segmenting Nonwords; and, Phoneme Reversal ("Ood", say "ood"; now say "ood" backwards").

An audiotape accompanies the test manual for standard of administration of a number of the subtests, practice items are presented for each subtest, and the administration time is generally about 30 minutes. It is only necessary to administer the core subtests in order to arrive at composite scores in Phonological Awareness, Phonological Memory, and Rapid Naming. Grade equivalent scores, percentiles, and standard scores conforming to those used with the various Wechsler scales are provided. As would be expected, a comprehensive discussion of norming procedures, demographics, and validity and reliability studies are presented in the manual as well.

Finally, while no measures assessing writing skills in adults exist, the Test of Written Language-3 (TOWL-3), which is normed on high school seniors, is still useful with college age young adults if one takes into account a degree of score inflation. The strength of the TOWL-3 is comprehensiveness as it covers both contrived and spontaneous writing. For a more detailed discussion of both formal and informal means of assessing writing skills in adolescents in particular, the reader is referred to the chapter by Wong (1996).

Selection of a Comprehensive Assessment Battery

We will not enter into a discussion of "the" appropriate assessment battery for use by clinicians. This issue is one that a competent professional should be dealing with on a daily basis, one that is driven by a solid knowledge base, consistent with standards of excellence and ecological validity, and grounded in ethics of practice. Further, the chapter by Beers (1998) provides a comprehensive discussion of a battery of neuropsychological and ancillary measures that were used to diagnose learning disabilities in a college age population and that were useful also in delineating the strengths and weaknesses in these students for the purposes of educational accommodations (Beers, Goldstein, and Katz, 1994). Similar approaches to neuropsychological assessment with adults seeking services from state vocational agencies have been previously documented by McCue, Katz, and Goldstein (1985), McCue (1994), and Michaels, Lazar, and Risucci (1997).

Comorbidity

There is one caveat to our disclaimer regarding the selection of an assessment battery with young adults. This is the necessity to select measures that recognize the prevalence of co-morbid disorders along with a reading and/or writing disorder. Among the various psychiatric disorders, the one with the highest rate of comorbidity with learning disabilities is attention-deficit hyperactivity disorder. Three to five percent of all school aged children are diagnosed with ADHD (American Psychiatric Association, 1987), with estimates of comorbidity reported in between 20 to 50% of children with ADHD. Also, some 30 to 70% of children with learning disabilities will experience ongoing symptoms of comorbid attention deficit disorder as they enter into adulthood (Weiss, Hechtman, Milroy, and Perlman, 1985; Barkley, Fischer, Edelbrock, and Smallish, 1990; Barkley, 1990; Bellak and Black, 1992).

In addition, Bruck (1986), in a review of the literature related to the social and emotional adjustment of children with learning disabilities, found that they were more likely to exhibit increased levels of anxiety, withdrawal, depression, and low self-esteem compared with their peers without learning disabilities. Hoffman *et al.* (1987) in their survey of adults with learning disabilities found that 13% had previously received therapy; 9% were currently receiving assistance from a counselor, and 5% had been in a mental hospital or psychiatric ward. McGuire, Hall, and Litt (1991) reported that approximately 21% of the 40 students with learning disabilities in their study at the University of Connecticut were currently receiving personal counseling (Price, Johnson, and Evelo, 1994). In a more recent review, Bender, Rosenkrans, and Crane (1999) reported that in the majority of studies they reviewed, students with learning disabilities demonstrated increased levels of depression compared to those without disabilities. Finally, since both learning disabilities and attention-deficit hyperactivity disorder (ADHD) maintain a high degree of comorbidity with other psychiatric disorders such as depression, conduct disorder in children, anxiety disorder, substance abuse, and Tourette's syndrome (Hooper and Olley,

1996), every comprehensive assessment should include a well-structured clinical interview and measures to rule out the co-existence of these other major disorders of mood and behavior.

INTERVENTION STRATEGIES AND REASONABLE ACCOMMODATIONS

Postsecondary Educational Settings

Ross-Gordon (1989) categorized intervention strategies for adults with learning/reading disabilities according to the goals driving the various models. These include (1) basic skills remediation, (2) subject-area tutoring, such as preparation for the General Educational Development Test (GED); (3) compensatory modification; that is a commitment to changing the environment or conditions under which learning takes place or helping the adult learner develop alternative means of accomplishing a goal; (4) cognitive or learning strategies training (learning to learn); (5) instruction in survival skills; and (6) vocational exploration and training.   We will limit our discussion of intervention strategies and accommodations around the issues of remediation, strategies training, and accommodations as they encompass the major approaches in the educational arena, whether provided through a tutorial model or in a group setting.

Remediation

The goal of remedial instruction for adults with reading disabilities is to help them to acquire reading skills that parallel those of their nondisabled peers. Regardless of the specific methodology employed, research in reading instruction based upon work with children would suggest that instruction must be more explicit and comprehensive, more intensive, and more supportive, both emotionally and cognitively (Torgesen, 1998). It would appear that these same guidelines should apply to adults as well. Even though adult basic education professionals involved in literary programs might differ from professionals in the reading disabilities field with respect to the definition of learning disabilities (Ross and Smith, 1990), common to both groups are core principles that include the importance of a trusting adult-to-adult, client-teacher relationship and the use of a variety of techniques and materials, particularly materials relevant to the life situations of adults (Ross-Gordon, 1996). In general, remediation efforts focus on those deficits known to be associated with reading disability while building on strengths.

Direct instruction in phonics and phonological awareness are two such methods. Explicit phonics training programs do not include specific training in phonological awareness, per se.   Clark and Urhy (1995) defined phonics as low level rote knowledge of the association between letters and sounds and phonological awareness as including a higher level metacognitive understanding of word boundaries within spoken sentences, of syllable boundaries in spoken words, and how to isolate phonemes and establish their location within syllables and words.

Reading remediation programs based on explicit phonics include the Orton-Gillingham approach (Gillingham and Stillman,1973), Alphabetic Phonics (Cox, 1985), Recipe for Reading (Traub and Bloom, 1975), and the Wilson Reading System (Wilson, 1988).   Among these, the Wilson Reading System is one of the few remedial programs developed specifically for adolescents and adults with dyslexia.   It, like many of the other programs listed above, is based on Orton-Gillingham principles, and as such is a multisensory, synthetic approach to teaching reading and writing (Church, Fessler, and Bender, 1998).

In terms of specific instructional approaches based upon the phonological awareness paradigm, Auditory Discrimination in Depth (ADD) was developed by Charles and Pat Lindamood (1975).   The aim of this program is to teach auditory conceptualization skills basic to reading and spelling.   It can be used with adults who fail to read and spell successfully because of a failure to acquire phonemic analysis skills. In a well-controlled remediation study comparing both an Embedded Phonics approach and an adaptation of ADD (Phonological Awareness Plus Synthetic Phonics) with 8 to 11 year old children, children in both groups moved from substantially below average in performance on measures of alphabetic reading into the average range.   At the end of the instruction period, a smaller of proportion of children in the ADD group remained substantially impaired (> one standard deviation below average) in alphabetic reading accuracy (9 vs. 26%). However, follow-up data were not yet available at the time of this writing to answer questions regarding the impact of stimulating alphabetic reading skills on subsequent growth in orthographic reading ability (Torgesen, 1998).   In the words of Torgesen: "Phonetic reading skills are probably a necessary but not sufficient cause of growth in sight word reading ability....We still do not have solid research evidence that explicitly phonetic methods produce greater gains in comprehension than those emphasizing whole word, or context oriented instruction" (p. 216).

Also in line with remediation interventions, in a recent study of college students from a technical institute and a western Canadian university, Leong (1999) was able to demonstrate quantitative and qualitative differences in processing morphological words and letter strings between students identified with reading disabilities and age matched contrast groups.   These results are in contrast to those reported by Bruck (1993) in her study with college students. However, the finding of deficits in rapidity of morphological as well as phonological processing, a previously well established finding, may have relevance in terms of intervention strategies.   Leong goes on to suggest that an approach to utilize with older learners is one that promotes systematic and explicit teaching of word knowledge and spelling based on morphological structure, word origin, and productive rules. "This approach emphasizes the interrelation of symbol-sound correspondences, syllable and morpheme patterns, and layers of language of Anglo-Saxon, Latin, and Greek origin (words of Greco-Latin origin occurring much more frequently in science texts)" (p. 236).

Remedial strategies directed specifically at spelling disorders have been addressed by Moats (1983; 1993a; 1993b; 1994). Her research has included high school level students diagnosed with dyslexia and she has described the nature of the persistent phonological and morphological spelling errors most typical of the population under study. In her text *Spelling Development, Disability, and Instruction* (1995) she details the elements essential to the remediation and teaching of spelling. Moats comments that "Adolescents and adults often view themselves as hopeless cases if they have spelling disabilities, especially if prior instruction has been haphazard or linguistically uninformed. Many of them, however, can make significant improvement if their disabilities are addressed systematically, sequentially, and logically over a sustained period of time" (p.107).

Finally, work by Klein and Hecker (1994) documents the use of kinesthetic and spatial strategies to teach essay writing to both college level visual thinkers and students formally diagnosed with dyslexia. In both cases models of how ideas relate w;re captured by the use of Tinkertoys, Legos, and colored pipe cleaners as well as choreographing ones ideas through whole body movement.

Strategy Training (Metacognitive Approaches)

A shift away from purely remedial models took place in the secondary schools in the late 1980s, based upon the work of educational researchers such as Palincsar and Brown (1984), Deshler and Schumaker (1986), McTighe and Lyman (1988). Others (Jones, 1988) were applying strategy instruction to text learning in the public schools and in the U.S. Army. These various strategy training approaches (e.g. reciprocal teaching, specific strategy procedures for teaching writing skills, word identification and paraphrasing, error monitoring and comprehension, and cognitive mapping) rely heavily on the individual student's ability to learn how and when to apply a specific problem solving strategy. Underlying the strategy training approach is an understanding among educational researchers that there are commonalities among individuals with a learning/reading disability. These include (1) difficulty organizing information on their own (especially abstract information), (2) bringing limited background knowledge to many academic activities, and (3) the requirement of feedback and practice to retain abstract information (Gersten, 1998).

Built into most of the strategic learning models is the notion that teachers and instructional materials need to be explicit about what is to be learned rather than "leaving it to learners to make inferences from experiences that are unmediated by such help" (Cazden, 1992, p.111). According to Gersten (1998), the principles of explicit instruction include the provision of a range of examples to exemplify a concept, models of proficient performance, experiences for student explanation of the how and why of decision making, frequent feedback on quality of performance, and adequate practice and activities that are interesting and engaging. These principles are operationalized through a series of cognitive strategies including procedural prompts, sometimes labeled scaffolds (Harris and Pressley, 1991; MacArthur, Schwartz, Graham, et al., 1996). These are defined as a series of questions and/or simple outlines of important structures (e.g., story grammar elements) that are used on a daily basis in the teaching environment. Additionally, cognitive approaches which are based on the precepts of explicit instruction include anchored instruction (linking explicitly taught academic concepts to authentic problem solving) and peer tutoring (Fuchs, Fuchs, Mathes, and Simmons, 1997). Finally, what all of these approaches have in common, according to Gersten, are two other critical aspects of cognitive strategy instruction. The first is the development of routine, or the "virtually automatic use of strategies" (p. 165), and the second is "an understanding of where and how to use it (metacognitive knowledge)" (Harris and Pressley, 1991, p. 398).

Reciprocal Teaching (Palincsar and Brown, 1984) has been used through the grade schools years and into college. It is deemed useful for students who have average reading decoding skills but below average comprehension. Four strategies are employed: summarizing, forming of potential test questions, clarifying ambiguities, and predicting. This intervention uses both media and materials and does not require extensive teacher training. The instructor initiates the dialoguing technique, which is gradually assumed by the students (Westberry, 1994). Hart and Speece (1998) evaluated the effectiveness of reciprocal teaching in a group of students at risk for academic failure in a community college setting, finding a positive effect for this structured reading comprehension approach. Their study was limited, however, in that the comparison condition was a nonreading intervention.

On the other hand, another approach, the Strategies Intervention Model (SIM), while validated by many researchers and applied in postsecondary settings, requires staff training as student gains are highly correlated with the level of training staff received who implement the program (Deshler and Schumaker, 1986; Deshler and Lenz, 1989). Two of the most widely used of the cognitive strategies developed by the Institute for Research in Learning Disabilities at the University of Kansas include COPS (Capitalization, Overall appearance, Punctuation, Spelling), a strategy for error monitoring in writing, and Multipass, a strategy aimed at enhancing reading comprehension (Schumaker, Deshler, Alley, Warner, and Denton, 1982).

Multipass is an adaptation of the SQ3R method developed by Robinson (1946) as a system for students to apply to their textbook chapters. Essentially the SQ3R method involves a quick survey (S) of the chapter, a second pass wherein subtitles are turned into questions (Q), reading to locate answers to the questions (R1), reciting and making notes of the answers (R2), and reviewing of the material (R3). The majority of the studies involving use of this stragegy have been with college students in general. The Kansas group adapted the strategy for high school level students with learning disabilities in particular.

While Berninger and her associates (Berninger, Mizohawa, and Bragg; 1991; Abbott and Berninger, 1993; Berninger, 1994) have written extensively on the diagnosis and remediation of writing disabilities in children, only more recently has the process of witing development been addressed in older individuals (Berninger, 1996). However, metacognitive and cognitive approaches have been used extensively in teaching writing to adolescents and postsecondary students with learning disabilities (Schumaker, Nolan, and Deshler, 1985; Wong, Wong, and Blenkinsop, 1989; Englert and Mariage, 1991; Graham, Schwartz, and MacArthur, 1993; Wong, 1996). Schumaker et al. (1985) developed the error monitoring strategy known as COPS. Wong and her associates used writing strategies that contained both cognitive and metacognitive components to teach the planning, writing, and revising of reportive, persuasive, and compare and contrast essays (Wong, Butler, Ficzere, et al., 1994; Wong, Butler, Ficzere, and Kuperis, 1996; 1997).

Gander and Shea [1998] have written an excellent chapter on the developmental writing classroom at the postsecondary level that incorporates strategies developed for individuals with writing disorders whether due to a specific learning disability or ADHD [at Landmark College in Putney, Vermont]. Their approach to writing instruction is one that incorporates both diagnostic and prescriptive components with particular emphasis on "fundamental neurocognitive processing...such as attention or memory" (p. 65) as well as an "accurate description of writing as a human activity that involves affective, social and linguistic elements" (p.65). They detail a framework for diagnosing writing problems as well as a thorough discussion of process-based instruction. A workbook entitled "Practical Strategies for Teaching Writing: Integrating Process, Form, and Student Metacognition" (Glennon and Kipp, 1997) is also available for those interested specifically in writing strategies with young adults and older students with disorders of written expression.

In summary, while no one intervention strategy has been found to meet the needs of young adults with reading and writing disorders, a series of overall techniques has been delineated (Ross, 1987; 1988; Clearinghouse on Adult Education and Literacy, 1989; Ross-Gordon, 1989) that are applicable across intervention models. These are summarized below.

- Assess individual learning styles and teach to the stronger modality or style
- Use multisensory techniques
- Create opportunities for concrete and experiential learning
- Give frequent, positive, and explicit feedback
- Teach transferable strategies (SQ3R, etc.)
- Teach memory techniques such as chunking and mnemonics
- Discuss cross-situational applications of strategies
- Use organizational techniques (color coding, margin noting, planning tools)
- Use compensatory techniques as needed

Compensatory Strategies: Assistive Technologies

Since the enactment of the Technology-Related Assistance Act of 1988 (P.L. 100-407), the use of technology to enhance the lives of individuals with disabilities has gained increased attention both in terms of research and public monies devoted to service. According to the Act, an assistive technology device is any item, piece of equipment, or product system that is used to increase, maintain, or improve the functional capabilities of individuals with disabilities. And while much attention has been drawn to its use with individuals with physical and/or sensory impairments, application of assistive technologies in the educational or work environments for individuals with learning disabilities has only recently begun to be addressed in the professional literature (Hebert and Murdock, 1994; Raskind, 1995; McNaughton, Hughes, and Clark, 1997; Raskind and Higgins, 1998; De La Paz, 1999; MacArthur, 1999), with most recent work conducted primarily with younger children.

Those assistive technologies that have been applied specifically to reading and written language disorders include word processing, spell checking, proofreading programs, outlining/brainstorming programs (e.g., Inspiration[R]), abbreviation expanders, speech recognition, speech synthesis/screen reading programs (e.g. Kurzweil Reader), word prediction, and variable speech-control tape recorders. Among these technologies, one of the earliest to impact the lives of individuals with reading disorders was Recordings for the Blind & Dyslexic (RFB&D). Created in 1948 for blinded World War II veterans who wanted to realize the benefits of the G.I. Bill (Kelly, 1998), the RFB&D has a tape library of more than 77,000 titles ranging from kindergarten through graduate school. The word "dyslexic" was added to its name in 1995, reflecting the increasing demand by individuals with learning disabilities for access to books on tape, currently 62% of its membership (Kelly, 1998).

More recently, RFB&D and the American Printing House for the Blind are producing books on discs, which make it possible for individuals with reading disorders to listen to text by means of a speech synthesis system (Raskind and

Higgins, 1998). OCR (Optical Character Recognition) systems permit the direct inputting of printed material into a computer by means of a scanner. Once scanned, the material can be read back by the user by means of a speech synthesis/screen-reading system. These systems can either be stand alone or are PC-based and have been developed by companies such as Xerox (Bookwise), Arkenstone (Open Book), and Kurzwweil (Omni) specifically for individuals with learning disorders. These systems provide the advantage of allowing the reader to highlight salient materials in the text and afterward produce a written outline of the highlighted materials. At the same time the reader can margin note while reading along with the speech synthesizer.

Elkind (1998) conducted a study with community college students in California who were diagnosed as "learning disabled" using a California system-wide discrepancy definition. Reading rate was a major problem for the majority of the students in the study with a median percentile ranking at the 12th percentile on a standardardized reading test, the Nelson-Denny. Results indicated that those who had poorer unaided scores obtained greater benefit from the use of the Kurzweil 3000 than did those whose unaided comprehension was better. Elkind wrote that: "...participants whose unaided comprehension is poorer than that of 10th graders are likely to experience gains in (timed) comprehension from the use of the Kurzweil 3000" (p.5). Only three of the participants (12%) indicated difficulty integrating the auditory and visual information provided by the reading machine. Elkind summarized his findings in terms of the characteristics of those individuals whose reading speed, comprehension, or endurance improves when they use computer reader technology as follow:

- Poor unaided reading rate, comprehension, or endurance
- Good oral language capabilities
- Good ability to integrate auditory and visual information

Hecker (1999) has reported on a pilot program for low decoders currently under investigation at Landmark College in Putney, VT. The program (Integrated Language Curriculum) was designed to allow adult students who read poorly to work on reading skills at two levels simultaneously: learning the fundamentals of decoding through remediation strategies and providing exposure to print that is intellectually challenging. The program has a 2-year baseline and comparative data that suggest remarkable progress in reading comprehension scores for the group with access to both remediation and text-to-speech software, specifically the Kurzweil Reader (Hecker, personal correspondence).

For those individuals with written language deficits, and depending upon the degree of severity of the deficit, various outlining programs, spell and grammar check capacities, and speech recognition systems that allow for dictation have been used successfully by individuals in postsecondary settings in conjunction with their personal computers. According to Raskind and Higgins (1998), systems such as Dragon Dictate™, Kurzweil Voice™, and IBM Voice Type™ used in conjunction with word processors enable the user to dictate to the computer at 40 to 70 words per minute, which then converts oral language into written text (Our usual rate of speaking is at a rate of 125 to 160 words per minute.) (De La Paz, 1999). However, as the technology now exits there is a considerable degree of training time required, anywhere from 3 to 6 hours, before an individual can work with the system independently. Training is essential in both basic operational procedures as well as training the system to recognize the user's voice.

As a result of a review of a number of studies comparing the use of oral composition devices such as dictation and speech recognition systems vs. written composition, whether by hand, typewriter, or word processor, (MacArthur and Graham, 1987; Burenstein, 1995; De LA Paz and Graham, 1995; Higgins and Raskind, 1995; Raskind and Higgins, 1995; Wetzel, 1996) De La Paz (1999) offers a number of recommendations with respect to the use oral composition devices. She points out that, as is the case for assistive technology in general, "these compensatory strategies must be combined with instruction to maximize their effectiveness" (p. 180). Instruction must include planning strategies in particular. Guidance in learning to use speech recognition systems must be scaffolded (e.g. building voice recognition templates, developing consistent vocabulary selection and pronunciation, error correction procedures). In addition, neither dictation nor speech recognition systems alleviate the need for individuals to compose using correct grammar and punctuation.

For individuals who have primary difficulty with initiating written output or organizing topics, categories and sequences, outlining programs such as Inspiration[R] enable the user to "dump" (Raskind and Higgins, 1998, p. 30) their ideas or thoughts in an unstructured manner that is later categorized and ordered. Systems are devised to allow automatic outlining as well as graphic capacities whereby semantic webs, mind maps, or cluster diagrams are produced prior to formulating an outline. Geometric shapes and lines allow for displaying and linking related ideas to a main ideas as well as reordering them throughout the process. A paper by McNaughton, Hughes, and Clark (1997) provides an excellent discussion of the variable impact of various proofreading strategies including a word processor with an integrated spelling checker on the spelling performance of college students with learning disabilities. And while the error detection provided by the word processor provided a statistically significant advantage over the four other independent conditions, the students still failed to detect a mean of 24.7% of the spelling errors in their written essays. Errors were evenly divided between homophones (their for there), errors related to meaning of the target word (run for ran), and errors unrelated to meaning (rain for ran).

In a study by Leyser, Vogel, Wyland, and Brulle (1999) (also discussed in Chapter 3) the practices and attitudes of faculty in higher education with respect to students with learning disabilities were examined. In response to a faculty survey, various factors were elicited that appeared to affect the willingness of those responding to provide accommodations either in the classroom or for examinations. The use of technology in examinations was a widely accepted accommodation, particularly use of a word processor with spell and grammar check capacities. Surprisingly, these faculty were less willing to permit students to answer test questions using a tape recorder, objecting to the time commitment involved in listening to the students' tape recorded responses.

Compensatory Strategies: Miscellaneous Accommodations

The issue of appropriate accommodations for students with learning disabilities at the college level was among the several issues addressed in *Guckenberger v. Boston University*. Students at BU claimed that the administration had significantly and abruptly changed its policy on accommodating individuals with learning disabilities, violating the ADA and creating a hostile learning environment. Among the issues was that of course substitutions in the areas of foreign language and math in particular. While math was not dealt with in the court's decision as none of the complainants were found to have a math disability, the issue of allowing a substitute for a foreign language requirement was addressed. The court found that it was reasonable to expect the university to substitute a foreign-culture requirement in place of a foreign language since it would not fundamentally alter its educational program (Rothstein, 1998).

There is, to date, "no empirical evidence about the accuracy of predictions with and without information about a student's performance in college language courses" (Shaw, 199, p. 326). However, Sparks, Philips, and Ganschow (1996) did report on a study following 97 students over a 10 year period, all of whom had received permission for course substitutions from a foreign language requirement in a midwestern university. Following their review, Sparks *et al.* recommended criteria for identifying students at risk for foreign language learning deficits. These included: a verifiable history of native language learning problems; a verifiable history of problems learning a foreign language; and recent testing which demonstrates at least average intelligence and low score on measures of foreign language aptitude and native language skill. Shaw (1999) would contend, however, that a thorough psychoeducational evaluation and the review of the student's previous educational history can be used to make a reasonable judgement about a student's success or lack thereof without requiring that the student fail the course first.

In addition to foreign language waivers, the use of extended or untimed testing for postsecondary students with reading and writing disorders has served as a standard accommodation for a number of years (Weaver, 1993; Mosberg and Johns, 1994). Discriminatory testing is prohibited under both the Rehabilitation Act and the Americans with Disabilities Act (ADA). Four questions must be answered to determine whether a test is discriminatory. Does the test measure a relevant academic skill or an irrelevant disability? If the test results may reflect the existence of a disability, is the measured skill one that is essential to obtaining the education offered? Are there alternative methods of measuring an essential academic skill, and is the process of providing alternative unreasonably expensive given the postsecondary institution's resources? (Latham and Latham, 1997). Thus, testing accommodations are required for individuals with disabilities unless the accommodations would alter the essential nature of the course materials or create an undue hardship.

Providing extended or untimed testing as a reasonable accommodation has been tested in the court at the professional and graduate school level with varying results. In *Price et al. v. The National Board of Medical Examiners*, Civil Action No. 3:97-0541 (S.D. W.Va. June, 6, 1997), two medical students were denied additional time and a private room from the National Board of Medical Examiners. Both students had been diagnosed with ADHD, Reading Disorder and/or Disorder of Written Expression as young adults and had not received any accommodations in college or earlier education. The Court ruled that the students were not individuals with disabilities under the ADA because their impairments did not substantially limit them in a major life activity, when compared to most people. In two other cases, the National Board of Medical Examiners agreed to terms set forth in a settlement stipulation and order and proceeded to grant double time testing (Latham and Latham, 1998). In both of these instances the individuals had been diagnosed with dyslexia as children and had received accommodations throughout their childhood.

In the case of *Bartlett v. New York State Board of Law Examiners*, 93Gv. 4986 (53) (S.D.N.Y. July 3, 1997), Ms. Bartlett, a law school graduate who had been diagnosed with a reading disorder as an adult, was found to be entitled to certain accommodations on the Bar Exam. These included double time, large print examinations, permission to circle multiple-choice answers, and the use of a computer. In distinguishing this decision from that taken in the Price case, the court found Ms. Bartlett substantially limited in the major life activity of working vs. education. Thus she was not able to read in the same condition, manner, or duration as an average reader when measured against the average person with comparable training, skill, and abilities (Latham and Latham, 1998).

While we have discussed a number of salient issues related to remediation interventions, compensatory strategies, and reasonable accommodations, ours has been a cursory review at best. If the reader is interested in a comprehensive discussion involving academic adjustments at the postsecondary level including programmatic and policy-related modifications as well as instructional modifications, he or she is referred to the chapter by Brinkerhoff, Shaw,and McGuire "Issues in Determining Academic Adjustments at the Postsecondary Level" (1993) in their book *Promoting Postsecondary Education for Students with Learning Disabilities*.

Accommodations in the Workplace

According to Reback (1996) the most important accommodation that employers must make is to have an Americans with Disabilities Act (ADA) coordinator on site if they employ more than 49 individuals and to insure that the coordinator is complying with all of the law's requirements. Equally important is an acknowledgment by the employer that hidden disabilities create difficulties in effective job performance much the same way that more visible disabilities do. Reback goes on to recognize that making appropriate accommodations requires that the individual with the learning disability self-disclose at times with some risk, and on the other hand, that accommodations that are made should not place undue burdens on other workers. The ADA provides for three categories of reasonable accommodations including change in method, orientation aids, and change in time, all of which are equally applicable to individuals with reading and writing disorders. Using computers vs. manual data entry, using icons as sequencing-task reminders, and using multi-modal procedures for on-the-job training programs are examples of accommodations that address a number of the issues raised by Reback.

On the other hand concerns raised by Beasley (1996), a training manager with Georgia-Pacific in southeastern Arkansas, go to the heart of the identification process itself, a precursor to the provision of reasonable accommodations in the work place. He wrote, "One of the key points that we need to examine is that most businesses and industries have no idea of the literacy levels of their employees. Cost control and profitability will suffer until we address the 10-15% of our work force with LD" (p. 143). In other words, how to assess the learning needs of the potential workforce with varying kinds of learning disorders remains a critical issue for trainers in business and industry settings.

According to Gerber (1997), learning disabilities are not easily understood in the workplace and are often grouped with other categories such as developmental disabilities, mental retardation, and sensory disabilities (Emily Hall Tremaine Foundation, 1995). "Moreover, invisibility causes the nature of learning disabilities to appear abstract" (Gerber, 1997, p. 4). Individuals need to be successful self-advocates in many instances, and self-advocacy goes beyond self-disclosure to an exact understanding of the nature of the underlying disability, how it manifests itself, and strategies to compensate for particular weaknesses while capitalizing on learning strengths. Gerber has labeled this process "reframing" (Gerber, Ginsberg, and Reiff, 1992; Gerber, 1996). (See

Chapter 3 for further discussion). The stages of the process of reframing, recognition, understanding, acceptance, and action are seen to apply to a model of employment success and have been previously identified as critical to vocational adjustment and success among individuals with learning disabilities by Spekman, Herman, and Vogel (1993) as well as Gerber and Reiff (1992, 1993). "Taking charge of one's life was a crucial first step to success and was accompanied by strong determination and desire, goal setting, and reframing" (Vogel, 1996).

Gerber (1997) goes on to say that because companies rely on training in order to be efficient and consequently competitive, training procedures are constantly under review. Thus an important focus would be to design training consistent with the ways all individuals learn, including persons with learning disabilities. A unique approach to helping trainers deal specifically with the issue of learning styles in the workplace is currently in progress by Sopper (personal correspondence) who is CEO of a newly formed corporate spin-off of Landmark College called Optimind. Optimind's purpose is to bring the best practices in working with adults with reading and writing disorders into the corporate/business training world based upon the assumption that all training efforts and thus workers with and without identified learning disabilities would benefit from such a highly explicated, multi-sensory and cognitively informed approach.

LONG-TERM FOLLOW-UP AND OUTCOME STUDIES

In their review of follow-up studies conducted on individuals with learning disabilities in 1983, Horn, O'Donnell, and Vitulano concluded that the choice of outcome variable significantly influences the conclusions one can draw. If a test of basic skill functioning is defined as the most important measure of outcome, then "clearly persons with learning disabilities suffer enduring deficits" (p. 554). If measures of educational/vocational attainment are more critical indicators of adult outcome, then persons with learning disabilities do not appear to have a particularly poor prognosis. "Finally, it is unclear whether LD (sic) persons are more likely to develop significant emotional/behavioral outcomes as adults than normal learners" (p.554). While the language of the 1980s is not particularly user-friendly, the message delivered forces us to ask whether these same results hold true some 17 years later.

A more recent review of the literature focused on long-term prognosis covering the year 1954 to 1993 has been reported by Satz, Buka, Lipsitt, and Seidman (1998). Twelve studies were identified that had been published since the previous review by Schonhaut and Satz (1983) which were then rated in terms of methodological criteria. Of the studies selected for review only 5 studies had follow-up intervals of 15 years or more. Three of these studies reported good outcomes and two poor outcomes. Outcomes were defined in terms of academic, occupational, social, and emotional parameters. In general, findings from this review suggest that while childhood reading or learning problems persist over time, the severity of the problems may decrease for some individuals who then proceed to pursue further schooling and occupational advancement. Whether these same individuals also experience fewer psychological problems remains an unknown.

Results from an even more recent review (Levine and Nourse, 1998) shed still less light on what we have learned from follow-up studies. Somewhat uniquely, the authors present aggregate outcome data concerning the issue of women with learning disabilities and suggest that the "uniformity of goals and school curricular interventions for youth, and for young females in particular" (p.230) are subject to challenge. In an earlier review (Levine and Edgar, 1995) the gender issue in long-term postschool adjustment of youth with and without disabilities was addressed. These authors concluded that the bulk of the literature would say that males and females with disabilities differ in their postschool outcomes in terms of employment, marriage, and parenting rates but not in terms of postsecondary attendance or independent residence. Earlier Bruck (1987) suggested that the poorer adjustments of females in the studies she reviewed might reflect differences in societal attitudes towards men and women who fail. "Females who fail may be more rejected by peers and less accepted by adults than boys who fail. These interactions may be the precursors of social and emotional problems of LD *(sic)* females" (p.260). In any case both sets of conclusions raise critical issues for any long-term follow-up study.

Numerous other studies have appeared in the literature regarding the educational, occupational, and social adjustment of young adults with learning disabilities (Spekman, Goldberg, and Herman, 1992; Vogel and Hruby, 1993; Lewandowski and Arcangelo, 1994; Greenbaum, Graham, and Scales, 1996; Goldstein, Murray, and Edgar, 1998; Witte, Philips, and Kakela, 1998). The topics range from job satisfaction of college graduates to employment earnings and from social adjustment and self-concept to factors related to "success" in the young adult years. As can be seen from the titles of the studies, there is a tendency to demarcate a specific area for outcome research vs. the previous look at numerous factors across the span of major life events and activities. It is too early to say whether this approach will yield more useful data with respect to outcome studies.

This concludes our review of outcome studies involving reading and writing disorders in the young adult population. What we have learned is that the field has far to go. The work of Shaywitz and her colleagues (1990) may well yield significant data in the years to come because of the rigorous design of their follow up study. On the other hand, the participant/ethnographic research paradigm which marks the work of individuals such as Gerber (1991) may make the content of outcome studies even richer and ultimately effect the nature of interventions and practices.   Bruck (1987) wrote that *the most important antecedents of positive outcome are early identification accompanied by early intervention.* It was the dimensions of intervention rather than dimension of IQ, socioeconomic status, and severity of childhood disability that had the greatest impact on positive outcome. We believe this message is still valid over a decade later and will be valid until our practices are congruent with the scientific knowledge base that we currently have at our disposal.

SUMMARY

The focus of this chapter was to present current thinking and research in the areas of reading and written language disorders as they present in a young adult population.   Our goal also was to incorporate psychoeducational and neuropsychological factors as they might impact the assessment process as well as co-morbidity status.   Clearly, however, controversy remains alive with respect to diagnostic and assessment procedures, the documentation of disability status, and justification for reasonable accommodations for young adults as well as for children.   Thus, a knowledge base by the clinician that is well grounded in research, theory, and practice remains critical.

2

MATHEMATICS DISORDER

INTRODUCTION

Considered as a learning disability, Mathematics Disorder is defined in DSM-IV (1994) terms as a condition in which mathematical ability, as measured by the appropriate tests, is substantially below that expected given the person's chronological age, measured intelligence, and education. In its pure form, this disorder is estimated to have a prevalence of 1% of school-age children (DSM-IV, 1994).   Therefore, Mathematics Disorder as a stand-alone condition is relatively rare in childhood, suggesting that the prevalence in adulthood is also quite rare. However, difficulties with mathematics in combination with other cognitive deficits or in a form that would not meet strict DSM-IV criteria are likely to be quite common. Normand and Zigmond (1980) and others have documented a prevalence rate as high as 6% in the school-age population of students with learning disabilities and, numerous other investigators have found that students with learning disabilities (the general prevalence of specific disorders of reading and written expression are discussed in Chapter 1) experience even greater difficulty in math than their peers without disabilities (e.g., Fleischner et al., 1982; Ackerman, Anhalt, and Dykman, 1986; Goldman, 1989).

Using the DSM-IV definition, adults with a mathematics disorder would be those with a developmental history of disability in mathematics that is not outgrown. If the disorder is still diagnosable despite special education, it would consist of individuals who retain the disorder despite such efforts as well. Throughout this volume we have provided evidence that specific learning disabilities often persist into adulthood, and may be identified during adulthood even when not diagnosed during childhood. Thus, such individuals exist and may continue to experience educational and vocational difficulties because of poor mathematical skills. However, it is probably unrealistic to assume that such a group constitutes all of the cases of specific mathematics disorder. As one gets into late adolescence and early adulthood, the incidence of acquired disability increases, initially because of the increased incidence of head trauma, and later in life, of stroke and other neurological disorders. A penetrating, focal head wound or a localized stroke can result in the acquisition of a reasonably specific, often severe mathematics disability.

In this chapter, we therefore will not limit our discussion to the developmental form of mathematics disorder but will provide some material on the acquired form, generally referred to as acalculia (Berger, 1926; Hecaen, Angelergues, and Houillier, 1961) or dyscalculia. In adults with the developmental form, the disorder becomes problematic when the cognitive demands of mathematics courses become too much for the student's limited capability. Thus, the disorder is commonly identified in college students (Morris and Walter, 1991). Vocational problems may emerge when the employee is transferred to a job that requires more mathematics than the previous job. The common scenario in the acquired case is the individual who is doing well in school or at work, gets into a car accident associated with head injury, and can no longer perform at the same level, as was the case prior to the injury. In effect, however, both groups have a common disability in the area of mathematics, and treatment and management considerations may have a great deal of overlap. The matter of whether there are differing optimal educational strategies depending upon whether one has lost an ability or has to be educated in ability that was never well developed is an open question. Most of the educational literature relates to developmental disability (Geary, 1990; Geary, 1993; Rivera, 1993; Jones, Wilson, and Bhojwani, 1997; Miller and Mercer, 1998; Rivera, 1998), and little has been done in re-teaching mathematics to individuals with dyscalculia.

Also related to education, there is a voluminous literature on strategies and educational technologies for mathematics instruction for normal individuals as well as for students with learning disorders (Schoenfeld, 1994). While this literature may have significant relevance for college students, it is less pertinent for most adults who have completed their educations, do not have the desire or resources to return to school, and who may have received maximum benefits from special programs provided while they were in school. In these cases, several other aspects of treatment and case management would appear to have priority. These include the following: (1) vocational counseling that guides the individual out of career choices that place heavy demands on mathematical abilities; (2) accommodation in educational and vocational settings such that the same goals can be accomplished through alternative routes; (3) instruction in the use of assistive devices that perform mathematical operations. (4) and, in the case of the individual with acquired severe disability in particular, counseling to assist in modifying level of aspiration and vocational goals in view of the changed circumstances. The accountant who has had a stroke may not be able to return to being an independent accountant.

DEFINITIONS

Acquired Mathematics Disorders in Adults: The Acalculias

The ability to do mathematical problem solving is often impaired following generalized brain damage, indicating that these abilities are highly sensitive to acquired damage in many parts of the brain over a wide range of severity. The impairment is often seen as part of a more global problem-solving deficit, and while mechanical arithmetic operations can still be performed, substantial difficulty may occur with word problems that involve numerical reasoning. Thus, some adults who experience mathematical difficulties do so as part of a more general problem-solving deficit because of the particular sensitivity of mathematics to brain dysfunction. This form of deficit tends to be more pronounced in reasoning than in performing calculations. Clinically, arithmetic tests are sometimes viewed as measures that particularly challenge sustained attention or concentration, and the individual with generalized brain dysfunction may often have significant impairment in those areas.

In acalculia, the deficit is typically severe and often isolated, with other abilities less impaired or intact. There is always inability to perform calculations, and the disorder is often quite profound. Acalculia is traditionally classified into subtypes including alexia or agraphia for numbers, anarithmetria, and spatial acalculia (Hecaen, Angelergues, and Houillier, 1961). There is also thought to be a developmental acalculia or dyscalculia, but it is not clear that this condition is different from specific mathematics disorder when it is characterized as a form of learning disability.

Alexia or agraphia for numbers is the inability to read or write numbers. Patients with this disorder are often also aphasic and have associated neurological dysfunction. This condition goes well beyond the bounds of what is generally characterized as learning disability. These individuals have frequently had major strokes or severe head injuries. In acalculia of the spatial type, oral calculation is normal, but numbers cannot be properly arranged during computation. There is, in particular, a difficulty in multiplication because of difficulty in positioning and alignment of numbers, and in making erroneous transpositions, as in reading 42 for 24. Patients with right hemisphere disease frequently have these difficulties. Anarithmetria is impairment in calculation secondary to alexia and agraphia for numbers or spatial disorganization of numbers. It typically exists in combination with numerous other cognitive deficits. Sometimes the deficit is selective with addition and subtraction preserved but division and multiplication impaired.

In working with adults with academic difficulties these syndromes generally represent end-state, extreme conditions, but they may be seen in young people who have suffered severe brain trauma or middle aged to elderly individuals who have suffered strokes involving either the posterior left or right hemisphere.

Moreover, the adult syndromes provide a rudimentary model for mathematical difficulties, indicating that the difficulty may be the result of an inability to interpret or produce numbers, an inability to organize numbers in space, or an inability to calculate based on these or other considerations.

Developmental Mathematical Disorders

There are a number of children who demonstrate calculation difficulties early in life, but who are otherwise cognitively normal. Using a traditional approach to identification, children with near average IQs who receive low achievement scores in the area of mathematics are diagnosed with a disability (Rivera, 1998). According to Geary (1993) given these criteria, at any given point 6% of elementary school and junior high school students would qualify for a diagnosis of a mathematics disorder. Conceptualization of the disorder in this manner appeared in an early publication by Spellacy and Peter (1978) who set specific psychometric requirements including a Wide Range Achievement Test (WRAT) (Jastak and Wilkinson, 1984) Arithmetic score that fell below the 20th percentile, a Full Scale Wechsler IQ score of above 80, and no disabling emotional disturbance. They were able to identify 14 such individuals in a sample of 430 children (3.26%).

At about the same time, Kosc (1974) argued that developmental dyscalculia was related to a specific brain dysfunction.

> Developmental dyscalculia is a structural disorder of mathematical abilities which has its origin in a genetic or congenital disorder of those parts of the brain that are the direct anatomico-physiological substrate of the maturation of the mathematical abilities adequate to age, without a simultaneous disorder of general mental functions (p. 47).

Kosc went on to define six subtypes including verbal, lexical, graphical, operational, practognostic, and idiognostic dyscalculia. According to Rourke and Conway (1998), operational dyscalculia appears to be roughly equivalent to Hecaen's anarthimetria, with the practognostic and ideognostic forms appearing to reflect impairments in more basic concept formation and nonverbal reasoning.

In more recent times, the term specific mathematics disorder (disability) appears to have replaced the terms "acalculia" and "dyscalculias", with these terms being largely reserved for the acquired disorders. However, the literature in this area has been based almost exclusively on children. Thus, while this volume has provided extensive documentation of the persistence of reading disabilities into adulthood, we will try to demonstrate here that a mathematics disability may present as a different clinical entity in adults than it does in children. To briefly summarize what will be detailed below the following considerations are raised.

(1) Adults with mathematical difficulties may have them on the basis of deficiencies in cognitive development; adult acquired neurological disorders, or a combination of the two. Even in young adults, the possibilities of head trauma, substance abuse with implications for the central nervous system, and neurological diseases that rarely but sometimes occur in young adults (e.g., brain tumors; stroke) need to be taken into consideration. Impairment of calculation ability is a very common symptom of a variety of brain disorders, and in that way calculation is different from reading, which may remain relatively intact despite the presence of substantial brain damage.

(2) The neurocognitive deficits that produced the mathematics difficulty during childhood may have disappeared after later development because of compensatory efforts, but the mathematics difficulty may remain. Thus, we may have an individual with academic difficulty but without the typically associated neuropsychological deficits, something that rarely appears in children. The processes involved in learning a skill are not necessarily the same as those that maintain it.

(3) Adults often go through a frustrating life long history of failure to achieve goals because of difficulty with mathematics. They therefore may build up substantial anxiety when doing mathematics, and even if they have acquired the capability of doing well they may fail to do so because of the anxiety. Anxiety may be a more significant consideration for mathematics than is the case for reading and other academic disabilities.

(4) Adults may have had the advantages of many of the educational strategies available for teaching mathematics to individuals with disability, and may have achieved optimal outcome from this instruction. They therefore may not be motivated, often appropriately so, to pursue further educational efforts. Accommodation and counseling then become more helpful than instruction.

(5) In children, difficulties with mathematics are often associated with difficulties in reading, producing a global subtype of learning disability. This combination is less frequently found in adults, and particularly in adult college students. That is likely to be the case because individuals with global learning disability may frequently not meet entrance requirements for college. Therefore the adult with an isolated mathematics disorder may less frequently have other academic skill disorders.

In summary, unlike what may be more prototypical for children, mathematics difficulty in adults is more likely to be an isolated deficit unrelated to other academic skills and presently existent neuropsychological deficits, more likely to be acquired as a result of structural brain damage or disease than is the case for children, and highly exacerbated by anxiety. Remediation utilizing career planning and accommodation is more likely to be pertinent than formal education. While some adults with mathematics difficulties may meet specific DSM-IV criteria for Mathematics disorder, in association with a specific pattern of neuropsychological deficits, substantial numbers of others may not.

Furthermore, part of so-called "nonverbal learning disability" (Rourke, 1989) involves poor mathematical abilities and nonverbal learning disability may persist into adulthood. Nonverbal learning disability is described elsewhere in this book. In addition to the mathematics problems, these individuals also have poorly developed social perception and skills, impaired spatial and problem-solving abilities, and numerous other deficits. Reading and spelling abilities are generally at least average. (See Chapter 3 for a comprehensive discussion.)

In view of these complexities, it might be best to describe adults with mathematics disability in two ways; first with regard to the nature of the difficulty itself and the second describing associated academic and neuropsychological deficits. With regard to description, the classification of the acalculias may be useful. That is, the individual may have difficulty in reading or writing numbers (alexia or agraphia for numbers), with spatial alignment or representation of numbers (acalculia of the spatial type), and basic calculation skills (anarithmetria) separate from the other two categories. We would suggest another category in which the individual does not have any of these mechanical difficulties, but lacks conceptual reasoning abilities, particularly with regard to varying levels of number concept. When the mathematics difficulty does not exist in isolation from other academic and cognitive skills, it is important to assess those skills for various diagnostic, planning, and intervention reasons.

NEUROPSYCHOLOGICAL ASSESSMENT

There are two major studies that deal directly with the matter of neuropsychological aspects of a specific mathematical disorder in adults, one by Morris and Walter (1991) based upon a sample of 104 college students and the other, by McCue, Goldstein, Shelly, and Katz (1986), based upon a more diverse sample of 100 mainly unemployed individuals seeking rehabilitation services. The studies were remarkably similar with regard to tests used and method of subtyping. Both used the Wide Range Achievement Test (WRAT), the Revised Wechsler Adult Intelligence Scale (WAIS-R) (Wechsler, 1981), and portions of the Halstead-Reitan Battery (HRNB) (Reitan and Wolfson, 1993). The system of subtyping was originated by Rourke (1982) and was based upon WRAT Results. One group is defined as being substantially better in Reading than Arithmetic based on grade level or standard score discrepancies, the second does better at Arithmetic than at Reading, and the third has a global disability, without a significant discrepancy between reading and arithmetic. Our major interest here would be in the first group.

The cognitive profile in the Morris and Walter study is characterized by the absence of a discrepancy between average level Verbal and Performance IQ scores, an uneven WAIS-R profile with relatively high scores on Digit Span and Vocabulary, and low scores on Block Design and Object Assembly, below average scores on the Rey-Osterrieth Complex Figure Test, and mildly reduced tapping speeds. In the study by McCue *et al.* neuropsychological data were obtained for the Rourke group characterized by poor arithmetic relative to reading, based upon WRAT scores. Their sample had a slightly lower Performance than Verbal IQ score, with general intellectual function falling into the low average range. The WAIS subtest profile had a configuration characterized by relatively high scores on Comprehension and Similarities and low scores on Block Design and Digit Symbol. We would note that the Arithmetic subtest score was 8.37 for Morris and Walter, and 6.75 for McCue *et al.* both reflecting low performance relative to other verbal abilities.

On neuropsychological tests, while the specific tests used differed, both studies found evidence of impaired spatial ability, in the case of Morris and Walter using the Rey-Osterrieth Figure, and in the case of McCue *et al.* using the Total Time and Location components of the Halstead Tactual Performance Test (Reitan and Wolfson, 1993). McCue *et al.* also compared the reading better than arithmetic with the other Rourke subtypes, finding that the reading better than arithmetic subtype was significantly better on WAIS Information and Vocabulary subtests and the Reitan Aphasia Screening Test, but significantly worse on the Total Time component of the Tactual Performance Test. Both studies described groups with low average to average general intelligence, good verbal abilities, and impaired visual-spatial and spatial-constructional abilities. This latter area is perhaps the most robust finding concerning individuals with mathematics disorder. Over a very large number of studies, these individuals often have been shown to have significant impairment of nonverbal skills measured with drawings, constructional tasks, and complex visual perception tasks such as identifying embedded figures. The McCue *et al.* study showed that the neuropsychological profile of individuals with specific mathematics difficulty had a different pattern of strengths and weaknesses from what was the case for subtypes with specific reading or global disability. The combined findings of Morris and Walter (1991) and McCue *et al.* (1991) confirm the existence of a pattern of intact verbal skills and relatively deficient spatial abilities in adults with specific mathematics difficulties. It is the same pattern as seen in children, but generally not in as extreme a form.

Aside from the Wechsler scales and the HRNB, research in adult learning disability (LD) has been accomplished with the Luria-Nebraska Battery (LNNB) (Golden, Purisch, and Hammeke, 1985). The LNNB is a standard, comprehensive neuropsychological test battery that contains individual scales for the major neuropsychological functions including Motor Function, Attention, Vision, Tactile Function, Receptive Language, Expressive Language, Memory, and Intelligence. Of particular interest for LD is that there are separate scales for Reading, Writing, and Arithmetic. It has been shown that these latter scales constitute a "mini-WRAT" since they are highly correlated with the comparable subtests of the WRAT (Shelly and Goldstein, 1982). Thus, the LNNB has the advantage of providing a set of academic achievement tests that can be given within the context of a broader neuropsychological assessment. All of the tests are placed on the same scale, and so are easy to evaluate relative to each other. McCue and Goldstein (1991) compared three LNNB studies (Harvey and Wells, 1989; Lewis and Lorion, 1988; McCue *et al.*, 1984) that reached remarkably good replication of each other. While overall level of performance differed, they all obtained profiles characterized by relative elevations on the Rhythm scale (thought to be an indicator of attention), and the academic scales. Thus, while the LNNB proved to be sensitive to learning disability, it did not delineate a profile of cognitive deficits associated with it. That is, with the exception of the Rhythm scale, which may have reflected the presence of ADHD in some cases, the remaining clinical scales tended to be normal. More detailed study utilizing cluster analysis did not reveal a subgroup characterized by specific academic impairment in arithmetic and an associated cognitive profile (McCue, Goldstein, Shelly, and Katz, 1986). The majority of subjects with learning disability in this study had profiles that were completely normal, or that had large elevations only on the academic scales from the LNNB.

These neuropsychological findings are characterized by a great deal of variability. The sources of variability are of substantial importance in contributing to the assessment process. First, some individuals with mathematics difficulties do not have identifiable neuropsychological deficits. This finding is apparent in the case of the LNNB, but is also obtained when the WAIS and HRNB are used. The anticipated spatial and motor deficits are found more often in individuals with well-diagnosed specific Mathematics Disorder. Other adults, who seek remediation for mathematics difficulties, may not exhibit these deficits, possibly because they were outgrown. One possible explanation is "math anxiety" and another is that the difficulty is so specific that it is not detected by standard tests. Thus, the individual case may have anxiety ranging from minimal to severe, presence of specific academic and neuropsychological deficits, presence of more generalized academic and neuropsychological deficits, or absence of neuropsychological deficits.

The other aspect of neuropsychological assessment in this area has to do with the specifics of the mathematics disability itself. This returns us to a consideration of the acalculias and their specific characteristics. As we have indicated above, the blatant inability to read or write numbers is rarely if ever seen except in the case of acquired brain damage. However, one might encounter individuals who make errors of the spatial type because of difficulty in lining up numbers in writing or in cognitive representation while solving a problem. More frequently, errors are conceptual in nature, marked by a failure to fully comprehend the number system. The meaning of subtraction or the other operations might not be fully developed such that the individual makes implausible solutions. That is, a subtraction problem may be solved by producing a larger rather than a smaller number. Additions may be made instead of multiplications. In some cases impairment of sense of direction might be involved. At one time it was thought that there was a condition called the Gerstman (1940) syndrome that involves inability to identify one's fingers, agraphia, acalculia and right-left confusion. While the construct validity of the Gerstmann syndrome has not held up well, there do appear to be individuals with fragments of it, who have a combination of mathematics difficulty and right-left confusion (Hartje, 1987).

An extensive treatment of the cognitive and behavioral bases for learning difficulties in mathematics is provided by Lerner (2000), who divides the problem areas into spatial relationships, body image, visual-motor and visual perceptual abilities, concepts of direction and time, memory, information processing, language and reading abilities, cognitive learning strategies, and math anxiety. She also gives specific behavioral examples of each of these areas, and takes note of the characteristics of the learner in development of a math curriculum. With regard to education, Lerner does not get into the more advanced specifics such as fractions or exponents, but does deal with the basics including placement of numbers, working from right to left, basic numerical operations, and the decimal system.

From a neuropsychological perspective, the work of Lerner is particularly pertinent because it implies that optimal education of the individual is ideally based on the cognitive profile of strengths and weaknesses, and there is no one method that works for everyone. Particularly in the case of individuals with developmental, and perhaps even more so with acquired learning disability, the key considerations determining the disability area may be specific cognitive functions. In mathematics it may be spatial abilities, or memory, or reading, or attention, or sequencing ability. When one gets into higher mathematics such as algebra or calculus, these matters become even more complex. Thus, for example, the calculation ability of an individual who sustained a head injury might benefit from a systematic program of memory training (e.g., Wilson, 1987) while direct training of mathematics may be of no help, because of failure to recall material presented or number facts, such as multiplication tables

In clinical assessment, arithmetic is often viewed as a measure of attention. The Arithmetic subtest of the Wechsler Intelligence Scales loads on the attention or "freedom from distractibility" factor (Cohen, 1957). Thus, in evaluating an individual with mathematics difficulties, it is important to assess attention, ideally with some instrument that does not involve numbers, such as the Rhythm Test from the HRNB or a continuous performance test. It is possible that the basis for the mathematics disability is a failure in concentration, possibly associated with frank ADHD or some other disorder that impairs concentration, such as depression. Elsewhere in this book we discuss the ways in which ADHD is manifest in adulthood. In these cases, there may be some hope that at least some portion of the difficulty with mathematics can be remediated with standard ADHD treatment. Mathematics difficulties are also associated with nonverbal learning disability, which is associated with disorders of white matter or the right cerebral hemisphere.

From a psychoeducational perspective, studies across countries found consistently that children with mathematical disorders have difficulties solving simple and complex arithmetic problems (Barrouillet, Fayol, and Lathuliere, 1997; Jordan and Montani, 1997) and that these difficulties involve both procedural and memory-based deficits. With respect to the procedural deficit, although some studies have attributed calculation difficulties to visuospatial deficits, this does not appear to be the case with the majority of children (Geary, Hamson, and Hoard, in press). Rather, they appear to have problems in monitoring the sequence of steps of the algorithm and poor skills in detecting and self-correcting errors.

In terms of retrieval deficits, it appears that the memory representations for arithmetic facts are supported partially by the same phonological and semantic memory systems that support word decoding and reading comprehension, and as such, might be the source for mathematical and reading disorders in the same children (Geary, 1993; Light, DeFries, and Olson, 1998). More recent studies suggest the presence of a second form of retrieval deficit (Geary *et al.*, in press) that relates to the inhibition of irrelevant associations during the retrieval process. Errors occur then because the individual cannot inhibit irrelevant associations from entering working memory, which then either suppress or compete with the correct association.

In the words of Geary (2000):

> Disruptions in the ability to retrieve basic facts from long-term memory, whether the cause is accessing difficulties or the lack of inhibition of irrelevant associations, might, in fact, be considered a defining feature of mathematical disorders....Moreover, characteristics of these retrieval deficits...suggest that for many children, these do not reflect a simple developmental delay but rather a more persistent cognitive disorder (p.8).

In like manner, Nolting (1988) has suggested that students who have learning disabilities often experience more difficulty learning mathematics than other subjects. He postulates that factors which may be relevant to diagnostics and interventions are those of linear learning and memory. Linear learning occurs when material learned one day is used the next day and the next and so forth. With nonlinear subject matter (social sciences, for example), material learned one day can be forgotten after the test and will not impact the learning of new material. With mathematics, if the first concept taught during a class period is misunderstood or not taught well, problems in understanding the remainder of the class material will be paramount. He suggests that the basis for the learning difficulty lies in problems either with short or long-term memory. In addition, with those students who also have a reading disorder, securing the missed information from textbooks will not be an easy task. Nolting (1997) has published an excellent manual appropriate for students at the college level in which he presents practical strategies for dealing with math anxiety, test-taking skills, studying for examinations, use of a calculator in class, with special references for students with LD, TBI, and ADHD.

In summary, description of the adult with mathematics difficulties is an exceptionally complex area for a number of reasons. In adults more than children, mathematics difficulties may be associated with acquired neurological disorders in both a specific and more general way. That is, there are cases of specific acalculia typically associated with left parietal lobe focal brain damage, but impairment of mathematical abilities is very commonly a result of generalized brain damage. Some, but clearly not all, adults have specific Mathematics Disorder in association with the characteristic pattern of neuropsychological deficits described in children. Most prominently, these individuals show deficits in visual-spatial and motor abilities. Other adults have the mathematics disability without the neuropsychological deficits. Some have their mathematics disability in association with attentional difficulties, if not frank ADHD. What often is a lifelong history of frustration and distress centering on the area of mathematics may produce severe "math anxiety" in adults. Various combinations of all of these considerations may exist in individual cases.

INTERVENTIONS

General Considerations

Based upon the descriptive and neuropsychological material we have been discussing, it is apparent that a broad range of interventions needs to be applied to mathematics disorders. Therapeutic and remedial interventions may range from basic reteaching a stroke patient to read and write numbers to advanced instruction for specific difficulties in some area of higher mathematics. In some cases, particularly those involving ADHD or severe anxiety disorders, pharmacological treatment may be indicated. There is an extensive educational technology for teaching mathematics to children, with some programs designed specifically for children with learning disability. There are issues associated with mental health interventions, accommodation, assistive devices, and vocational choice.

Educational methods proposed vary greatly in content and orientation. Some of them focus on strategies and emphasize such considerations as planning without specific regard to the specifics of the mathematics areas or deficits themselves (Naglieri & Johnson, 2000), some on behavioral techniques such as modeling and demonstration associated with use of reinforcement, some on use of advanced audiovisual technologies such as videodiscs with specific applications in fractions, equations, roots, and exponents (Kitz and Thorpe,

1995), and some on computer instruction (Wilson, 1993). A number of these programs are designed for general use and others for individuals with learning disability. In general, these innovative methods were found to be better both in terms of student support and objective indices of improvement than were traditional methods. However, traditional course work may be associated with subsequent mathematical achievement, but in a complex way depending upon grade in school and level of the course (Xin, 2000).

Dixon (1994) presented a series of six research-based guidelines for selecting mathematics curricula that appear to be particularly critical for teaching individuals with a mathematics disorder at whatever stage of development or educational level. First is the concept of teaching "big ideas"—important math concepts that will facilitate the greatest amount of knowledge acquisition across the content being taught (i.e., basic operations, place, value, fractions, estimations, probability, volume and area, and word-problem solving). The second guideline is that explicit strategies should be included in the instructional process. Third, the use of mediated scaffolding should be included to allow learners to obtain support while performing new skills. Fourth, after skills are taught in isolation, opportunities should exist for students to integrate problem types (e.g., adding and multiplying fractions). Fifth, new learning should be primed by reviewing prerequisite skills for a substantial period of time before introducing new and more complex skills. And last, opportunities should exist for review, sufficient for obtaining fluency, distributed over time, cumulative as new skills are learned, and varied to promote generalization.

Adults with Mathematical Disabilities: Subgroups and Remediation

For practical purposes, there appear to be two large subgroups of adults that seek assistance. One of them consists of college students who are having difficulties with their mathematics courses, and the other group consists of nonstudents who are seeking employment or who are having on the job difficulties involving mathematics. For example, individuals who are on a new job or who have been reassigned and find themselves in work situations that require more mathematical skill than was the case previously. Through contrasting the studies of McCue et al. (1991) and Morris and Walters (1991), and, in a more direct way, through a study of Beers (Beers, Goldstein, and Katz, 2000), it seems to be the case that there are relatively high functioning and low functioning subgroups of adults with learning disability. Beers has shown that their cognitive profiles are similar, but that the high functioning group has an overall higher level of cognitive ability than the low functioning group. Morris and Walter (1991) as well as Beers et al., both of whom studied the high functioning group, remarked on the extremely small number of high functioning individuals who were in the Rourke reading worse than arithmetic and global disability subtypes. In our own work (Beers, Goldstein and Katz, 2000) we found college students in all three subtypes, but showed that there were substantial differences in the proportion of Rourke subtypes between college student and vocational rehabilitation client groups. The vocational rehabilitation clients were predominantly in the global subtype, while the college students were predominantly in the poor arithmetic subtype. Thus, college students who seek remediation very frequently tend to have specific difficulties in mathematics, with normal or better reading and spelling. On the other hand, McCue *et al.* found adult subjects in all three subtypes.

These considerations would appear to have major implications for direct remediation. For example, in the relatively low functioning group, remediation could be based upon the underlying cognitive deficit area such as spatial abilities, with the strategy being that improvement in these abilities generalize to mathematics. However, high functioning individuals may not exhibit these spatial deficits but still have mathematics problems, suggesting that a different approach would be more productive. These individuals may benefit from a more expanded assessment in which it is determined whether the mathematics problem is attributable to anxiety, to some general difficulty such as poor capacity to attend or bad study habits, or to some specific deficit in conceptualization. Such an assessment should establish the best alternative or combination of alternatives for treating the anxiety, providing more generic remediation regarding attending, organizing material, and maintaining an adequate study schedule, or providing highly specific training using an educational technology that addresses the specific problem area. For example, with respect to the latter deficit, some modification of the use of manipulatives used with young children who have difficulties with forming abstract representations of problems (Marsh and Cooke, 1996). Treatment planning of this type is greatly benefited from an analysis of errors, which should provide important information as to the spatial, mechanical arithmetic, or conceptual source of the disability. For example, Wong (1996) has distinguished calculation errors due to partial completion of the given problem, errors due to incorrect placement and regrouping, errors due to incorrect procedures in computation, and errors due to failure in mastering the concept of zero.

It is possible, but not thoroughly demonstrated, that the more low functioning adults may benefit from neuropsychological rehabilitation. The question is, Will training programs available for such abilities as memory, various language skills, and spatial abilities help these individuals with their mathematics? There is some support for the view that use of memory aids or training is useful in mathematics instruction of individuals with mental handicaps (Judd and Bilsky, 1989). Often these individuals cannot read well and so mathematics problems are presented orally, but such presentation requires memory, which may be deficient. In a similar way, reading ability may provide a source of difficulty. If normal reading is defined on the basis of the WRAT Reading score that could be misleading because the WRAT only assesses mechanical reading (word recognition), which may be intact in the presence of serious reading comprehension deficits. Thus, some individuals have mathematics difficulties because they fail to fully comprehend written problems (Zentall and Ferkis, 1993). Greene (1999) has demonstrated that mnemonic-based memory training of the type used with brain-damaged patients may be helpful to students with learning disability in learning mathematical facts. It is possible, but not well demonstrated, that established cognitive rehabilitation methods might be suitable for re-teaching individuals with acquired acalculia and substantial associated cognitive deficits basic numerical skills such as reading, writing, and aligning numbers.

With the exception of college students having academic difficulties, formal interventions of this type are rarely accomplished with adults, particularly those who have completed their educations. They may hire a tutor if they have sufficient income, utilize services provided by the local Learning Disabilities Association (LDA) or related organizations, or return to school. Aside from the lack of appropriate resources, there are several reasons for this lack of participation in formal education. In our experience, adults with learning disability who have completed their education do not look forward to more of it. School has generally been an unpleasant experience for them, often filled with frustration, disappointment, anxiety, and depression. As special education becomes increasingly available, growing numbers of these individuals will be provided with remediation, and many will reach optimal benefit while in school. In these cases, further formal educational efforts would appear to have a good chance of being unproductive. In essence, the very reasonable process of providing formal special education in specific academic areas for children with learning disabilities seems very worthwhile, but that same activity in adults may be less viable.

Individuals with adult learning disability often express the need to be in job situations that do not expose their academic deficiencies or where the deficiencies impair work performance. They may often have difficulties in obtaining jobs or fail at jobs they get because of disabilities in reading, writing, or calculation. While they may not wish to engage in activities that seem like a return to school, they would like to be productive in situations in which they can function up to expectations. Therefore, they may wish to obtain jobs in which they feel comfortable, and that do not require much in the way of deficient academic skills, or they may want to receive appropriate accommodation.

Interventions with College Level Students

While the clinical and research work of Davidson (1983) on "learning differences" (Marolda and Davidson, 2000) in students' acquisition of mathematics has focused primarily on children before the college age, frequently for those with a diagnosed mathematics disorder the problems continue well into the post-secondary setting. The work of Marolda and Davidson is useful for the clinician attempting to delineate the nature of the disorder as it manifests in a given individual and what interventions or accommodations might then be appropriate.

According to Marolda and Davidson (1994), students tend to process mathematical situations following two distinct patterns. One is linear; the other is global or gestalt. Both patterns have been incorporated in learning profiles by these researchers: *Mathematics Learning Style I* and *Mathematics Learning Style II*. Both styles must be available for successful acquisition of mathematical operations and concepts. However, often students with a diagnosed mathematics disability are limited to one or the other learning style and thus are unable to utilize strategies available to the other style. These styles, their cognitive and behavioral correlates, and the implications for teaching/intervention strategies are reprinted from an article by Marolda and Davidson as described below. As will be seen, they are transferable to work with college students who require remediation or developmental course work in the area of mathematics.

MATHEMATICAL LEARNING PROFILES AND DIFFERENTIATED TEACHING STRATEGIES

MATHEMATICS LEARNING STYLE I

A. Cognitive and Behavioral Correlates
  1. Highly reliant on verbal skills
  2. Tends to focus on individual details or
     single aspects of a situation
     Sees the "trees," but overlooks the "forest"
  3. Prefers HOW to WHY
  4. Relies on a defined sequence of steps to
     pursue a goal
     Reliant on teacher for THE approach
     Lack of versatility
  5. Challenged by perceptual demands
  6 Prefers quizzes or unit tests to more
     comprehensive final exams

B. Mathematical Behaviors
  1. Approaches situations using recipes; "talks
     through" tasks
     Interprets geometric designs verbally
  2. Approaches mathematics in a mechanical,
     routine based fashion
     Overwhelmed in situations in which there
     are multiple considerations, such as in
     multi-step tasks
     Can generate correct solutions, but may
     not recognize when solutions are
     inappropriate

Difficulties "checking" work; must re-do
    entire problem
Difficulties choosing an approach in word
    problems
Difficulties appreciating larger geometric
    constructs because of an emphasis on
    component parts

3. Prefers numerical approach over manipulative
    models
    Needs drill and practice to establish procedure
       before considering applications or broader
       conceptual meaning

4. Prefers explicit delineation of each step of a
    procedure and linkage of steps one to another
    Vulnerable when there are multiple approaches to
       a single topic
    Overwhelmed by multiple models or multiple
       approaches
    Prefers linear approaches for arithmetic topics

5. Difficulties with more sophisticated perceptual
    models, such as Cuisenaire rods
    Geometric activities may be challenging,
       especially in three dimensions
    Difficulties interpreting analog clocks
    Difficulties distinguishing coins, especially nickel
       and quarter
    Difficulties organizing written formats

6. May be able to complete the most difficult example
    in a set of examples relying on the same concept/skill,
    but has difficulty switching to a new topic or new approach

C. Teaching Implications and Strategies

1. Emphasize the meaning of each concept or procedure in
    verbal terms
    Build on subvocalization strategies to direct procedures

2. Highlight concept/overall goal
    Break down complex tasks into salient units and make
       linkage between units explicit
    Build simple estimation strategies; encourage two final
       steps to each calculation problem: "Does this answer
       the question?" and "Does the solution seem right?"
    Encourage students to rewrite or state problems in their
       own words
    Develop metacognitive strategies to analyze word problem
       situations
    Encourage parts to wholes approach in building geometric
       figures and explicit descriptions of the overall design that
       emerges

3. Link manipulative model on a step-by-step basis to the
    numerical procedure
    Once procedure is secure, relate math topics to relevant real life
       situations

4. Offer flow chart approaches
    Help students create handbooks with procedures described in

their own words

Choose one manipulative model or approach to develop
a wide range of topics; avoid switching models or
approaches too quickly

Don't emphasize special cases; rather develop an over-
riding rule that applies to all cases; e.g. for the addition
and subtraction of fractions with unlike denominators,
develop a single process using the product of the
denominators in all cases, even if it is not the least
common denominator

Give explanations before or after procedure, but not
while student is pursuing procedure

Use counting on techniques for addition facts and
missing addend techniques for subtraction facts.

Interpret multiplication as successive additions

5. Emphasize set (discrete) models for counting, such as
money or counting chips

Translate perceptual cues in terms of verbal
descriptions

6. Spiral all topics to keep them current

MATHEMATICS LEARNING STYLE II

A. Cognitive and Behavioral Correlates
1. Prefers perceptual stimuli and often reinterprets
abstract situations visually or pictorially
2. Likes to deal with big ideas; doesn't want to be
bothered with details
3. Prefers WHY to HOW
4. Prefers nonsequential approaches, involving patterns
and interrelationships
5. Challenged by demands for details or the requirement
of precise solutions
6. Prefers performance based or portfolio type assessment
to typical tests
Prefers comprehensive exams to quizzes and unit tests
More comfortable recognizing correct solutions than
generating them

B. Mathematical Behaviors
1. Benefits from manipulatives
Loves geometric topics
2. Prefers concepts to algorithms
Tolerates ambiguity and imprecision
Offers impulsive guesses as solutions
Uses estimation strategies spontaneously
Skims word problems first but must be encouraged
to re-read for salient details
Perceives overall shape of geometric configurations
at the expense of an appreciation of the
individual components
3. Requires a definition of overview before dealing with
exacting procedures

Requires manipulative modeling before developing a
  concept or algorithm
Likes to set up problems, but resists following through to
  a conclusion
4. Prefers successive approximations approach to formal
  algorithms
Addition and multiplication facts involving 9s more readily
  generated because of underlying patterns that are
  recognized but not verbalized
Not troubled by mixed practice worksheets
Comfortable with horizontal formats for long calculations
Can offer a variety of alternative answers or approaches
  to a single problem
Can appreciate operation needed in a word problem but
  has difficulty following through to an exact solution
Likes logical problem solving in the form of general reasoning
  problems
5. Difficulties with precise calculations
Difficulties offering rationale for correct solutions
6. May be overwhelmed when faced with multiple examples

C. Teaching Implications & Strategies
  1. Offer a variety of models; introduce perceptual models,
     such as *Base Ten Blocks* or *Cuisenaire Rods*, to support
     calculations
  Emphasize geometry as a vital part of the curriculum
  2. Relate manipulative models to procedures before practicing
     algorithms
  Reward approach as well as precise solutions
  Develop an appreciation of how much precision a situation
     warrants
  Reward/encourage estimation strategies as first step
  Encourage diagrams as a technique to organize data in
     problem solving situations
  Allow calculators to support problem solving
  Encourage multiple refinements when building geometric
     designs in order to incorporate all the individual parts
  3. Offer opportunities to work in cooperative groups
  4. Allow alternative calculation procedures
  Help students to create their own handbooks of typical
     problems
  Generate arithmetic facts through relationships to known
     facts; e.g. doubles for + facts
  Emphasize area model for multiplication
  Start with real-life situation and tease out more formal
     arithmetic topics
  Use simulations, relating similar concepts/approaches in a
     variety of different situations
  Model complex problems with similar problems in simpler
     forms
  Give two grades on word problem activities; one for correct
     approach; one for exact final solution
  Include general reasoning examples in logical problem solving
     activities

5. Encourage students to describe the approach or conceptual
   underpinning even if they cannot mobilize an exacting
   procedure
6. Consider a variety of assessment techniques
   Allow oral presentations
   Do not always require exact solution but sometimes grade
      homework and tests only for correct approach
   Include some multiple choice items on tests

Reprinted , not in its entirety, with permission from The International Dyslexia
Association quarterly newsletter, *Perspectives*, Summer 2000, Vol. 26, No. 3,
pp. 13-14, M. R. Marolda and P. S. Davidson.

In addition, Morris and Walter (1991) suspect that math anxiety may be a
major source of academic dysfunction in college students.   The disruptive
effects of anxiety on cognitive function are well known, and can be quite
disabling.   One can treat math anxiety in a number of ways including
psychotherapy, cognitive behavioral interventions (e.g., desensitization, anxiety
management), and pharmacological treatment.   Perhaps a desensitization
procedure would be particularly effective, accomplished through specifically
reducing anxiety responses to situations related to mathematics. There does not
seem to be any specific treatment for math anxiety except to possibly consider it
as a form of phobia, perhaps a form of school phobia, that may be treated in a
targeted manner, such as with the use of desensitization, cognitive therapy, or
relaxation.   The use of anti-anxiety medication might be considered in
appropriate cases.

ASSISTIVE DEVICES

Another approach to remediation and/or accommodation involves the use of
assistive devices.   Since the use of hand calculators and computers is so
commonplace, we rarely think of these devices as remedial tools or training
devices. Furthermore, allowing an individual with a mathematics deficit to use
such a device at work or in school is no longer a major event. The point to be
made here about assistive devices is that it is typically not sufficient to simply
make the device available, or to allow the individual to use one. In order to use
an assistive device as a remediative tool, two considerations are pertinent. First,
the device must be designed so as to be "user-friendly" to the person using it.
There are obviously the physical characteristics, such as the weight and size of
the device, and its use by individuals with various motor and perceptual
handicaps. For example, the individual with acquired acalculia resulting from
stroke may only have the use of one arm.   For individuals with cognitive
impairment, the display portions of devices must often be designed more simply
than is the case for normal individuals. Keyboards should have a minimum

number of keys, graphics should be as simple as possible and instructions for use and maintenance should be written in basic, simple terms. For individuals with perceptual and motor handicaps, visual displays need to be adequately large and illuminated. For the person with motor difficulties, the device must be adapted to the individual's deficit. For example, keys should be sufficiently large and widely spaced. It is generally necessary for the best work in this area to use individually designed or modified devices, or devices that have been specifically designed for use by individuals with physical, perceptual, or cognitive disabilities. It is exceptional for a commonly available commercial product to be an optimal assistive device. However, commercial devices may be used as "platforms" with modifications made through the use of rehabilitation engineering technology.

The other consideration revolves around the general principle that it is not sufficient to offer the individual an assistive device, provide information concerning how to operate it, and then leave the individual on her or his own. It is generally necessary to provide training in use of the device, ideally in the form of a systematic training program. We know of no formal programs in the area of mathematics with the exception of the specific procedures outlined by Nolting (1997) for use of a calculator while note-taking in the classroom. However, there are several programs available in the area of memory. For example, we effectively trained patients with severe amnesia to use a very basic personal reminder device to access items of information that they could not recall (Goldstein, Beers, Shemansky, and Longmore, 1998). The training involved meeting with a therapist over several sessions to provide training to use the device to obtain requested information. A conditioning program was used, initially associating a tone with a question and then gradually fading the tone to the point at which the patient would spontaneously take out the device and use it to look up requested information.

Several points from this research can be generalized to mathematics. First, it is often necessary to encourage the individual to use the device when needed in a natural environment. There is an extensive literature on characteristics of the environment in relation to the use of prosthetic aids and assistive devices. Rogers and Holm (1998) said, "The presence of a grab bar on the bathtub is a safety feature, but if it is not used when entering and exiting the bathtub it does not serve this purpose" (p. 103). The same may be said for cognitive function assistive devices. Clinically, rejection of prostheses such as hearing aids is not uncommon. We have recently published a case report of a patient with amnesia who "lost" a reminding device he was given to use, apparently because it represented something of a security threat (Goldstein, 1999). Indeed, the training might involve practice runs in which the student is called and asked to solve a problem. She or he may be questioned about using the device and encouraged to use it if it is not being used. That procedure should be followed by hopefully *in vivo* instruction in use of the device in educational or vocational settings. The basic point is that the individual with a mathematics difficulty may not be able to make full utilization of a hand calculator to the extent that an individual without a disability can, without special instructions. With regard to design, it may be necessary to use specially modified hand calculators engineered to accommodate the specifics of the deficit. For example, with new developments in voice technology, it may be possible to utilize auditory as opposed to visual calculators for people who do better with hearing than with seeing information. For example, some individuals with mathematics difficulties may do better by presenting problems through speaking into a device and receiving spoken answers. Speech may also be employed by individuals whose physical disabilities prevent use of a keyboard.

Assistive Devices as a Means of Accommodation

The use of assistive devices may be viewed as part of the process of accommodation. Accommodation often involves the use of devices such as calculators or tape recorders, allowance of increased time to perform a task, or receiving and transmitting information in other than the conventional modality. The question then becomes one of determining the most productive accommodations for the individual with mathematics disability. Very few jobs now require hand calculation without the use of even a simple calculator. Perhaps an appropriate question for contemporary times would involve whether or not individuals with mathematical difficulties also have difficulties with learning how to use modern computers. If they do, while assistive devices may get the individual beyond the limitations imposed by being able to do basic calculations, they may not help with more advanced mathematics or mathematical problem solving. Computers may do your work for you through solving exceedingly complex mathematical problems and performing complex operations, but they may not improve conceptualization of the mathematical aspects of the problem. On the other hand, defining assistive devices and accommodation as remediative procedures has philosophical implications since to some extent the functional handicaps associated with mathematics difficulties may have diminished substantially since we now have machines that can perform mathematical functions more quickly, precisely, and accurately than the human brain. It may be reasonable to suggest that calculators and computers may be used as assistive devices when appropriately applied within the context of a more comprehensive program, but serve other purposes as well. It may be analogous to the idea that a lens may be used in microscopy, astronomy, or other scientific endeavors, but can also assist people with their vision. To draw the analogy further, this latter application is best done by a clinician skilled in optometrics.

Nevertheless, there are now many people with significant calculation difficulties that can perform work-related tasks requiring calculation through the use of calculators or computers. Only rarely, if ever, are they required to do mental arithmetic of the type assessed with the Wechsler Intelligence Scales. The choice therefore arises in intervention as to whether to teach mental arithmetic or to optimize utilization of calculators and related assistive technologies. Future research might address itself to a number of issues in this area including such matters as whether it is really true that people who have difficulty with mechanical arithmetic and related skills are as adept at using calculators or computers as are people who do not have these difficulties, and does the failure to attempt to teach mental arithmetic and only focus on better use of assistive devices compromise the development of problem-solving ability and analytic reasoning in other areas?

Vocational Choice

Appropriate vocational choice is also a major consideration. There appear to be a number of occupations, notably architecture and engineering for which mathematical and associated spatial skills are crucial. Even if mathematics is remediated, it is exceptionally difficult to develop the spatial skills with which successful engineers and architects are apparently gifted. Appropriate guidance and career counseling may be quite helpful here. A different set of problems arises for the individual who, for example, wants to become a physician, and probably has the ability to do so except for difficulty with the mathematics courses needed to get into medical school. In these cases, one might consider favorably the potential benefits of an aggressive remediation program in mathematics. Still another consideration involves the individual with acquired brain damage who can no longer function adequately in a previously held occupation. Here, the major issues often involve modification of level of aspiration and vocational placement that is viable in consideration of the permanent residual disability. The period during which there is consideration of returning or not returning to work is typically stressful, and supportive treatment is often need for individuals who try and fail or who have a future characterized by inability to function at a previously held level. Early disability retirement or return to employment at a lower level are generally the major alternatives, with the outcome often depending on a complex combination of motivation, status of residual abilities, and vocational opportunities.

A CASE STUDY

Mathematics is in one respect a language that uses numbers and symbols rather than words, a system of logical operations, such as dividing and subtracting, and an analytic method that serves in problem solving. It has been described as a "handmaiden to the sciences" since it supports such major scientific areas as chemistry, physics, and some of the life and social sciences. Some individuals have major difficulties in studying science because they can't handle the mathematics. They may have excellent language skills, reasoning ability, ability to learn in areas other than mathematics, and excellent memory.

The case presented here is that of an individual who wanted to be a scientist and possessed many of these positive cognitive characteristics. However, from early in school, he did poorly at mathematics, with recollection of failure going back to the first grade. Other schoolwork was performed at an average or better level, but poor mathematical abilities compromised achievement in such areas as physics and chemistry when he was in high school. It was noted early in school that he had not developed a clear hand preference. He was primarily left handed, but would write with either his left or right hand. Over time, he remained predominantly left-handed, but increasingly wrote consistently with his right hand. He was right eyed, making him crossed eye-hand dominant, and possibly efforts to convert him to right-handedness were owing to the belief that existed at the time of his education that not to do so would impede his ability to learn to read. Ultimately, his reading turned out to be normal.

The quality of his mathematics education was high, and he could recall having excellent, interesting teachers throughout school. He experienced understanding everything during the lectures, but did exceptionally poorly in solving problems at home and on tests. He minimally passed courses up to elementary algebra, but failed intermediate algebra. Exponents, complex equations, and related matters were not at all well-learned. Repetition of intermediate algebra led to a minimal pass. Since his other grades were good, he was admitted to an academically prestigious college, and since he had passed intermediate algebra in high school, he was immediately placed into a required two-semester calculus course. The first semester was failed, repeated and minimally passed, and the second semester was minimally passed. However, he had little real understanding of calculus. He was required to take a course in statistics, and although the mathematics involved were less demanding than calculus, he achieved a minimal pass.

Other grades still being good, he was admitted to graduate school where he was required to take advanced statistics. Surprisingly, he got straight A's in both statistics courses, marking the beginning of a series of unexpected developments. During graduate school and following completion of a Ph.D., he became heavily involved in research. Most of the research involved quantitative analysis of data, with a heavy emphasis on advanced multivariate statistics. These methods involve use of matrix algebra, simultaneous equations, and related advanced mathematical methods. However, when he read journal articles, he had extensive difficulty in following mathematical arguments based on sets of formulas and equations. Fundamental mathematical ability did not appear to improve at all. Nevertheless, he authored a book in research design and statistics, and has published numerous scientific papers involving application of advanced statistical methods.

This case is of particular interest because it is illustrative of how an individual with substantial mathematical disability can use mathematics in his everyday life. He never received special education or tutoring in mathematics since these options were not available to him during the period of his education. It is likely that with or without his awareness, he spontaneously employed a number of learning strategies and that he was able to use some better than average abilities for compensatory purposes. With regard to calculation, he rarely did mental arithmetic and always had available some form of hand calculator or computer for his work. In initial learning of statistics he accepted the common wisdom that one could not do statistical analyses without learning and understanding the underlying mathematical basis. He eventually discovered that, at least for him, that was not the case, and that statistical analyses could be accomplished without any basic understanding of the relevant mathematics. Computation was always done with a calculator, but everyone uses a calculator to do statistical computations, and it was never viewed in terms of accommodation or use of an assistive device. He was greatly benefited by the development of the "statistical packages" associated with the then evolving high-speed computers. He was able to use these packages and do some of the necessary programming for them, since that did not involve mathematics. He learned that the really important matter was a conceptual understanding of the substantive problem rather than the specifics of the mathematics used in solution. The disability apparently did not extend to interpretation of statistical results but mainly to the mechanical and conceptual elements involved in obtaining them, some of which may involve matrix algebra and geometry, and other forms of higher mathematics. Good writing skills allowed him to translate these interpretations into scholarly and readable prose.

This individual has not outgrown his mathematics disability and still has problems with more than the simplest algebraic equations. He cannot solve them nor can he follow a mathematical argument based upon a series of equations. Hand calculation is slow and often inaccurate. Such concepts as negative exponents are difficult for him to grasp. His reading comprehension of statistics and mathematics books is limited to the description of the procedures and the mechanical formulas used for computation. Material on derivation of these formulas is beyond him. Nevertheless he has developed skills needed to use mathematics in his occupation through a combination of identifying areas in which he can function well, using technology that serves as assistive devices, and exploiting his good skills as a method of compensation.

Perhaps this case can be more fully explained by revealing the identity of the individual. He is one of the authors of this book (GG). Having revealed myself, I can make some additional comments. I do not completely understand the basis for my mathematics disability. There is a family history of left-handedness and associated awkwardness, but I know of no relatives with notably poor mathematics ability. My spatial and motor abilities are not as good as my verbal skills, and my left-handedness may be associated with crossed cerebral dominance for language.   It is also not clear to me whether special education efforts accomplished during my early childhood would have significantly improved my basic mathematical abilities. I doubt that they would have because I worked very hard at mathematics and had excellent teachers. There was no lack of opportunity for special attention when needed. The adjustments I made were not specific, intentional efforts but seemed to be more driven by my ambition to enter a scientifically oriented occupation. Perhaps the major general consideration here is that one can use mathematics without "doing" mathematics, particularly with the technology we now have available.

SUMMARY

Consistent with the other disorders and disabilities discussed in this volume, mathematics disability exists in adulthood. We use the term "exists" rather than "persists" because there is a greater prevalence of acquired mathematics disability in adulthood than is the case for reading or writing. We also use the term "disability" rather than "disorder" because many adults with mathematics difficulties would not meet DSM-IV criteria for Mathematics Disorder or any of the academic skill disorders. In brighter adults, notably college students, the distribution of academic skill subtypes is different from what is the case for children and lower to average ability adults. That is, in college students one seldom sees individuals with global disability or the reading worse than arithmetic subtype, but the reading better than arithmetic subtype is quite common. Unlike children, there appears to be a high prevalence of adults with substantial mathematics disability who either do not have the typically associated spatial and motor neuropsychological deficits or who do not meet DSM-IV criteria for Mathematics Disorder or other academic skill disorder. Many adults who sustain diffuse brain damage or focal damage particularly to the left posterior hemisphere may acquire mathematics disability. An unknown but apparently substantial number of individuals have mathematics anxiety either as the source of the disability or a reaction to it. Interventions may cover a broad range including formal specific remediation, general remediation of study habits and organizing skills, cognitive rehabilitation of attention, memory, and problem solving ability, use of accommodation and assistive devices, anti-anxiety treatment, and vocational counseling particularly with regard to occupational choice.

3

NONVERBAL LEARNING DISABILITY

INTRODUCTION

Myklebust (Johnson and Myklebust, 1971; Myklebust, 1975) coined the term nonverbal learning disability to describe children with disturbed social relationships, poor social skills, difficulty in interpreting the meanings of actions of others, arithmetic deficits, and functional difficulties such as distinguishing left from right, telling time, reading maps, and following directions. This chapter begins with a description of nonverbal learning disability that considers diagnostic considerations, epidemiological aspects, and proposed biological mechanisms for the disorder. The neuropsychological aspects of nonverbal learning disability are discussed, framing the subsequent consideration of psychosocial and vocational function. Next, various treatments are reviewed, again within the framework of the neuropsychological strengths and weaknesses associated with this disorder. This chapter concludes with suggestions for future work.

CHARACTERISTICS OF NONVERBAL LEARNING DISABILITY

Individuals with nonverbal learning disability (NLD) are characterized by problems in the organization, analysis, and synthesis of nonverbal information. The concept of NLD emerges from a long and somewhat controversial history (Feagans and McKinney, 1991; Hooper and Willis, 1989; Torgeson, 1991). Today, NLD is becoming more fully characterized in children, but the topic continues to stimulate much discussion. While the purpose of this chapter is not to resolve this debate, it is important to acknowledge the historical "evolution" and the various diagnostic labels for this group of primary disabilities that are generally classified under the rubric of "nonverbal" deficits.

Before 1970, educators assumed that learning disability was a homogeneous entity, most relevant to the school setting, and "outgrown" by adulthood. Based on this assumption, researchers employed comparative-population or contrasting groups methodology to determine the specific strengths and weaknesses of children with learning disabilities (Beers, 1998). In the 70s, however, both clinical and empirical models of learning disability raised the possibility of several relatively discrete constellations of symptoms and learning patterns.

Feagans and McKinney (1991) acknowledge the importance of the search for subtypes of learning disabilities as a way to clarify the theoretical framework and adequately reflect the multidimensionality of learning disability in general. As these authors note, early subtype investigations were grounded in carefully considered clinical observations regarding children with LD. Most particularly, this work documented the developmental variability of these children. Research generally compared and contrasted various patterns on IQ tests (e.g., Bannatyne reclassification, ACID cluster), attempted to identify and describe "academic" subtypes associated with various reading problems, or explored patterns based on the IQ-achievement discrepancy then used to identify children with LD. At the same time, neuropsychologists and neurologists also began to compare children with various learning disorders on neuropsychological constructs such as memory, learning, and attention. While these clinical studies did much to advance knowledge of LD in general and subtypes of LD in particular, Feagans *et al.* applaud rigorous empirically-based methods such as factor analysis and cluster analysis as providing the firm methodological foundation for subtype research. They note, "...empirical classification demonstrates the importance of creating more homogeneous subtypes of specific leaning disabilities since it clearly shows the intra-individual differences of children with learning disabilities." (p. 24).

Much early classification research focused on defining subtypes of children with reading disorders. More recently, however, attention has turned to children who display deficits in nonverbal learning. In their cogent review, Semrud-Clikeman and Hynd (1990) discuss the similarities and differences of six classification methods used to characterize children with NLD. As might be expected, the over riding difficulties in visual-perceptual skills, social skills, motor development, and arithmetic are marked with labels that generally reflect the research background of the investigators. Several subtypes are classified according to the area of the brain felt to be affected: right hemisphere syndrome (Voeller, 1986; Voeller and Heilman, 1988), left hemisyndrome (Denckla, 1978), and right parietal lobe syndrome (Weinberg and McLean, 1986). Others base classification upon clusters of more diverse symptoms including Asperger Syndrome (Asperger, 1979; Gillberg, 1985; Shea and Mesibov, 1985; Wing, 1985) and, albeit of questionable validity, Developmental Gerstmann Syndrome (Kinsborne, 1968; PeBenito, 1987; PeBenito, Fisch, and Fisch, 1988). Another classification schema, and one of the few that has extended research into adulthood, is based on a disorder of central processing that is descriptively labeled as a nonverbal perceptual-organization-output disorder (Rourke and Fisk, 1981). While the reader is referred to the Semrud-Clikeman and Hynd review and the other references listed for a comprehensive discussion of classification methods, research within each category has identified several unifying constructs. For example, almost every study has identified delays in arithmetic, poor motor development, and visual-spatial problems. In contrast, no matter how classified most subjects showed relatively strong vocabulary skills but disorders in higher order language skills (e.g., pragmatics). Subjects within the various classifications also showed remarkable and striking similar difficulties in social understanding, interpretation of gesture, and discrimination of the nuances of speech. As Semrud-Clikeman and Hynd caution, "All of these classification schemes should be viewed as exploratory.... replication and refinement is needed..." (p. 205). Of the investigations discussed, the work of Rourke and his colleagues address these concerns in both children and adults and will be discussed in some detail here.

During the 1980's, the seminal work of Rourke and his colleagues provided major support for the characterization of what has come to be termed NLD syndrome. This syndrome describes a constellation of deficits that co-occur at a rate greater than chance and disrupt abilities generally felt to be subsumed by the right hemisphere of the brain (Petrauskas and Rourke, 1979; Rourke, 1985). Interestingly, these researchers were among the first to add comprehensive neuropsychological assessment to the more standard psychoeducational evaluation (i.e., intellectual ability and academic achievement tests) in order to describe the cognitive deficits and strengths of children with learning disability. (For a complete review of this literature, see Beers, 1998). Based on these early studies and further work done across developmental levels, Rourke (1989a) developed a dynamic picture of NLD. In Rourke's model, children with NLD syndrome performed better on neuropsychological measures associated with the left hemisphere while the converse was true in children with reading disorders. In contrast children with NLD had more difficulty on tasks measuring tactile and visual perception and attention, performed poorly on tests requiring complex psychomotor skills, and demonstrated problems in abstract concept formation and problem solving.

Definition and Diagnosis of Nonverbal Learning Disability

As with other subtypes of learning disability, evidence suggests that NLD persists into adulthood (Denckla, 1993; Rourke, Young, Strang, and Russell, 1986b); and, in fact, NLD may not be diagnosed *until* adulthood. Later in this chapter we will review case material illustrating such an example. Two problems relating to the diagnosis of NLD are considered here. The first is that of the lack of diagnostic specificity in the general classification method employed by mental health professionals and sometimes educators. The second is that of differential diagnosis.

Although the work of Rourke *et al.* has taken major steps in defining the disorder, there is little consensus as to the definitive, operationalized definition of NLD. As discussed in Chapter I, the specific characteristics of the descriptive term "learning disability" usually reflect the perspective of the professionals involved, be they educators, neuropsychologists, psychiatrists, behavioral neurologists, or rehabilitation specialists. Although the literature is beginning to report more concise and concrete definitions of various reading disorders, NLD lacks what Stanovich (1999) terms a "domain specific" diagnosis that enables researchers to address the issues of identification, diagnosis, intervention, and prognosis. This may be because the problems with arithmetic so often noted in children with NLD are frequently attributed to motivational or cultural factors and thus tend to be overlooked rather than conceptualized as a single feature of a more over riding cognitive disorder (Fletcher, 1989).

Within the mental health system, assigning a formal medical diagnosis to a person having a "learning disability" is rendered even more problematic by the inability of the *Diagnostic and Statistical Manual of Mental Disorders, 4th Edition* (DSM-IV) (American Psychiatric Association, 1994) to adequately characterize NLD. Indeed, when an actual diagnosis is required, that of Learning Disability Not Otherwise Specified (LD-NOS) with the addition of Cognitive Disorder NOS is probably the most appropriate. Certainly these catchall categories fail to elaborate the principle identifying cognitive patterns and symptoms, discussed later in this chapter, that represent the defining characteristics of NLD. Finally, because the diagnosis of LD-NOS also fails to reflect the emotional and social ramifications so frequently associated with NLD, any appropriate Axis I diagnosis (e.g., Major Depressive Disorder; Adjustment Disorder) should also be assigned if the individual meets those particular criteria.

Differential Diagnosis

According to DSM-IV coding procedures, certain diagnoses must be excluded or "ruled-out" before the diagnosis of a developmental disorder is appropriate. The differential diagnosis section for learning disability in the DSM-IV again reflects a poor understanding of the complexity of learning disability in general, and NLD in particular. For example, rule out diagnoses are usually education-ally focused, including mental retardation and other specific learning disabilities such as Disorder of Written Expression. Kinsborne's (1997) recommendations reflect a better understanding of the complexity of NLD. Below are aspects of particular disorders that Kinsborne feels may lead one to misdiagnose symptoms as consistent with NLD.

1. Attention Deficit Hyperactivity Disorder
   • Difficulty with "automatized" learning such as multiplication tables and number facts
   • Social insensitivity associated with poor impulse control
2. Depression
   • Impaired visuospatial performance
   • Mild left-sided neurological signs
3. Over focused attention (e.g., Obsessive-Compulsive Disorder)
   • Slowed information processing
   • Perseveration or rigid fixation of problem-solving techniques
   • Overly focused on individual standards to the point of ignoring social conventions
4. Autistic spectrum disorders (e.g., high functioning autism, Asperger Syn-drome)
   • Rigid problem-solving abilities
   • Circumscribed interests
5. Anxiety Disorder
   • Arithmetic skills disrupted by heightened anxiety
   • Interpersonal difficulties
6. Social Learning Disability
   • Poor social skills

The diagnosis of social learning disability and Asperger Syndrome warrant discussion here because they both illustrate not only the controversial aspects of NLD but also how the professional's perspective is sometimes reflected in the diagnostic label. Voeller (1991, 1997) considers children and adults who evi-dence chronic difficulty relating to others to have another variant of "nonverbal" learning disability: social-emotional learning disability (SELD). Noting that these individuals usually present to psychiatrists and psychologists with anxiety, depression, and school problems, Voeller posits that this group is united by their incompetencies of social communication. Although Voeller readily notes the cognitive investigations that raise the possibility of right hemisphere dysfunc-tion with attendant attention and visual-spatial deficits, she describes the social communication deficit as the *defining* or overarching characteristic of the disorder. In contrast, Rourke (Rourke and Fisk, 1992) argues that the social, emotional, and academic manifestations of NLD are a result of the interaction between neuropsychological deficits and preserved areas of cognitive function. While Voeller discusses various DSM-based diagnoses that more or less successfully capture the defining characteristics of SELD, the pervasiveness of social deficits across disorders, however, does not support the argument that SELD is a *primary* disability. For example, in Gresham and Elliott's view, specific social skill deficits are not unique to persons with learning disabilities (Gresham and Elliott, 1989). Reiff, Gerber, and Ginsberg (1997) remind us that the NJCLD definition for learning disabilities specifically states, "Problems in self-regulatory behaviors, social perception and social interaction may exist...but do not *by themselves* constitute a learning disability." (p. 59) (Emphasis added.). Thus, while the diagnosis of SELD might facilitate mental health services by acknowledging the severity of social deficits, this label may actually restrict other appropriate interventions. In order for these individuals to obtain appropriate treatment within the school system (for younger persons) or at vocational rehabilitation agencies, psychoeducational and/or neuropsychological testing must confirm deficits in *cognitive* abilities.

Later in this volume we will discuss the relationship between high functioning autism and severe verbal learning disability. As noted by Rourke (1989a) and others (Semrud-Clikeman and Hynd, 1990; Gillberg, 1983; Weintraub and Mesulam, 1983), another autistic spectrum disorder, Asperger Syndrome bears a rather striking similarity to NLD and may represent a more severe expression of the same syndrome. In fact, Asperger Syndrome is distinguished from high functioning autism by some of the defining characteristics of NLD. That is, the normal development of language coupled with marked visual-spatial deficits and motor clumsiness in the context of generally normal intellectual function. While everyday language function is intact, as with NLD pragmatic interactive language skills are usually deficient. In addition, individuals with Asperger Syndrome display social impairment and as adults are frequently overwhelmed by the complex demands of adult life.

A study by Klin, Volkmar, Sparrow, Cicchetti, and Rourke (1995) investigated the validity of Asperger Syndrome in adolescents, comparing neuropsychological performance to a group with high functioning autism. Noting the similarities in presentation between Asperger Syndrome and NLD, the authors hypothesized that the pattern of neuropsychological test scores in the AS group would be similarly to that associated with NLD. Subjects who met rigorous diagnostic criteria for either high functioning autism or AS were selected from consecutive admissions at a treatment center. Neuropsychological testing was completed without knowledge of the psychiatric diagnosis. Using these results, subjects were classified as meeting neuropsychological criteria for NLD by experienced clinical neuropsychologists after review of test results and behavioral assessment (e.g., articulation, prosody, verbal content, empathy). Interrater reliabilities for both the psychiatric and neuropsychological classifications were evaluated and found to be excellent for diagnostic assignment and very good for the LD characterization. Groups were compared in terms of Verbal vs. Performance IQ difference, the overlap between psychiatric diagnosis and LD characterization, and a broad range of *a priori* defined cognitive characteristics. Although Full Scale IQ did not differ between groups, the AS group demonstrated a higher VIQ and lower PIQ when compared to the autistic group. The degree of overlap between psychiatric diagnosis and NLD was minimal with only 1of 19 of the autistic individuals meeting criteria for NLD but almost all (18/21) of the AS group meeting that criteria. The neuropsychological profiles were also compared with respect to 22 identifying characteristics of NLD. For each characteristic the frequency of individuals in the two groups who exhibited deficits was compared. The AS group evidenced a significantly higher frequency of individuals deficient in the following areas: visual-motor integration, visual-spatial ability, visual memory, and nonverbal concept formation. The autistic group showed a significantly higher number of individuals deficient in the areas of auditory perception, verbal memory, articulation, vocabulary, and verbal output. Frequencies were not different with respect to novel material, rote learning, verbal content, and verbal concept formation. Based on these results, the investigators concluded that NLD can serve as a marker of AS, and that the neuropsychological deficits associated with AS are distinct from those associated with high functioning autism, especially when stringent psychiatric diagnostic criteria are applied. In spite of the diverse neuropsychological characterization of these two disorder, the authors caution that further research must be completed on the developmental, genetic, and neuroantonomic aspects of the two conditions before further conclusions can be drawn regarding etiological similarities or differences. In any event, these findings suggest that the interventions and vocational training appropriate for adults with NLD might have some clinical utility for individuals with Asperger Syndrome as well.

Incidence and Prevalence

As noted in Chapter 1, approximately 50% of the children receiving special education services in the United Sates have a learning disability of unspecified subtype (U.S. Department of Education, 1989). Expressed differently, approximately 1.3 million students between the ages of 12 and 21 with LD received special education services (Dowdy, Smith, and Nowell, 1996). More recent data indicate that between 5 to 20 percent of the general population has some type of LD (Gadbow and DuBois, 1998; Gerber and Reiff, 1994). However, there is little discussion of the incidence and prevalence of NLD in either children or adults in the literature. This fact is probably not surprising due to the historical emphasis on reading disabilities, the continuing controversial nature of NLD, and the lack of a clearly operationalized definition of this disorder. Early work by Denckla (1979) identified a 1% prevalence of right hemisphere learning disability in a general clinical LD sample. More recently, Rourke (1995) estimated that the prevalence of NLD within the general LD clinical sample is from 5% to 10%, an increase that perhaps is due to the somewhat better characterization of NLD. Based on a conservative estimate of the 10% rate of unspecified LD in the general population, Rourke's data suggest the population prevalence of NLD is between .5 and 1.0%. These statistics indicate that NLD is less prevalent than internalized disorders such as Major Depressive Disorder and Generalized Anxiety Disorder that occur in approximately 15% and 5% of the general population, respectively (American Psychiatric Association, 1994). In contrast, NLD is as prevalent as Schizophrenia, a thought disorder that also occurs in between .5 and 1.0% of the population (American Psychiatric Association, 1994).

Etiology and Neurobiological Correlates

The processing deficits associated with NLD suggest that dysfunction in the right, or nondominant, hemisphere of the brain may account for this disorder. However, as with definition, the etiology of NLD remains controversial. Some like Hiscock and Hiscock (1991) assert that NLD is a variant of "normal" learning while others speculate regarding genetic and/or encephalopathic origins of the disorder (Denckla, 1983; Pennington, 1991; Rourke, 1988; Semrud-Clikeman and Hynd, 1990; Voeller, 1997). These encephalopathic or environmental etiologies of NLD are considered variable and include pre- and perinatal complications, acquired insults such as early head trauma, untreated hydrocephalus, cranial radiation, and agenesis of the corpus callosum. Rourke (1988; Tsatsanis and Rourke, 1995) has developed a "white matter model" to describe the brain mechanisms responsible for NLD. This model is based on the assumption of the divided responsibilities between the two brain hemispheres, with the right hemisphere being more involved in the intermodal integration and sharing processed information with the left hemisphere. In contrast, the functions of the left hemisphere are more intramodal and discrete. In more everyday terms, the right side of the brain appears to be specialized to synthesize diverse information, process novel stimuli, and develop novel concepts. As Rourke notes, all these activities depend on the greater density of white matter or the myelinated fibers that are responsible for communication within the brain. Thus, the mechanism of NLD may be the changes in particular brain circuits that are disproportionately represented in the right hemisphere and are in this altered state "...less evolved and less specialized" (Tsatsanis and Rourke, 1995, p. 481). As noted above, these changes in white matter occur for various reasons such as abnormal development, degenerative processes, or injury. This, in fact, may account for the numerous syndromes (e.g., Fetal Alcohol, Asperger, Williams) that demonstrate the NLD syndrome to a greater or lesser degree. (See Rourke, 1995 for an extensive discussion of this topic).

Until recently the evidence suggesting that learning disabilities are associated with neurological dysfunction has been inferred from correlation studies. While the literature exploring the right hemisphere function on learning and behavior is extremely limited, advances in technology have allowed for interesting studies that are applicable to the mechanisms of NLD and validation of the white matter hypothesis. An early study by Gur *et al.* (1980) measured regional cerebral blood flow and found a greater gray to white matter ratio in the left hemisphere, confirming differences in the distribution of white matter between the two hemispheres. Voeller (1986) identified a group of children from clinical referrals who demonstrated right hemisphere findings on either a neurological examination or a CT scan who also showed neuropsychological deficits suggestive of right hemisphere dysfunction. These groups also had the typical NLD intellectual ability profile (i.e., VIQ>PIQ) and variable academic skills showing reading ability stronger than math ability. Nichelli and Venneri (1995) studied a 22-year-old man who demonstrated neuropsychological and academic deficits highly consistent with NLD as described by Rourke. Although structural imaging studies were normal, a positron emission tomograph (PET) scan indicated a marked hypometabolism in the right hemisphere. This finding provides preliminary evidence to suggest NLD might reflect *functional* abnormalities in the brain even when *structural* abnormalities are not appreciated.

CONTRIBUTIONS OF NEUROPSYCHOLOGICAL ASSESSMENT

Neuropsychological assessment for individuals with learning disability has met with controversy over the years. When considering these disabilities in children, some have argued that neuropsychological batteries lacked validity when used for this population (Coles, 1978). Others have successfully refuted this conclusion with respect to the both children (Rourke, 1989a) and adults (Beers, Goldstein, and Katz, 1994; Goldstein, Katz, Slomka, and Kelly, 1993; McCue, Goldstein, Shelley, and Katz, 1986; Oestreicher and O'Donnell, 1995). In spite of these studies confirming the construct and discriminant validity of the neuropsychological methodology, some educators continue to strongly criticize these techniques, feeling they have little to offer either in understanding the etiology of the disorder or the effect of deficits on everyday functioning.

Calling into question the "disease model" of LD that emphasizes the source of learning problems, Hiscock and Hiscock (1991) challenge the educational utility of neuropsychological data in relation to academic problems. In a comprehensive discussion of this issue these authors posit that LD is a normal variation of skills rather than a reflection of subtle neurological deficits. They charge that the disease model justifies gathering extraneous information regarding perception, attention, memory, motor skills, language, and reasoning that from an educational perspective has little value. In fact, these authors feel that the application of neuropsychological findings may actually distort the nature of the learning disorder and contribute to unrealistic expectations regarding treatment and outcome. As an alternative, Hiscock and Hiscock propose that investigations of LD should focus on the learning problem *per se*, with an emphasis on academic remediation (For further discussion of the interface between special education, neuropsychology, and neurobiology, also see Kershner, 1991 and Duane, 1991). While we agree that early neuropsychological investigations focused almost exclusively on localization and lateralization (Morrow and Beers, 1995), the field has evolved from this narrow perspective. Based on both our clinical experiences, the validation of neuropsychological methodology with respect to LD (Selz and Reitan, 1979a, 1979b; O'Donnell, 1991), and recent advances in neuroimaging, we feel that a comprehensive neuropsychological assessment provides essential information for the accurate development of individualized academic and psychological interventions. A neuropsychological evaluation, based on the biopsychosocial model, actually seeks explanations "other than" neurological impairment. When these other explanations are ruled out, the evaluation synthesizes information regarding the integrity of the central nervous system across the cognitive domains in order to develop effective remediation and compensatory strategies. The next section of this chapter illustrates neuropsychology's role in defining and treating NLD in particular.

Neuropsychology's Role in Defining the NLD Syndrome

As noted earlier, NLD—at least as conceptualized by Rourke—evolved from the methodology of neuropsychology. Because his early studies of children are reviewed elsewhere (Beers, 1998), they will not be discussed in detail here. Based on these and later investigations, Rourke has developed a dynamic picture of the neuropsychological strengths and weaknesses and emotional sequelae associated with NLD. Although not discussed in this chapter, Rourke's schema includes a hierarchy of neuropsychological deficits and strengths that are related to academic performance and to social functioning (Harnadek and Rourke, 1994). When considering this list of NLD symptoms and intact abilities, one should note that this classification is based on shared features and that all aspects of the classification are not necessary to define any individual case (Fletcher, 1989).

1. Generalized tactile-perceptual problems and bilateral tactile-perceptual deficits that may be disproportionately affected on the left side of the body;

2. Generalized psychomotor coordination problems again with the possibility of more deficiency noted on the left side;
3. Deficient visual-spatial abilities;
4. Relatively preserved rote memory skills;
5. Deficits in nonverbal problem solving and difficulty discerning cause and effect relationships;
6. Inability to benefit from feedback in novel and/or complex situations;
7. Lack of appreciation of humor at an age-appropriate level;
8. Rigidity and a general inflexibility resulting in an over reliance on routine;
9. Language deficits that include verbosity, lack of prosody in speech, and impoverished content of language;
10. Relative deficits in mechanical arithmetic and reading comprehension;
11. Intact reading recognition and spelling (spelling may be deficient but it is usually phonetic); and
12. Impaired social functioning (e.g. perception, judgment, and interaction), with a tendency toward social withdrawal.

Evidence from the few extant longitudinal studies suggests that there is a developmental aspect to these deficits; that is, the cognitive and socioemotional deficits become more debilitating as the child grows older (Casey, Rourke, and Picard, 1991). This fact is particularly intriguing with respect to NLD as it manifests in adults. However, a literature search conducted for the years 1997 though mid-2000 identified over 300 empirically based studies of adults with LD but only three of these investigations differentiated between NLD and other subtypes. Comprehensive adult studies of NLD are long overdue.

Neuropsychological Aspects of Adult Studies

As learning disability subtypes gained empirical validation in the pediatric population, researchers turned their attention to validity and stability of these subtypes in older individuals. Rourke's group (Rourke *et al.*, 1986b) compared the neuropsychological test performance of adults (age range: 17 to 48) and children exhibiting the NLD pattern, finding almost identical cognitive profiles pattern but a general worsening of deficits. That is, adults were shown to have greater performance deficiencies relative to their age-matched peers. Interestingly, all of these adults had a history consistent with NLD as children (e.g., awkward and poorly coordinated, academic problems in mathematics, geography, science; relative success in language-based subjects; poor social skills), although none had received learning support in school.

Considering that the early investigations of NLD were stimulated by academic problems, it is not surprising that research has extended into the area of higher education. In his 1991 chapter, O'Donnell summarizes his own studies and those of others that investigated the construct and discriminate validity of the Halstead-Reitan Neuropsychological Test Battery (HRNB) in young adults with LD. Based on a sample of 233 young adults applying for college admission, his work demonstrated that HRNB factor scores were correlated with academic skills (i.e., reading, spelling, and arithmetic computation) and thus demonstrated the test's construct validity. In addition, the HRNB successfully differentiated normal young adults from those with LD or head injury, supporting the discriminate validity of the instrument. In fact, results indicated that approximately 42% of the young adults with LD experienced mild cerebral dysfunction, suggesting that the neuropsychological evaluation serves as an appropriate tool for planning interventions and accommodations in young adults. Finally, cluster analysis techniques were applied to neuropsychological data, resulting in homogeneous and valid LD subtypes. That is, the LD subtype with computational deficits in mathematics was associated with visual-spatial and abstract reasoning deficits.

Other, smaller studies, have also explored the validity of LD subtypes within the college population. For example, Morris and Walter (1991) applied Rourke's classification methods to study college students participating in a remedial mathematics class. Results indicated that 21% of these students met criteria for the arithmetic deficit subtype (21%), with the remainder exhibiting no learning disability at all. In our own work with a group of college students with previously unclassified LD, a group with mild head injury, and controls, we regrouped all students using a modification of the Rourke procedures (Rourke and Finlayson, 1978) into either a no LD or LD subtype (Beers, 1993; Beers et al., 1994). The majority of students who met LD criteria (46%) were found to have a global learning disability as defined by Rourke (Rourke and Finlayson, 1978). That is, they showed similar deficiency in the three academic areas of reading, mathematics, and written expression. Almost as many (43%) met criteria for an arithmetic disability and exhibited the pattern of neuropsychological deficits consistent with the more broadly defined NLD. A disability specific to reading and writing was not as frequently identified, occurring at the rate of approximately 10%.

Although the pervasive and persistent aspects of LD were pointed out in a position paper by the National Joint Committee of Learning Disabilities as early as 1985 (Smith, 1996), by the year 2000 very few studies had focused on homogeneous groups of adults with LD outside the academic setting. In 1986, Spreen and Haaf investigated the stability of three LD subtypes in an adult cohort (Mean age = 24 years) that they had evaluated during childhood (Mean age = 10 years). In both phases of this research the subjects were grouped using cluster analytic techniques. While there was not complete concordance with cluster classification at the two study points, visual-perceptual and graphomotor subtypes persisted into adulthood. Important to the present topic is the finding that subjects with LD displaying visual-spatial deficits in childhood maintained their level of impairment over the course of the study.

Our own group completed a series of investigations of older adults with LD who had been referred for vocational rehabilitation services. These studies demonstrated the utility of the Halstead Reitan Neuropsychological Battery and the Luria Nebraska in diagnosing and characterizing adult learning disability (Goldstein et al., 1993; Goldstein, Shelly, McCue, and Kane, 1987; McCue, Goldstein et al., 1986; McCue, Shelly, and Goldstein, 1986; McCue, Shelly, Goldstein, and Katz-Garris, 1984). McCue, Goldstein, et al. (1986) compared the neuropsychological test profiles of 100 adults having a mean age and education of 24.4 years and 10.5 years, respectively. The entire sample was learning disabled. Applying a rule-based method similar to that of Rourke and his colleagues, subjects were classified into three groups: Reading Disorder, Global Disorder, and Arithmetic Disorder. Findings indicted that only small proportions of the sample exhibited either a Reading or Arithmetic Disorder comparable with Rourke's groups. Most of the adult sample showed poor performance on both reading and arithmetic similar to Rourke's Global Deficit subtype. These results must be interpreted cautiously, however, as the sample was referred by the Office of Vocational Rehabilitation and may not be representative of the adult LD population as a whole.

A 1994 controlled study by Shafrir and Siegel is another of the large-scale investigations (N = 331) that explored the validity of LD subtypes in an older, nonacademic population (e.g., approximately 40% of this sample had not participated in postsecondary education). These researchers investigated adolescents and adults with LD (age range 16 to 72 years) classified by subtypes based on the pattern of academic achievement as described in children by Rourke (reading disability, arithmetic disability, reading and arithmetic disability) to determine the presence of discrete patterns with respect to cognitive tasks requiring attention, memory, and visual-spatial ability. The results of this study supported the hypothesis that homogeneous groups of learning disabled adults show similar cognitive or neuropsychological patterns as children with similar academic deficits. Specific to this discussion of NLD, is the finding that adults in the arithmetic disabled group did not show differences from normal controls with respect to phonological processing but performed at a lower but not deficient level on measures of vocabulary and reading recognition. In contrast, clear group differences were noted with respect to visual-spatial abilities. On this construct, the arithmetic disabled adults performed more poorly than both the normal control and the reading disabled groups.

A more recent study also applied a neuropsychological testing to classify individuals with LD receiving vocational rehabilitation services (Michaels, Lazar, and Risucci, 1997). Earlier work had described adults with LD involved in the governmental vocational rehabilitation setting as a *homogeneous group*, particularly as compared to college students with LD and individuals with LD already in the work force. The goal of this study was to provide more focused rehabilitation services. Comprehensive neuropsychological testing delineated within group differences in abilities in the domains of visual and auditory perception, verbal and nonverbal reasoning, and learning and memory. Subjects also completed instruments measuring more general constructs such as intellectual ability, academic achievement, and psychological adjustment. Measures of central tendency documented the low function of this group, particularly with respect to language, verbally mediated learning, and both verbal and nonverbal reasoning. Clinically significant Verbal versus Performance IQ differences were noted in 20 subjects (65% of these with PIQ > VIQ). However, the two IQ profiles did not relate to significant differences in cognitive functioning or language ability, a finding that suggests this comparison does not provide particularly relevant information at least in the OVR population. As the authors point out, neuropsychological testing did describe particular patterns of strengths and weaknesses of this vocational rehabilitation group. The investigators present the distributions of scores in the various cognitive domains grouped according to the following classifications: deficient, impaired, low average, high average, and superior. Visual inspection of these data indicated divergence from normality on several of the constructs. For example, a weakness was noted on several language dependent measures, including verbal learning, verbal reasoning, and verbal learning and memory. While this might suggest more evidence of verbal LD in this group of subjects, distributions also identified particular weaknesses in the domains of visual perception, nonverbal memory, and semantic language, areas often noted to be impaired in adults with NLD. From an overall standpoint, these individuals manifested a generally low level of function similar to the subjects in the McCue study (McCue *et al.*, 1986) discussed earlier. However, the variability noted within this sample does suggest that vocational decisions that are individualized based on neuropsychological assessment may have a better outcome. As Michaels *et al.* note, " [Neuropsychological] constructs...have the potential for being powerful predictors of service needs when combined with ...more direct indicators of competency" (p. 551).

An Assessment Model

Adults with LD often have difficulty understanding particular aspects of their learning disability and more broadly, how that disability actually affects their lives (Buchanan and Wolf, 1986). As noted earlier in this chapter, one assessment goal for adults with NLD is to understand how the disability interacts across life settings, including educational, vocational, family, and social. Rather than a narrowly focused assessment that attempts the identification of dysfunction in particular or even more general areas of the brain, results of a neuropsychological evaluation should also provide information relevant to the areas outlined in Table 1. As McCue (1993) notes, "Central to the task of providing services to persons with learning disabilities is obtaining a clear understanding of how the disability impairs the ability to function....in employment, in higher education, and in independent living" (p. 56). Contrary to the conclusions of Hiscock and Hiscock (1991), we assert that a comprehensive neuropsychological evaluation can delineate the impairment or underlying mechanisms of the disability, suggest appropriate remedial and or compensatory educational strategies, and provide the foundation for career counseling or vocational rehabilitation services (Beers, 1998). Various components of LD assessment including the clinical interview, functional assessment, psychoeducational assessment, and neuropsychological testing are demonstrated in the following case presentation. Essentially, a carefully considered neuropsychological assessment *begins* the actual intervention process and guides the further efforts of remediation, compensation, accommodation, vocational rehabilitation, and individual psychotherapy as well.

TABLE 1. ASPECTS OF TREATMENT ADDRESSED BY COMPREHENSIVE NEUROPSYCHOLOGICAL ASSESSMENT

Intervention
- Capitalization on strengths
- Remediation
- Compensation
- Avoidance
- Individual/group psychotherapy
- Support Groups
- Vocational rehabilitation

Accommodation
- Academic
- Workplace

Case Study: "How do I get to the bank from the grocery store?"

RS is a 48-year-old, married, Caucasian female referred for a neuropsychological evaluation by her neurologist. While the patient's neurological examination and a recent magnetic resonance imaging scan were unremarkable, the referring physician noted a history of academic problems characterized by reported difficulties in reading comprehension, mathematical operations, and visual-spatial orientation.

RS described a long history of "learning disabilities" that were noted in school when her teachers realized she was "different." Apparently never formally diagnosed with LD, RS states that her parents told her she was "stupid." RS indicated that she has always read fluently, but with poor comprehension. Math was consistently her most difficult subject. She described long-standing difficulty working puzzles, poor coordination, difficulty learning new procedures, and problems finding her way around shopping malls and the city in general. When describing her navigation problems, RS indicated that she had to return home between each errand, otherwise she lost her way. RS also described feeling extremely uneasy when the furniture is rearranged in her home. She reported the recurring dream of being blind and in a state of complete hopelessness and panic. In spite of these problems, RS recounted her assets as successfully completing a nursing program. She has been steadily employed and reported that she is successful in her profession. However, RS noted that she has particular difficulty with unpredictable situations or when over learned sequences change. At these times she indicated that she experiences heightened anxiety that in turn further compromises her effectiveness. RS recounted her problems working with unfamiliar medical equipment, stating that she has much difficulty learning how to set up a piece of equipment by watching a demonstration.

The patient's medical history is essentially unremarkable. She had a breast biopsy (benign) approximately 10 years earlier and a tonsillectomy and adnoidectomy in the remote past. She had hepatitis as a child. RS did not endorse the current use of alcohol but felt that she has used alcohol as a means to alleviate her anxiety in the past. She described attention and concentration problems that have worsened over the past 5 years or so, reporting a somewhat cyclical pattern. RS was treated by a psychologist for depressive symptoms approximately 5 years ago. According to the patient, she was diagnosed with PTSD secondary to her ridicule by her parents and with a "visual agnosia." RM is prescribed Wellbutrin, 75mg three times a day by her family physician. The patient described learning problems in her mother and her siblings that are similar to her own. Her father was described as dysthymic.

While tearful at times during testing, RS appeared motivated to do her best. Test results, shown in Table 2, appear to present a valid measure of the patient's current level of cognitive function.

TABLE 2. SUMMARY OF TEST SCORES

Wechsler Adult Intelligence Scale-Revised

FSIQ: 98	VIQ: 107	PIQ: 87	
Information	12	Picture Completion	06
Digit Span	09	Picture Arrangement	06
Vocabulary	13^S	Block Design	08
Arithmetic	10	Object Assembly	06
Comprehension	12	Digit Symbol	07
Similarities	09		

Academic Achievement

Wide Range Achievement Test-Revised
Reading	109
Spelling	105
Arithmetic	102

Nelson-Denny Reading Test
Reading Comprehension 30th percentile (Finished early but did not check work)

Woodcock Johnson Psychoeducational Battery
Word Attack   27/30

Language

Controlled Word Association Test
F	18
A	18
S	15
Total	51 (z = +.88; Spreen and Strauss norms)

Speech Perception (Heaton norms)
T Score	52

Attention

Stroop Color/Word Test (T scores)
Word	51
Color	42
Color/word	36
Interference	41

Rhythm Test (Heaton Norms)
T score	49

Learning and Memory

California Verbal Learning Test
Trial 1	07 (z = -1)
Trial 2	10
Trial 3	08
Trial 4	08
Trial 5	09 (z = -3)
Total List A	42 (T = 27)

Digit Symbol Incidental Memory
4/9   z = -1.56 (Ryan norms)

Wechsler Memory Scale-Revised
Logical Mem. Immed.	53rd %ile
Logical Mem. Delay	17th %ile

List B	07 (z = 0)
Short Delay Free Recall	06 (z = -3)
Short Delay Cued Recall	08 (z = -2)
Long Delay Free Recall	08 (z = -2)
Long Delay Cued Recall	09 (z = -2)
Recognition	13 (z = -1)

Visual-Spatial Skills

Rey Complex Figure (Spreen and Strauss norms)		*Embedded Figures Test*	
Copy	34/36 (z = -2.07)	7/10	z = -.06
Recall	5.5/36 (z = -1.68)	Av. time	6.56 sec
		(POET norms)	

Motor and Psychomotor Function

Lateral Dominance Examination		*Grip Strength* (Heaton norms)	
Hand	7R/0L	Dominant (R)	31 kg (T = 51)
Foot	3R/0L	Nondominant	27 kg (T = 54)
Eye	7R/3L		
Name	Right		

Grooved Pegboard (Heaton norms)		*Finger Tapping Test* (Heaton norms)	
Right	62" (T = 50)	Right	32.4 (T = 32)
Left	77" (T = 41)	Left	26.3 (T = 25)

Problem Solving and Abstract Reasoning

Category Test (Heaton norms)		*Trail Making Test* (Heaton norms)	
Total Errors	54 (T = 38)	A	35", 0 errors (T = 41)
Perseverative errors	12	B	89", 2 errors (T = 38)

Tactual Performance Test (Heaton Norms)
(Unable to complete test, very tearful, upset by inability to complete test)

Dominant hand	15.0', 07 blocks (T = 29)
Nondominant hand	10.0', 02 blocks (T = 13)
Both hands	04.9', 02 blocks

Memory (Able to name 7 blocks, was not asked to draw)

Level of Performance

RS obtained a WAIS-R Verbal IQ score of 107, a Performance IQ score of 87, and a Full Scale IQ score of 98. She is therefore functioning in the average range of general intelligence, but a great deal of scatter was noted among the verbal abilities. Performance tests were all done below average levels. Her general academic achievement, as evaluated with the WRAT-R, was at an average level for word recognition, spelling, and mathematics. Reading comprehension, however, was performed more poorly than reading recognition. RS does not appear to have a discrepancy between IQ and achievement that is sometimes seen in individuals with academic skill disorders.

Language

No significant impairment of basic language abilities was noted. Fluency, phonetic analysis, and auditory discrimination all appear to be within normal limits. As indicated above, there was scatter on the WAIS-R Verbal scale marked by above average performance on tasks assessing semantic knowledge and fund of information, and relatively poor performance on linguistic tasks requiring attention and problem solving. That is, RS has an excellent vocabulary and general knowledge of facts, but is relatively deficient with respect to verbal problem solving.

Attention and Memory

RS had difficulty repeating digits, with a marked discrepancy noted between the scores for the forward and backward conditions (10 vs. 4, respectively). Again, a good performance was noted for an overlearned activity, but with relative deficit indicated when more complex processing was required. Other tests of attention, including the Rhythm Test and the Stroop Color/word Test, demonstrated essentially the same phenomenon; normal performance on basic tasks but mild impairment on more complex procedures. Memory function reflected a similar pattern. RS preformed normally on immediate recall of stories, but there was a substantial loss of information on delayed recall. On the California Verbal Learning Test she did not appear to improve significantly over learning trials for the first word list, and she demonstrated substantial susceptibility to interference. Her delayed recall of nonverbal material was also poor. In general RS appears to have a significant impairment of complex memory functions with normal basic associative processes.

Perceptual and Motor Skills

Basic sensory-perceptual tests were not accomplished for this patient, but there was no apparent evidence of neglect or significant tactile, visual, or auditory dysfunction. On motor tasks, RS had normal strength of grip, but mild bilateral slowness of tapping speed. Dexterity was normal with her right hand, but mildly impaired with her left.

Spatial Abilities and Problem Solving

These two domains showed a strong interaction and thus, will be discussed together. Based on her educational level, RS performed below expectation (i.e., 11th percentile) on the Category Test. She performed even more poorly on problem-solving tasks with perceptual-motor demands. As perceptual-motor demands increased, she performed progressively worse. On visual-spatial tasks RS generally performed poorly regardless of whether or not there was a constructional component. On Block Design, she made several configuration errors (i.e., breaking the contour of the design) that are frequently seen in patients with frank right hemisphere disease. Her performance on the Tactual Performance Test, which is done blindfolded, strongly suggests that her spatial deficit is not restricted to the visual modality, but is a more generalized deficit of spatial cognition. She was able to correctly place 7 of 10 blocks after 15 minutes with her right hand, but could only place 2 blocks with her left hand. She was not asked to draw the blocks from memory because she seemed so upset about this task, but was able to correctly name the shapes of most of the blocks. It would therefore appear that RS could identify the blocks tactually, but could not match their configurations with the corresponding recesses in the formboard.

Discussion and Recommendations

RS appears to meet criteria for a nonverbal learning disability. While RS does not manifest basic academic skills deficits, her weakness in reading comprehension is consistent with the NLD academic pattern. The visual-spatial and complex problem-solving components of NLD are most prominent in this patient and appear to be of sufficient severity to be substantially disabling. While the presence of active right hemisphere disease is unlikely, there would appear to be significant dysfunction in that hemisphere of the brain. RS did substantially less well with her left hand than her right on the tactual performance and manual dexterity tasks, and obtained a lower Performance IQ than Verbal IQ. Perhaps most significantly, her error performance on Block Design was of a type demonstrated in patients with frank lateralized right hemisphere disease.

The spatial disability as demonstrated by RS could be viewed as a subclinical form of spatial agnosia, or as a developmental spatial agnosia. That is, it appears to go beyond difficulties with representational spatial cognition and may also impact on her topographical orientation in daily living. She would certainly be an interesting individual to evaluate further with more specialized tests of route-finding, facial recognition, and related tasks. Management of this condition would involve taking precautions in unfamiliar environments and conversely, making optimal use of over-learned spatial routines. Cognitive rehabilitation directed toward spatial deficits is available in some rehabilitation programs. RS appears to utilize verbal mediation appropriately and efficiently, and can deal with spatial structures by naming them, as we saw on the Tactual Performance Test. It appears that her problem is not so much temporal sequencing as it is organizing objects in a representational spatial array. She did well on temporal sequencing tasks, but not on tasks in which she had to spatially organize information. It might therefore benefit RS to try to learn new information in step-by-step temporal sequences rather than all at once.

PSYCHOSOCIAL CONSIDERATIONS

It is now appreciated that learning disabilities impact most, if not all, aspects of everyday life. As Smith (1988) summarizes, "...adults with learning disability are actually challenged and frustrated by their difficulties in achieving valued cultural standards of *literacy, job performance, social skills, and communication skills*" (p. 22). (Emphasis added). This statement is supported by the results of a needs assessment of 381 adults with LD (mean age = 23.2 years) (Hoffmann *et al.*, 1987). Accomplished within a vocational rehabilitation setting, the survey included the areas of daily living, social skills, and personal problems and was completed by clients with LD, service providers, and advocates and/or parents. Not surprisingly since 64% of the LD sample was either unemployed or working only part time, all three groups concurred that adults with LD have major vocational needs. Interestingly, both the service providers and advocates perceived the LD sample as having significantly more social problems than did the adults with LD themselves. All three groups agreed that personal problems were prevalent, with all indicating that low frustration tolerance, poor self-confidence, and poor control of emotions and temper were particularly problematic. This survey also demonstrated that few adults with LD had ever participated in any form of therapy (i.e., 13%) and that none had ever participated in a social skills or self-help group. In summary, these results not only strongly confirm the psychological difficulties in adults with LD but also suggest that adults with LD either do not avail themselves of such therapeutic services or do not know of their availability.

Although a comprehensive discussion of the psychosocial aspects of LD is beyond the scope of this chapter, we refer the interested reader to a poignant chapter that discusses in the most concrete of terms the social/emotional and daily living issues faced by adults with LD (Reiff and Gerber, 1993). In spite of a growing awareness of the pervasive implications of learning disabilities on psychological function, it is our own clinical experience that adults with NLD are frequently incorrectly diagnosed as having a primary psychiatric disorder. There is often little or no appreciation of pre-existing learning deficits or the continuing impact of these deficits on socio-emotional functioning.

Psychological Adjustment

Most studies of the psychological status of adults with LD are cross-sectional and completed within the academic setting. However, an early longitudinal study completed by Peter and Spreen (1979) provided not only evidence that learning disability extends into adulthood but also that the significant behavior problems and emotional maladjustment of this groups persists as well. This investigation followed 177 children with LD who initially completed neuropsychological testing between the ages of 8 and 12. Subjects were followed for varying periods, some for as long as 12 years. In this follow up study adolescents and young adults were grouped according to CNS status (brain damage, minimal brain damage, no neurological signs) and compared to a control group with no history of learning problems or brain injury. After adjustment for differences in age, gender, and IQ, all three groups with learning problems demonstrated significantly more behavior problems and psychological distress than the normal control group. Although this early study strongly suggests a meaningful relationship between learning deficits and later emotional problems, as noted above only a few studies have investigated the course of learning disabilities through adulthood and even fewer have explored the psychosocial functioning of this group. One more recent study (Lapan, Koller, and Holliday, 1991) of clients with LD referred for vocational rehabilitation services found that almost one-third met DSM criteria for a psychiatric diagnosis, including adjustment disorder, mood disorders, and personality disorders.

In spite of the growing recognition that LD affects psychological functioning in both work and family life, the psychosocial status of adults in academic settings continues to be the most frequently studied area. Saracoglu, Minden, and Wilchesky (1989) investigated the general adjustment to college of students with LD. As might be expected, this investigation documented significantly poorer academic and emotional adjustment in the LD sample in comparison to a peer group with no LD. However, the positive correlation between measures of self-efficacy and self-esteem in both groups suggests that students with LD as well as those with other academic difficulties demonstrate similar emotional and adjustment problems. While another study comparing LD and nondisabled adult students showed only a trend toward between-group differences in the *level* of reported depression, depressive *symptoms* were significantly correlated with dysfunctional cognitions in the LD group (Mattek and Wierzbicki, 1998). Other investigations have identified differences in the type of symptoms manifested by adults with LD. Hoy and colleagues (Hoy, Gregg, Wisenbaker*et al.*, 1997) compared two groups of adults with LD not classified by particular subtype. In this case, college students with LD showed more symptoms of anxiety than a group of student controls. Adults with LD in a rehabilitation setting were the only study group to demonstrate significant differences with respect to level of depression. Although this study suggests that psychological function in adults with LD may be closely related to the particular demands of the environment, another study provides evidence to dispute this conclusion. A study of adults with LD who had obtained at least a baccalaureate degree and maintained a minimum of one year of successful employment found a greater degree of depression than noted in the general population (Stafford-Depass, 1998).

NLD, in particular, is frequently associated with affective disturbances in children that become more salient during adulthood (Casey, Rourke, and Picard, 1991; Rourke et al., 1986b; White, Moffitt, and Silva, 1992). Semrud-Clikeman and Hynd (1990) summarize several physiological studies of depression, speculating that problems in the regulation of affect noted in children with NLD may be directly associated with right hemisphere dysfunction.

Cognitive-behavioral theories suggest that difficulties in perceiving or reacting to the environment are associated with a higher risk for depression (Mattek and Wierzbicki, 1998). These theories considered within the context of the problem-solving and social skills deficits noted in NLD may have influenced Rourke to hypothesize that NLD is associated with the increased likelihood of social withdrawal, isolation, and depression in both children (Rourke and Fuerst, 1996) and adults (Rourke, Young, and Leenaars, 1989; Rourke et al., 1986b). Rourke et al. (1986b) conducted a descriptive study of 8 adults (age range: 17 to 48) who exhibited a neuropsychological pattern consistent with NLD. These subjects exhibited a pattern of deficits similar to children with NLD but what is relevant to this discussion is the level of psychological problems. Serious occupational maladjustment was manifested in 75% of the sample, with more serious psychopathology noted in the remaining two individuals. All of these patients exhibited psychological difficulties associated with depression; and 4 of the 8 were in active treatment at a psychiatric clinic. Discussing the adult consequences of NLD, Rourke et al. (1989) focuses on the "practical, concrete ramifications" (p. 171) of the syndrome. They predict underemployment in jobs that tax already compromised motor skills, an inability to adapt with new and/or complex situations, an inability to recognize the significance of job problems, and an inability to appreciate nonverbal communication. Taken together, these deficiencies place the adult at great risk for emotional disturbance, including an increased risk for suicide (Also see Bigler, 1989; Fletcher, 1989; Kowalchuk and King, 1989; and Rourke, 1989b for an extensive discussion of this topic.).

Noting that NLD appears to lead to the development of depressive symptoms, Cleaver and colleagues completed a study of adolescents and young adults hospitalized for psychiatric illness (Cleaver and Whitman, 1998). Based on academic achievement score comparisons, the 484 subjects were classified into four groups: arithmetic disabled, reading disabled, generally disabled, and non-disabled. Subjects were classified with respect to psychiatric diagnosis and the presence or absence of suicidal ideation defined as either spoken or written evidence of a wish to commit suicide. The reliability of the psychiatric diagnosis was confirmed by a secondary study using the Structured Interview for the DSM-III-R (SCID) (Spitzer, Williams, Gibbon, and First, 1992). Analyses indicated that the arithmetic disabled group showed a significantly higher level of depression than the remaining study groups but the groups did not differ significantly with respect to suicidality.

Our own group (Katz, Kelly, Goldstein, Bartolomucci, and Comstock, 1992) investigated incidence and prevalence various LD diagnoses, including those defined by visual-spatial and perceptual/motor deficits, associated with three distinct MMPI profiles. In this study, subjects were not necessarily defined by a single diagnosis. A cluster analysis of the MMPI scores identified three valid clusters of varying severity: 1) high levels of psychiatric distress, primarily with features of neurotic depression and anxiety; 2) similar neurotic features but with lower levels of psychological distress, and 3) a normal MMPI profile. The various subtypes were not differentially represented in any of these MMPI clusters. That is, visual-spatial disability did not predominate in one MMPI cluster and reading disability in another. The *number* of LD diagnoses, however, was significantly different among the subtypes, with Cluster 1 containing individuals with the most diagnoses. This finding suggests a positive relationship between number of cognitive deficits and level of psychological distress. These results are highly consistent with Peter and Spreen's (1979) early study that indicated overall intellectual level moderated the degree of psychological distress in their learning handicapped subjects.

Rourke's hypothesis of increased psychological dysfunction associated with NLD has recently come under scrutiny. White, Moffitt, and Silva (1992) studied teens with various LD subtypes (i.e., specific reading disability, specific arithmetic disability, and global LD), comparing them to a group of nondisabled controls. While they noted that the group with specific arithmetic disability had a neuropsychological profile consistent with NLD, all three disabled groups showed similarly poor social-emotional adjustment. O'Donnell (1991) reports unpublished data by Leicht (1987) who performed a subtype analysis of personality function of young adults with LD based on a brief personality inventory. Some but not all adults with LD exhibited "maladjustment," but this was not related to either academic skills or neuropsychological status. While these results do not support the conclusion that some LD subtypes are more apt than others to show particular patterns of emotional symptoms, they must be viewed as tentative. The assessment of emotional status was apparently completed with a self-report instrument and not supplemented with a comprehensive psychiatric interview such as the SCID.

Two more recent studies, however, support the findings of Leicht. A study by Waldo et al. (Waldo, McIntosh, and Koller, 1999) compared the personality profiles of 3 LD subtypes defined by Wechsler IQ differences. All participates were in a vocational rehabilitation setting. Although no statistically significant between group differences were identified between the LD subtypes, 20% of their adult sample displayed significant clinical elevation on at least one MMPI scale. As the authors point out, these finding argue for attention to the emotional consequences across all aspects of LD. Likewise, a study that defined subtypes by cluster analysis found no differences in the prevalence of psychiatric diagnosis by subtype (Dunham, Multon, and Koeller, 1999).

Vocational Function

Because vocational rehabilitation services to individuals with LD have increased dramatically over the last 10 years (Dunham *et al.*, 1999; McCue, 1993), the vocational functioning in LD adults has become a topic of particular interest. As early as 1984 Kite stressed the importance of assessment and accommodation, noting the heterogeneous nature of this population. In a needs survey Hoffman *et al.* (1987) elaborated on the particular problems of adults with LD in the vocational rehabilitation setting. Survey results indicated that very limited vocational and career education had ever been provided, usually one high school course. Only a quarter of the sample had participated in post-secondary technical, vocational, or trade school training. The need for career counseling in the LD group is best highlighted by the problems noted. The most frequently endorsed problems included locating a job or appropriate job training, filling out job applications, and reading classified advertisements. As in other studies, individuals with LD often perceived themselves to have fewer problems than actually reported by their supervisors or service providers.

Research indicates that less than half of high school graduates having LD make the successful transition into employment (Faas and D'Alonzo, 1990). A recent descriptive study compared vocational functioning of adults with LD of nonspecific subtypes and nondisabled peers two years after high school graduation (Rojewski, 1999). This author noted that vocational goals were lower for the LD group, with that cohort generally aspiring to moderate or lower level occupations, depending on gender. In addition, the LD group was more apt to be employed, at the expense of pursuing higher education. A second study (Witte, Philips, and Kakela, 1998) investigated job satisfaction in college graduates (mean age: 25 years) and a control group matched in gender, major, degree, and graduation year. The LD group took more time to graduate and obtained a lower GPA. This study again highlights the fact that individuals with LD often have difficulty with self-perception, as these individuals perceived themselves as getting paid less, having fewer promotion opportunities, and less job satisfaction. Interestingly, no salary differences existed between the groups.

A descriptive study by Holliday, Koller, and Thomas (1999) investigated the long-term vocational outcome of a unique group of adults with LD. While all were identified as gifted based on IQ scores (Verbal, Performance, or Full Scale IQ $\geq$ 120), they experienced vocational problems consistent with other individuals with more typical LD. All met state and federal Rehabilitation Services Administration criteria for a specific learning disability. In spite of expressed educational goals (e.g., 48% of the sample had expressed the goal of at least 2 years of education past high school), the sample showed limited post-secondary education. Only 21% completed more than 4 semesters of college. Serious under employment was indicated by frequent job changes, limited earning capacity (e.g., 76% earned less than $6 per hour), and participation in unskilled jobs (52%). Thus, although these individual possessed definite assets, their vocational functioning was highly limited, suggesting an inability to capitalize on strengths or perhaps, the tendency to overlook strengths in vocational planning.

In spite of this increased interest in the vocational functioning of persons with unclassified LD, information regarding the vocational functioning of individuals with NLD is sparse. Rourke *et al.* (Rourke, Del Dotto, Rourke, and Casey, 1990) provide anecdotal evidence of vocational difficulties in a young woman, discussing her limitations in judgment and reasoning and their effect on her vocational functioning. We located only one empirical study that addressed the occupational function of individuals grouped according to homogeneous categories. Dunham *et al.* (1999) noted that the verbal vs. nonverbal LD distinction might be too simplistic to capture the cognitive, academic, and occupational complexities of different jobs. They classified a group of 613 adults with LD, using cluster analysis to group individuals according to their IQ (Verbal and Performance IQs from the Wechsler Adult Intelligence Scale-Revised (Wechsler, 1981) and academic achievement (reading, mathematics, and writing summary scores from the Woodcock-Johnson Psychoeducational Test Battery [Woodcock and Johnson, 1990]). They identified three meaningful and valid clusters labeled as "Linguistically/globally academically impaired," "Linguistically/writing impaired," and "Eclectic." The latter group did not display the language problems of the other groups, but nevertheless showed the VIQ<PIQ pattern and mild academic deficits in reading and writing. While none of these groups seem to capture the essence of NLD, this study did identify important differences in vocational outcome for the three verbal LD clusters, suggesting that a similar analysis with an NLD sample might elaborate differences in vocational function for this group as well. In contrast, there were no significant between group differences with respect to psychiatric diagnosis, including anxiety and mood disorders, with 30% of all the subjects evidencing the presence of a secondary psychiatric disability. These data replicate the more recent work in this area with respect to subtypes and suggest that in adults, psychiatric involvement is relatively common in *any* LD subtype.

In summary, adults with NLD often exhibit psychological, social, and occupational problems. Typically, they exhibit low self-esteem, social isolation, depression, and withdrawal. Their lack of problem-solving skills is attributed to difficulties that range from under appreciation of the significance of a problem to over reaction to minor inconveniences.

INTERVENTIONS

It is suggested that the careful delineation of LD subtypes will result in more informed interventions, directed at particular aspects of the noted disability and refined based on individual needs (Hooper and Willis, 1989; Rourke and Fuerst, 1996; Torgesen, 1991). This section will briefly discuss the aspects of treatment outlined in Table 1. While a more through discussion of this important area is outside the scope of this chapter, we invite the interested reader to consult the references cited for more information. Of course many treatments developed for children with LD are also applicable with adults. While the following section does review some particularly relevant aspects of the pediatric literature, more detailed information is available regarding general intervention techniques (Hooper and Willis, 1989) and those neuropsychologically-based approaches that are directed toward NLD (Foss, 1991; Rourke, 1995; Rourke, Fisk, and Strang, 1986a; Rourke, Bakker, Fisk, and Strang, 1983). Finally, few of these interventions discussed below are associated with empirical research that evaluates outcome. There is much work to be done in this area.

Capitalization on Strengths

A recurrent theme in the intervention literature is the use of career counseling to encourage realistic educational and vocational goals. As Holliday et al. (1999) note, to be successful this experience must be based on the foundation of well understood strengths as well as deficits. However, this understanding may not come easily for individuals with LD (Kronick, 1981). An early study of adults with LD by Buchanan and Wolf (1986) demonstrated that some but not all subjects could identify personal strengths. However, their perceptions were often inaccurate. Reiff, Gerber, and Ginsburg (1997) discuss "learned creativity" as a way that successful individuals with LD adapt to the demands of their environment. This concept builds on personal areas of strength to develop the strategies and techniques that enhance performance. These highly personal strategies involve the avoidance of weaker areas in favor of developing unique ways of accomplishing necessary tasks. However, key to this creativity is the anticipation of problems, an activity that is sometimes highly demanding and involves the introspection that is often difficult for individuals with NLD in particular. Acknowledging this, Reiff and colleagues have developed a therapeutic model that is addressed in detail later in this chapter.

Remediation

Remediation implies treatment with the goal of curing or diminishing deficits. As noted throughout this chapter, adults with NLD demonstrate social difficulties that include poor social and conversational skills, the inability to negotiate personal space, and difficulty interpreting novel or highly complex social situations. These social deficits are coupled with a remarkable lack of understanding and insight into the functional effects of their disability (Denckla, 1993). Several studies have addressed the social skills deficits manifested by adults with LD (Holliday, Koller, and Thomas 1999; Ryan and Price, 1992; Sitlington and Frank, 1990), but few have addressed the efficacy of various treatment strategies. A recent study (Michie, Lindsay, and Smith, 1998) compared outcome of adults (age range 19 to 63 years) with unclassified LD who participated in a 2-year community living skills training program. The study groups included a classroom training module, in vivo learning setting, and untreated controls. After the treatment period, assessment of living skills and adaptive behavior indicated that those individuals participating in vivo training performed significantly better than the two other groups.

Denckla (1993) notes lack of empirical data to assess outcome of similar interventions with adults with NLD. However, she cites anecdotal evidence that indicates further research should be completed to assess the efficacy of various remedial techniques. These include remedial academic approaches that use verbal mediation to develop step-by-step formulas to encode and process complex problems as well as cognitively based social skills training programs that address problems in interpreting facial expression, body language, and tone of voice.

Difficulties with novel problem solving and abstract reasoning are probably the hallmark of NLD. A study of high school students investigated a graduated teaching sequence as a way to increase problem-solving skills (Maccini and Hughes, 2000). This technique progressed from concrete applications through semi-concrete procedures, in order to accomplish the ultimate goal of abstract understanding of a mathematical concept. Importantly, students were taught an explicit strategy to cue problem-solving procedures. Study results indicate that both the use of strategy and performance improved across the instructional levels. Generalization of this treatment effect was also noted.

When discussing effective remedial interventions for NLD, Foss (1991) notes that they must address problems in the areas of planning and organization, social cognition, and interpersonal communication directly and explicitly. She asserts that the most effective procedures provide verbal labels and descriptions for concrete objects, actions, and experiences with instruction heavily dependent on verbal mediation and verbal self-direction. Several researchers and academicians have developed metacognitive treatment programs that might be applicable to NLD based on this group's difficulties with novel problem solving in general. However, few of these programs are based on the results of empirical research.

Hooper and Willis (1989) compare and contrast three metacognitive approaches that emphasize training in academic strategies, but note that none are refined enough to address the rather specific deficits associated with the various LD subtypes. Bireley's 1995 chapter on academic interventions, while generally addressing childhood learning problems, outlines a metacognitive model that may be particularly applicable to adults with NLD. This 6-step program depends on mulitsensory input, group discussion to facilitate elaboration, guided practice and feedback, and generalization activities. Unfortunately, data on the efficacy of this intervention are apparently lacking. Other models use neuropsychological data to direct remediation (Hooper and Willis, 1989), offering the advantage of providing a means to conceptualize a realistic treatment program that compensates for weaknesses and builds on strengths. One recent and promising development are investigations that explore the efficacy of subtype-to-treatment matching. However, upon review of these studies one notes that most involve children who have subtypes of dyslexia.

Compensation

Compensation usually involves instruction and practice in the use of alternate strategies in a particular cognitive domain or social skill. While the pediatric literature in this area is extensive, little work is available that directly addresses the problems of adults outside the academic setting.

Levine (1987, 1994) discusses several compensatory strategies that have applications in the adult population. Bypass strategies are based on the combination of functional and neuropsychological assessment and provide a means to circumvent cognitive deficits or underdeveloped skills. These strategies are usually applied in the educational setting. Examples include adjustments to the rate and/or volume of learning, the provision of multiple examples of complex concepts, an emphasis on key learning points, the use of assertive devices, and the alteration of standard classroom routines. Levine also discusses building on strengths, stressing that individuals with LD should be provided the opportunity to exploit, enhance, and demonstrate their preserved learning abilities.

Compensatory techniques have also been related to employment issues. An article by Kohaska and Skolnik (1986) provides suggestions that are applicable to adults with NLD. These include selecting a career that emphasizes cognitive strengths, choosing a job that enables the individualization of work techniques, obtaining social skills training to support interpersonal interactions, expending more effort for success, and tolerating a realistic assessment of work performance.

Avoidance

The self-imposed avoidance of problematic areas is probably the most univer-
sally applied intervention in NLD. For example, when discussing specific learning problems with a college sample, we found that many students with math difficulty avoided those subjects if at all possible (Beers *et al.*, 1994). This being
the case, it is surprising that the topic of avoidance is rarely addressed in the
literature. Rourke's treatment program for children with NLD (1995) encour-
ages the adoption of specialized learning procedures (e.g., concrete step-by-step
teaching, teaching specific strategies for recurring problematic situations) rather
than the avoidance of the difficult material

Counseling and Psychotherapy

Effective participation in counseling or psychotherapy may be particularly difficult for persons with NLD who often experience low self-esteem, loneliness,
depression, isolation, and withdrawal (Rourke *et al.*, 1986b). While these are
challenging problems within any patient group, the neuropsychological ramifications of NLD, particularly the difficulties with novel problem solving and deficits in understanding social nuances such as facial expression and body language further complicate the therapeutic process. Certainly it behooves the
treating professional to develop comprehensive understanding of the deficits
associated with NLD before attempting treatment. It is particularly important for
treating professionals to appreciate that NLD extends beyond the educational
realm, as there is indication that many young adults with LD fail to understand
how their learning problems interact with other aspects of their lives. A descriptive study by Blalock (1987) found that young adults with LD who completed
counseling or psychotherapy saw no relationship between their "other problems"
and their actual learning disability. Individuals with nonverbal problems were
especially noted to have little awareness of the functional significance of their
learning problems.

Effective psychotherapy for adults with NLD depends on moving away from
educationally grounded definitions and assuming a developmental lifespan approach (Bassett, Polloway, and Patton, 1993; Smith, 1996). This perspective
appreciates how NLD interferes with the multidimensional demands of adult
developmental stages that include moving away from home, establishing an occupation, selecting a life partner, and parenting. Holliday *et al.* (1999) point out
the need for therapies that strengthen self-confidence and interpersonal skills. In
their study of high IQ adults with LD, an important goal was that of helping deal
with the frustration produced by discrepant abilities. A recent controlled study
by Wachelka and Katz (1999) reported the effectiveness of an 8-week treatment
for reducing test anxiety in individuals with LD. Although all participates were

involved in the pursuit of secondary or post-secondary education, the age range reached well into adulthood, from 17 to 52 years. Specific treatments included the cognitive-behavioral techniques of progressive muscle relaxation, guided imagery, and self-instructional training coupled with more academically based instruction in study and test-taking skills.

In an effort to understand the ramifications of LD in the workplace and how disabilities were overcome, Reiff and colleagues completed ethnographic interviews with 71 adults with LD. All of these adults had become highly or moderately successful from a vocational standpoint (Gerber, Ginsberg, and Reiff, 1992; Reiff, Gerber, and Ginsburg, 1997). Through this process, the investigators compiled a model elaborating the interplay of factors that contributed to the success of these individuals. Although this model generally focuses on vocational outcome, we briefly discuss the model in this section because we feel that it can inform the therapy process, in a sense outlining an Individual Educational Plan (IEP) for adults. Reiff *et al.* found that successful adults with LD were able to gain control of their lives by focusing on internal decisions and external manifestations of success. According to this model, individuals made highly personal, explicit, and focused decisions that related to the desire to attain practical, realistic and attainable goals. Inherent in this process is reframing, or "reinterpreting the learning disabilities experience from something dysfunctional to something functional"(p. 105). The process of reframing is an integral aspect of treatment because it involves self-perception as well as *change*. Successful reframing works toward the recognition, acceptance, and understanding of the disability. Finally, a conscious decision must be made to take action, or to address interpersonal and vocational goals. Once these internal decisions are clarified, the model focuses on the external manifestations of success, translating internal decisions into actual behaviors. These so-called action strategies focus on the adaptability and creativity of the individual with LD and considers persistence; environmental fit that maximizes strengths and downplays weaknesses; creativity in the use of strategies, techniques, and devices that enhance performance; and the willingness to establish support networks and mentors. In summary, vocational, and in turn, personal success in individuals with LD appears to depend on a process that requires learning about the disorder, learning about the self, and developing a realistic action plan.

Support Groups

Brown (undated) describes support groups as a useful counseling strategy for young adults with LD, providing a way for individuals to share successful coping skills and become more informed about learning disability in general. Somewhat surprisingly, we were able to locate little information regarding support groups with the specific focus on LD. A consumer survey indicates that young adults with LD, approximately 35% of whom had been diagnosed with nonverbal problems, expressed the desire to participate in groups composed of others with LD who were experiencing similar problems. While most viewed this interaction as beneficial, it was generally not characterized as a long-term intervention (Blalock, 1987).

Vocational Rehabilitation

According to Dunham *et al.* (1999), persons with learning disability make up the fastest growing population served by the vocational rehabilitation system. Vocational rehabilitation services provide counseling, rehabilitation, and placement services to persons with learning disability whose functional abilities such as communication, self-direction, and social skills are severely limited (Dowdy *et al.*, 1996). In this case the focus moves from educational issues to that of employability. The need for such transitional programming and vocational counseling for young adults with LD is frequently noted (Holliday *et al.*, 1999; McCue, 1993; Rojewski, 1999), with studies identifying traits that predict vocational success. For example, attainment of higher level vocations is associated with personal characteristics such as motivation, persistence, and the realistic ability to develop compensatory strategies (Reiff *et al.*, 1997; Stafford-Depass, 1998). Interestingly, the possession of knowledge about LD in general and an appreciation of ones strengths are also traits associated with vocational success.

ACCOMMODATIONS

As with interventions, a review of the literature found little discussion of accommodations for adults outside of the educational setting and even fewer, if any, discussions aimed at addressing domain-specific disabilities as recommended by Stanovich (1999).

Academic

In response to Rehabilitation Act of 1973 and the Americans with Disabilities Act in 1990, educational settings from elementary school though postgraduate institutions have provided academic accommodations for students with LD. For example, a survey of 105 medical schools in the United States and Canada reported that 96% admitted students with learning disabilities (Faigel, 1998). All reported academic accommodations with the most frequent being tutoring (93%), untimed examinations (91%) computer-assisted learning (83%), and decelerated curriculum (79%). Few medical schools, however, indicated a willingness to adjust the curriculum to meet the special needs of students with LD. Only 14% of the schools provided curricular exemption or alternative courses.

The Rehabilitation Act of 1973 provides for a variety of accommodations or "academic adjustments" in the post-secondary setting (Brinckerhoff, Shaw, and McGuire, 1996). The major accommodations are adaptations in the *manner* of teaching, modifications in academic requirements (e.g., changes in time limit to complete degree; substitution of courses), and the use of auxiliary equipment or technology (word processors; proofreading programs; outlining devices; personal data managers). As Raskind notes, this last category of accommodations is particularly appropriate for adults with LD as it moves away from the remediation model that seeks to cure or instruct (Raskind, 1993). Although outcome research is needed in this area, by building on strengths and enabling the individual to attain at a level more commensurate with intellectual ability, assistive technologies provide a way for adults to compensate for their deficits and thus lead a more productive life.

In spite of these mandated procedures, accommodations remains controversial (Stanovich, 1999) and problems remain in their application. Difficulties are associated with both student and faculty *perceptions*. A small sample of college students with LD was interviewed to discover the students' perceptions of the faculty attitudes toward accommodation for persons with hidden disabilities (Beilke and Yssel, 1999). This paper identified instructional accommodations such as extended time on exams and special seating arrangements that are often made reluctantly and within a "less than positive classroom climate" (p. 364). Problems were also noted from the faculty perspective. A paper by Bourke, Strehorn, and Silver (2000) discusses the actual *practices* of instructional accommodations for college students with LD. A large group of faculty members were surveyed about their perceptions regarding accommodations that included untimed, proctored, and alternate-form examinations, note taking assistance, and additional time for assignments. As might be expected, the faculty who understood the need for accommodation and who believed that accommodations would be effective tended to provide them. In addition, support from academic departments also influenced faculty involvement in the program. As Bourke *et al.* note, their findings indicate that close communication among with faculty, administration and service providers is essential in providing effective accommodations at the secondary level. Another large study also investigated faculty attitudes regarding accommodations across multiple sites (Vogel, Leyser, Wyland, and Brulle, 1999). Table 3 shows more and less favored teaching and examination accommodation procedures that relate to various academic needs. As noted in the previous study, certain faculty characteristics were associated with more or less willingness to provide accommodations. At first look, these studies indicate progress in attitudes toward academic accommodations at institutions of higher learning. However, the results are probably skewed by the low return rate by faculty. For example, in both studies the response rate was approximately 35%.

TABLE 3. FACULTY VIEWS OF ACCOMMODATION PROCEDURES

LESS FAVORED	MORE FAVORED
Teaching Accommodations	
-Provide lecture outlines	+Tape record lectures
-Assignments in alternative form	+One-on-one assistance
	(e.g., clarification and review)
Examination Accommodations	
-Altered exam format	+Extended time
-Paraphrase questions	+Change venue of exam
	+Assistive technology
	(e.g., word processor, spell check,
	taped answers)

Note: Adapted from Vogel *et al.* (1999).

One of the most commonly applied accommodations in the academic setting is the provision of extended time on tests and research suggests that this procedure is well founded. A recent multi-site controlled study (Alster, 1997) indicated that a heterogeneous group of college students with LD obtained significantly lower scores than their nondisabled peers on a timed algebra test. However, students with LD were able to improve their scores to a level comparable to the control group under the extended time condition. Interestingly, the control group scores did not differ by testing condition. That is, the provision of extended testing time did not result in any significant improvement in test scores.

Workplace

Information regarding workplace accommodations comes from the consumer as well as the scientist. Based on their study of the consumers of vocational rehabilitation services, Michaels *et al.* (1997) strongly recommended the application of neuropsychological testing to understand the abilities and deficits of each individual with LD. Brown and Gerber (1991), in a practical discussion, illustrate how neuropsychological constructs such as visual perception, spatial ability, and memory function can inform the accommodation process in the workplace. Taking a somewhat different approach to accommodation, Reiff and colleagues (Reiff and Gerber, 1993; Reiff, Gerber, and Ginsberg, 1997) used ethnographic interview techniques to provide comprehensive information regarding the success, or lack thereof, in adults with LD at work. While a comprehensive discussion of their interesting and informative research is beyond the scope of this

4

ADHD

INTRODUCTION

Attention-deficit hyperactivity disorder as a disorder of childhood has been extensively documented in the research literature. However, since it has been recognized as a disorder that continues into the adolescent and adult years, the diagnostic process has taken on some significant dimensions that bear discussion. Thus, we will examine the diagnostic process in some detail in this chapter including the role of neuropsychological measures in the assessment process and the saliency of comorbid conditions. In addition, we will address issues involving incidence and prevalence and the roles that referral source and gender play in setting these parameters. Etiological factors including genetics will be addressed as well as theoretical perspectives on the neurochemistry and physiology of the brain's attention system that may underlie ADHD as a disorder. The various research studies involving brain scans and mapping techniques that shed light on the disorder will be included. The issue of comorbidity and its relationship to personal adjustment and therapeutic interventions will also be discussed in some detail as will adjustments to the college environment and work place. Intervention strategies and treatments including the critical role of medications, coaching, and reasonable accommodations will be addressed as they relate specifically to young adults. And, finally, the relevance of previous outcome studies to the young adult population, which are highly suspect on account of past diagnostic and referral biases, will be critically examined, in light of our current knowledge base.

DEFINITIONS

Historical Foundations

At the present time in order for a diagnosis of ADHD to be made, diagnostic criteria as set forth in the Diagnostic and Statistical Manual (DMS-IV) of the American Psychiatric Association (1994) must be met. Six or more symptoms of inattention and/or hyperactivity/impulsivity must be present and must have persisted for at least 6 months to a degree that is maladaptive (clinically significant impairment) and inconsistent with developmental level. In addition, some of the symptoms must have been present before age 7 years, some impairment from the symptoms is present in two or more settings, and there is evidence of clinically significant impairment in social, academic or occupational functioning. Finally, the symptoms do not occur exclusively during the course of another disorder or are not better accounted for by another mental disorder. These criteria are applied whether the individual presenting for evaluation is a child, adolescent or adult, even though the studies utilized to empirically establish these criteria were conducted primarily with male children and the history of the diagnostic process is steeped in the medical treatment of children, again primarily males.

That this should be the case is not surprising given the history of the disorder first described in 1902 (Still,1902) and later reported by Bradley (1937) who treated the male children he saw with Benzedrine. Following that early work, ADHD became associated with "minimal brain damage" (Strauss and Lehtinen, 1947) as the children they observed resembled children who survived the 1917-1918 encephalitis epidemic in terms of their behavioral and cognitive problems. Then in 1968, the hyperactive component of the behavioral observations made about these children came to the forefront and the new label "hyperkinetic reaction of childhood disorder" was coined by the American Psychiatric Association in their diagnostic manual.

It was not until 1972 that Virginia Douglas reported that level of activity alone could not differentiate children with ADHD from those without the disorder. Her focus included the importance of attentional components as a distinguishing factor. The ability to use time efficiently, screen out distracting stimuli, concentrate on tasks, and sustain focus with minimal external reinforcers became the focus of much of her later research (Douglas, 1983). Her work and the numerous studies of attention, impulsiveness, and other cognitive variables eventually led to renaming the disorder "attention deficit disorder" (ADD) when the DMS-III appeared in 1980 (Barkley, 1997a). Triolo (1999) suggests that this shift from activity levels to an assessment of cognitive deficits may be at least indirectly "responsible for the consideration of ADHD as a lifelong condition" (p. 4).

When the DSM-III-R was published (American Psychiatric Association, 1987) a distinction was then made between two types of ADD: one with hyperactivity and one without. However, concerns then arose that the problems of hyperactivity and impulse control which were deemed critical to a differential diagnosis and also to predicting later developmental risks needed to be formally recognized, hence a renaming of the disorder in DSM-IV to ADHD (Barkley, 1997a). In addition, three subtypes were now identified, ADHD, predominantly Inattentive Type, ADHD, Combined Type, and ADHD, Predominantly Hyperactive/Impulsive Type. A fourth category, ADHD NOS (not otherwise specified) is provided for disorders with prominent symptoms of inattention or hyperactivity-impulsivity.

While Barkley's *Hyperactive Children: A Handbook for Diagnosis and Treatment* (1981) established his place as a major researcher in the field and he continues in this capacity at the present time, his work focuses on children and his latest work sets forth the proposition that children who present primarily with attentional difficulties are not properly classified as ADHD but rather constitute a distinct disorder (Barkley, Duple, and McMurray, 1990; Barkley, 1997a). In defending his model of core deficits in self-regulation and executive functions (mental activities he categorizes into four groups: working memory, internalization, self-control of emotions, motivation and state of arousal, and reconstruction), Barkley writes: "the conclusion is unavoidable that ADHD is far more a deficit of behavioral inhibition than of attention" (p. 313), based again on research conducted in the area of child psychopathology. Further, "Many... researchers seem to be coming to view it (ADHD, Inattentive Type) as probably a deficit in focused or selective attention and speed of information processing that may have distinctive features from the other two types of ADHD and may be more akin to internalizing rather than to externalizing disorders" (p. 9). As a consequence, his theoretical model applies primarily to those children having hyperactive-impulsive symptoms, whether inattention is a factor or not.

Thus, in addition to the question of how much emphasis to put on hyperactivity vs. inattention, we are now confronted with whether one or both of these factors should take a second seat to the issue of "developmental deficiencies in the regulation and maintenance of behavior by rules and consequences...which give rise "to problems with inhibiting, initiating, or sustaining responses" Barkley, 1990, p.71). Barkley goes so far as to suggest renaming the disorder, "Behavioral Inhibition Disorder" (1997a, p.313). That these controversies are still surrounding the diagnosis and definition of the disorder(s) in children should give us pause as we attempt to define and diagnose the disorder in adults.

DSM-IV Criteria and the Diagnosis of ADHD in Adults

First, we must consider the impact of the DSM-IV criteria on diagnosing adults with ADHD. If the diagnosis has not been made during the childhood years, consideration must be given to the initial manifestation of symptom behaviors, the presence of co-morbid disorders as suggested by Triolo (1999), and the presence of particular coping strengths, environmental supports, and strategies which have played major roles throughout the developmental years. Problems with the criterion "some symptoms causing impairment were present before 7 years of age" immediately comes to the fore. Unless a child is presenting substantial management problems to his or her parents prior to the kindergarten years, this child will not be referred to the pediatrician or child psychiatrist. Thus, this criterion would seem best to apply to those children presenting with hyperactivity almost exclusively, and this DSM-IV subtype (Predominantly Hyperactive/Impulsive) was found primarily among preschool children in the DSM-IV field trials (Applegate *et al.*, 1995). According to Barkley (1997b), symptoms of inattention associated with the Hyperactive-Impulsive Subtype emerge later in the development of the disorder and primarily manifest as problems with sustained attention (persistence) and distractibility. The types of problems with inattention seen in the Predominantly Inattentive Subtype "appear to have their onset even later..." (p.67). If age of symptom onset is a limitation of the criterion with children, then it certainly becomes a limitation in the diagnostic process when working with adolescents and adults.

With respect to meeting the criterion "some impairment is present in two or more settings" when the initial diagnosis is made in adolescence or adulthood, comorbidity may indeed be a salient issue. A number of years ago, researchers such as Shaffer and Greenhill (1978) and Stewart, Cumming, Singer, and Deblois (1981) reported that the diagnosis of ADD closely overlaps that of Conduct Disorder. Thus, one could speculate that if, as a child, observed behavior at the beginning of his or her school years did not meet criteria for a Conduct Disorder or a juvenile presentation of Bipolar Disorder, then his or her level of activity could well have seemed within the bounds of appropriate classroom behavior particularly if the child were able to control energy levels until after the classroom day, having then the opportunity to engage in fairly rigorous physical activity such as that presented by competitive sports. By the time evenings were spent in the home environment, hyperactive motor behaviors may well have been substantially diminished due to physical exhaustion. On the other hand, if these same adults were dysthymic as children, typically the classroom teacher or the parent would not have found their level of low arousal or shyness especially noteworthy. Also, they may well have been judged to be less bright than their peers, and as such, their quiet nature and poor academic performance inaccurately attributed to this (Triolo, 1999).

Once entering the adolescent or adult years undiagnosed, the individual "has most likely traveled a path to other pathologies" (Triolo, 1999, p. 66). The presence of comorbid disorders in the adult ADHD population has been well documented (Biederman, Newcorn, and Sprich, 1991; Biederman *et al.*, 1993; Hallowell and Ratey, 1994; Wender, 1995; Katz, Goldstein, and Geckle, 1998). But, often adults will seek professional interventions because of secondary issues such as marital conflicts, alcohol and other drug abuse, anxiety, depression, etc., unaware of the possible co-existence of ADHD. As a result, they will most likely be treated for these common adulthood problems (the presenting problem) vs. a disorder which traditionally has been linked with childhood even though evidence of "clinically significant impairment in social, academic or occupational functioning" comes closest to defining the nature of the disorder in the young adult and adult population. Again, criterion B (some symptoms causing impairment present before 7 years of age) may not be part of the developmental history in many cases.

Further, it has been demonstrated that ADHD symptoms tend to decline in number during the growing years (Achenbach and Edelbrock, 1981). While reduction of symptoms does not stop at adolescence, core impairments remain prominent and stable (Barkley, Fischer, Edelbrock, and Smallish, 1991), although more disruptive behaviors tend to be less overt in adulthood. Here, the capacity of individuals to develop compensatory strategies is limited only by the extent of the individual's own creative potential. Thus, when reviewing the symptoms of inattention or hyperactivity-impulsivity with the individual, often times, responses will include what he or she has done to cope with distractibility, forgetfulness, lack of organization, fidgeting, interrupting, rapid speech, etc. vs. the perceived impact of the symptom on functions in the home, on the job, or in school. Years of employing strategies result in a tendency to minimize possible negative consequences. Behaviors are viewed as problematic only when the external environment does not reinforce the efficacy of such strategies (e.g. poor performance appraisals on the job, near-failing grades, marital discord).

For example, take the bright student who up until his freshman year in college sailed through high school with minimal effort both in terms of input and output, but whose parents provided the regulating, monitoring, and structuring of his external environment on a daily basis. Failing out of a prestigious school is a blow to the ego, can make one quite depressed, and the process of self-doubt begins. When asked if there were problems with time management, organization, distractibility, lack of follow through, or forgetfulness during his earlier years in school or while growing up, the answer may just as readily be "no" as "yes". If his parents are available for collateral information, they may well testify about their efforts. On the other hand, if one or both of them also have undiagnosed ADHD, then their efforts may well be par for the course rather than out of the ordinary.

A final issue with respect to using DSM-IV criteria relates to the nature and severity of current symptoms.   Individuals may have significant difficulty sustaining attention in a lecture hall or when reading required texts or when filling out routine forms, while at other times they report no problems with inattention or sustained focus when reading for pleasure, surfing the Internet, or tackling a highly challenging and /or competitive endeavor. The DSM-IV does not take into account this vacillation between "hyperfocus" and lack of focus often seen in adolescents and adults with ADHD. Parents will confirm the hours spent and degree of intensity maintained by the young adult engaged in playing with legos or computer games as a child playing hockey or watching sports programs as an adolescent. At the same time, they will report that their child is unable to sit quietly during a TV show in which other members of the family are interested if the demands for attention are greater than 10 minutes. Adults often incorporate the attributional labels given them on account of this waxing and waning of attention and assign moral judgments to the perceived voluntary nature of their behaviors. Thus, the symptom becomes a character trait, most often a negative one, and again is not thought of as a characteristic symptom of a disorder.

Subtyping

While the DSM-IV provides three subtypes and a "not otherwise specified" category" (p. 85), a number of clinical researchers have begun to examine subtypes based on brain imaging studies as well as neurochemical hypotheses. Amen and Goldman (1998) have posited five clinical subtypes of ADHD for both children and adults to which they have linked psychopharmacological therapies based on SPECT studies. These include ADHD, combined Type, ADHD, primarily inattentive type, Overfocused ADD, Temporal Lobe ADD, and Limbic ADD. Both ADHD, Combined Type and ADHD, Predominantly Inattentive Type show decreased activity in the basal ganglia and prefrontal cortex during a concentration task.   Overfocused ADD is identified with increased activity in the anterior cingulate gyrus and decreased prefrontal cortex activity and is associated with obsessive type behaviors. Temporal Lobe ADD is associated with increased or decreased activity in the temporal lobes and decreased prefrontal cortex activity and linked to aggressive behaviors. Limbic ADD shows increased central limbic system activity and decreased prefrontal cortex activity on SPECT and is associated with low arousal.

The theoretical work of Hunt (1997) attempts to link ADHD subtypes in adults to four brain systems and disturbances in these multiple pathways and their respective neurotransmitter networks (cognitive, arousal, behavioral inhibition, and reward) resulting in four subtypes: Subtype I-Cognitive Processing Deficit; Subtype II-Excessively Aroused ADD; Subtype III-Impaired Behavioral Inhibition System; Subtype IV-Deficient Reward Systems.

Faraone, Biederman, Mennin, *et al.* (1997) presented data to suggest that comorbid ADHD with Bipolar Disorder (BPD) is a familially distinct and nosologically discrete form of ADHD and may be related to childhood-onset BPD. In other words, these researchers suggest that ADHD+BPD and childhood-onset BPD may be the same disorder with a significantly younger age of onset, a strong familial link, and the predominance of males (four times greater than the rate in females, consistent with the literature on childhood BPD). However, no adult subject data are available because at this point follow-up studies of hyperactive children have not addressed the issue by assessing for "a lifetime history of BPD (Weiss, Hechtman, and Perlman, 1985) or (have) excluded children if the primary reason for referral involved aggressive behavior, a prominent feature of juvenile BPD (Mannuzza, Klein, Bessler, *et al.*, 1993)" (Faraone *et al.*, p.1385).

This same group of researchers (Faraone, Biederman, Mennin, *et al.*, 1998) has published results from a four year follow-up study of children from antisocial-ADHD families. Their findings confirm and extend previous work and support their contention that Antisocial ADHD may be a nosologically and clinically meaningful subtype of ADHD, distinct from other forms of ADHD. These results are in keeping with the earlier behavioral subtyping work of Dykman and Ackerman (1963).   In their study, children with ADDHA (hyperactive/aggressive) were found to be at increased risk for oppositional and conduct disorders vs. those without hyperactivity or with hyperactivity and no aggression.

While research into subtypes continues to occur and work such as Amen's and Hunt's with adults remains somewhat controversial and/or theoretical, the clinician must supplement DSM-IV criteria in a way that is clinically useful and empirically sound if the various confounds described earlier are to be weighed into the decision making process. In summary, in the words of Triolo (1999), "the DSM-IV is a long way from providing the diagnostician all of the necessary criteria for reliable and valid diagnosis of ADHD in adults" (p.70).

INCIDENCE, PREVALENCE, AND COMORBIDITY

Given what we know about the history of the diagnostic process and the problems inherent when attempting to apply current criteria to an adult population, information about incidence and prevalence rates as well as comorbidity can be somewhat problematic. What we do know from clinical studies is that approximately 40% to 50% of children with ADHD have symptoms persisting into adulthood (Gittelman, Mannuzza, Shenker, and Bonagura, 1985; Weiss, Hechtman, and Perlman, 1985), which allows us to project that impairment in some level of functioning exists in some 1.5% to 2% of the adult American population (Hunt, 1997).   It has been estimated also that

1% to 3% of the college age population has ADHD with symptoms severe enough to warrant treatment and/or accommodations (Barkley, 1993). Community studies of children have yielded prevalence rates between 1.7% and 16% depending on the population and the diagnostic methods used (Goldman, Genel, Bezman, *et al.*, 1998). These authors go on to report, "The evolution of criteria from DSM-III to DSM-IV, although based on a progressively larger empirical base, has broadened the case definition....This is largely a function of the increased emphasis on attentional problems as opposed to a more narrow focus on hyperactivity....As a result, girls have been diagnosed more frequently...than they were in the past" (p.1102)." Historically, women have been underdiagnosed or misdiagnosed with sex ratios of 9:1 and 6:1 reported in clinically referred samples (Gittleman *et al.*, 1985; Weiss *et al.*, 1985; DSM-IV, 1994) and 3:1 in population-based samples (DSM-III-R, 1987; Szatmari, 1992).

Gender Issues

In a meta-analysis of research literature available between 1979 and 1992, Gaub and Carlson (1997) were able to locate only 18 studies on ADD, that specifically included samples of females. While their analysis suggested some gender differences between girls and boys, many of the differences were clearly mediated by source of referral and methodological limitations. In the few studies available involving rating scales and structured interviews (Achenbach, 1991; Bauermeister, 1992; Eme, 1992; Zocccolillo, 1993; McDermott, 1996), community based investigations (Berry *et al.*, 1985; Breen, 1989; Horn *et al.*, 1989) and brain metabolism research (Ernst *et al.*, 1994), findings are divergent with respect to gender differences, with some studies suggesting that women have a greater prevalence of comorbid internalizing and learning problems.

Beiderman *et al* (1994), in a systematic study of the differential expression of ADHD between the sexes, found women to have equal rates of major depression and anxiety disorders as their males counterparts. The referred adults in their sample had not been identified or treated for ADHD as children, and the authors commented that "the lack of childhood recognition of ADHD among these adults is consistent with findings reported by Shekim (1989) and Zametkin *et al.*, 1990)" (p.26). Using self-report and interview data, Rucklidge and Kaplan (1997) found that women in their sample who were diagnosed with ADHD in adulthood were more apt to report depressive symptoms, were more stressed and anxious, had more external locus of control, lower self-esteem, and engaged in more emotion-oriented vs. task-oriented coping strategies than women who did not meet diagnostic criteria for ADHD.

Similarly, in our recent work, (Katz, Goldstein, and Geckle, 1998) we found women, again identified in adulthood, to have a far greater degree of psychological distress than males with ADHD but more efficient cognitive strategies. However, there were no significant differences between the genders on account of age, race, IQ, level of education, or comorbidity for either learning disabilities or depression. Taken together these studies highlight the possible risks of not being diagnosed with ADHD until adulthood, including depressive symptomatology, anxiety symptoms, and lowered self-esteem, that are based solely on one's gender.

Comorbidity Factors

Complicating the establishment of prevalence rates further is the issue of comorbidity, which we have touched on in our previous discussion of gender issues. Reported overlap rates between the various disorders and ADHD in children in a community sample between the ages of 9 and 16 were 50% for depression, 22% for anxiety disorders, and 36% CD/ODD (Conduct Disorder/Oppositional Defiant Disorder) in children diagnosed with ADHD. In those diagnosed with depression, 27% had ADHD, 51% with anxiety disorders had ADHD, and 93% of the children with CD/ODD had ADHD (Bird, Gould, and Staghezza, 1993). In a recent study of 8 to 18 year old twins with and without ADHD results indicated that all three DSM-IV ADHD subtypes were associated with significant elevations of comorbid symptomatology as reported by parents, teachers, and the children themselves (Willcutt, Pennington, Chhabildas, *et al.*, 1999). Biederman *et al.*'s (1993) data found rates of 31% for major depressive disorder, 25% for substance abuse, 43% for generalized anxiety disorder, and 52% for overanxious disorder in their sample of adults diagnosed with ADHD, two-thirds of whom were males. In addition, having a comorbid condition with ADHD contributes significantly to the persistence of ADHD into adulthood (Biederman *et al.*, 1996; Gittelman *et al.*, 1985).

In an attempt to account for this substantial overlap between ADHD and other disorders, Biederman, Newcorn, and Sprich (1991) have put forth six competing hypotheses:

> 1) The comorbid disorders do not represent distinct entities but rather, are the expression of phenotypic variability of the same disorder, 2) each of the comorbid disorders represents distinct and separate clinical entities, 3) the comorbid disorders share common vulnerabilities..., either genetic (genotype), psychosocial (adversity), or both, 4) the comorbid disorders represent a distinct subtype (genetic variation) within a heterogeneous disorder..., 5) one syndrome is an early manifestation of a conduct or mood disorder..., and 6) the development of one syndrome increases the risk for the comorbid disorder...(p.565).

As a consequence, Biederman and his colleagues have published numerous studies on major depression, bipolar disorder, and anti-social disorders and their co-existence with ADHD attempting to parse out the possibility of a familial link in addition to the previously established high levels of comorbidity seen in both clinical and epidemiological samples in children and adolescents

(Milberger, Biederman, Faraone, *et al.*, 1995; Faraone and Biederman, 1997; Faraone, Biederman, Mennin, *et al.*, 1997; Biederman, Russell, Soriano, *et al.*, 1998).

Comorbidity with Learning Disabilities

In their text, *ADHD with Cormorbid Disorders*, Pliszka, Carlson, and Swanson (1999) write, "There is probably more confusion over the comorbidity of learning disorders (or disabilities; LDs) and ADHD than any other topic we will address" (p. 188). They suggest that the confusion may have originated with the term "minimal brain dysfunction," which included both children with learning problems and those with hyperactivity. By far the vast majority of studies support a higher prevalence rate for learning disabilities in reading, spelling, and arithmetic in children with ADHD than in controls (Pliszka, Carlson, and Swanson, 1999). However, prevalence rates vary depending on whether one is talking about LD as the initial diagnosis or ADHD as the initial diagnosis. In the Cantwell and Baker (1991) study, 37% of the sample of children diagnosed with early speech and language impairments met criteria for ADHD at a five year follow-up. Of those who met criteria for a comorbid psychiatric disorder (70%), ADHD was the most common comorbid condition. Similarly, in the Shaywitz and Shaywitz (1988) study, while 11% of ADHD children met criteria for LD, 33% of the children with LD also had ADHD. Dykman and Achkerman (1991) reported that over half of their clinic-referred ADD sample met criteria for a specific reading disorder (RD).

In general, both RD and ADHD are more prevalent among boys than among girls when the samples are based upon clinic participants. Taking this finding as a given, Willcutt and Pennington (2000) examined the comorbidity of the two disorders differentiated by gender and subtype in a large community sample of twins between the ages of 8 and 18. Their findings indicated that (1)individuals with RD were more likely than individuals without RD to meet criteria for DSM-IV Inattentive Type and Combined Type; (2) the phenotypic relationship is different in boys and girls, with the association between RD and ADHD restricted to the ADHD, Inattentive type in the females; and (3) when the sample was subdivided by FSIQ, both the high and low IQ groups of boys with RD exhibited a significantly higher frequency of both Inattentive and Combined Type ADHD than did boys without RD. However, boys with low IQ RD were significantly more likely to meet criteria for ADHD, Inattentive Type. They concluded, "Taken together, these results suggest that higher intelligence may represent a protective factor against symptoms of inattention for individuals with RD, but does not affect the association between RD and H/I" (Hyperactivity/Impulsivity) (p. 188). "And while the phenotypic analyses reported support the hypothesis that RD and ADHD co-occur "significantly more frequently than would be expected based on chance" (p. 188), they do not shed light on a possible etiological association between the two disorders, although this has been suggested in the past (Stevenson, Pennington, Gilger, *et al.*, 1993) and also disputed (Faraone, Biederman, Lehman, *et al.,* 1993).

With respect to a mathematics disorder, several studies have reported an association with ADHD, Inattentive Type in particular (Ackerman, Anhalt, Dykman, *et al*, 1986; Carlson, Lahey, and Neeper, 1986; Hynd, Lorys, Semrud-Clikeman, *et al.*, 1991; Zentall, 1993). Marshall, Hynd, Handwek, and Hall (1997) suggest that although there is evidence to suggest a relationship between ADHD and a math disability, the relationship is under-reported because it has been under-investigated. Secondly, it has been found that math deficits are more pronounced in older than in younger elementary school students (Ackerman *et al.*, 1986), and that older children with ADHD are more likely to have a math disorder (Nussbaum, Grant, Roman, *et al.*, 1990). However, both referral source and test selection could explain math test performance differences to some degree in these reported studies (Marshall *et al.*, 1997).

Tourette's Syndrome

Finally, we refer the reader to the Pliszka, Carlson, and Swanson (1999) text for an in-depth discussion of comorbid disorders and ADHD. In particular, there are chapters devoted entirely to medical disorders, mental retardation and pervasive developmental disorders, and tic and obsessive compulsive-disorders as well as the more commonly discussed mood and anxiety disorders, although the focus is on children rather than adults. In addition, the text edited by Leckman and Cohen (1999) details the comorbidity and prevalence of Tourette's Syndrome (TS), tics, obsessions, and compulsions with ADHD and other learning disorders. The chapter by Walkup, Khan, Scherholz, *et al.*, (1999) is devoted to *Phenomenology and Natural History of Tic-Related ADHD and Learning Disabilities*, and in it the authors present data which estimate the frequency of ADHD in Tourette's Syndrome to be anywhere from 25% to 75%. In a review of nine reports of 1500 cases of TS in individuals of all ages, ADHD was present in approximately 62% of the cases (Comings and Comings, 1988). Findings suggesting a relationship between the sequence of onset of Tourette's Syndrome and ADHD (earlier-onset ADHD being more etiologically independent of Tourette's Syndrome and later-onset ADHD being secondary to the expression of Tourette's) are regarded as hypothesis generating only at this point in time (Pauls, Alsobrook, Gelernter, and Leckman, 1999). The text by Fisher (1998) also devotes a chapter to comorbid disorders associated with ADD including various neurobehavioral and neurological disorders including Parkinson's Disease, multiple sclerosis, epilepsy, neurofibromatosis, and toxicity, among others.

ETIOLOGY

Genetic Studies

Twin and Adoption Studies

According to Tannock (1998), "ADHD is a paradigm for a true biopsychosocial disorder, raising critical questions concerning the relations between genetic, biological, and environmental factors" (p. 65). That there is considerable evidence that ADHD is a heritable disorder is based upon data retrieved from twin and adoption studies. Over ten years ago, Goodman and Stevenson (1989) investigated a large sample of children with ADHD who were identical or fraternal twins. They reported a concordance rate among monozygotic twins of approximately 50% and a 33% rate for dyzygotic same sex twins. Stevenson (1992) found heritability for mothers' but not teachers' ratings of hyperactivity and a laboratory measure of attention; Gillis, Gilger, Pennington, and DeFries (1992) found a high degree of heritability using a parent interview instrument designed to measure problems of attention and hyperactivity. Both research groups studied large samples of MZ and DZ twins using multiple regression procedures. Family studies consistently support the assertion that ADHD runs in families (Farone and Biederman, 1994a; 1994b).

Adoption studies of ADHD also implicate genes in its etiology. The first study of foster children was conducted by Safer (1973) and investigated the psychological status of maternal full and half siblings of children with minimal brain dysfunction (MBD) who had been placed in different foster homes. Fifty percent of the full siblings were diagnosed with MBD vs. 25% of the half siblings, a finding compatible with genetic transmission. Boreland and Heckman (1976) indicated a greater occurrence of ADD symptoms in the biological siblings of diagnosed ADD children as did Cantwell (1975) and Morrison and Stewart (1983). McGuffin, Owen, and O'Donovan (1994) also reported significantly higher rates of hyperactivity (7.5% vs. 2.1%) in biological parents of children with hyperactivity compared with adoptive parents.

A study by Van der Oord, Boomsma, and Verhulst (1994) provides even more convincing evidence for the heritability of ADHD symptoms. Their study involved biologically related and unrelated sibling pairs of international adoptees (111 pairs and 221 pairs, respectively) as well as a group of adoptees who grew up alone. The study is unique in that both the controls and the study group (biologically related siblings) were raised by adoptive parents. Also, the influence of multiple children within one family could be compared with children raised as singletons. Their results indicated that a strong genetic component (47% of the variance) was obtained for parental ratings of attention problems on the Child Behavior Checklist (Achenbach, 1991), with no significant sibling interactions or shared environmental effects.

Molecular Genetic Studies

According to Biederman and Spencer (1999):

> Although the segregation analyses of ADHD suggest that a single gene is in
> the etiology of ADHD, the differences in fit between genetic models were
> modest....This suggests that ADHD may be caused by several interacting
> genes of modest effect. This latter idea is consistent with ADHD's high
> population prevalence and high concordance in monozygotic twins but modest
> recurrence risks to first degree relatives" (p. 1235).

Molecular genetic studies have produced mixed results to some extent.
However, one of the first association studies based on the dopamine transporter
gene DAT1 was reported by Cook, Stein, and Krasowski, *et al.* (1995). A
significant increase in the frequency of the 480 base pair allele of the dopamine
transporter gene DAT1 was found in a case-control study of 49 patients with
ADHD as defined by DSM-III-R criteria. Gill, Daly, Heron, *et al. (1997)*
replicated their findings in an Irish family-based association study of 40 children
with ADHD.

Some promising data have emerged from studies of the dopamine D4 receptor
(DRD4) gene as well. This gene encodes one of five known protein receptors
that mediate the postsynaptic action of dopamine (Tannock, 1998). The DRD4-
repeat region of the dopamine receptor gene, associated with the personality trait
of high novelty-seeking behavior, is thought to influence "postsynaptic
sensitivity" largely in the dorso-lateral prefrontal cortex, which is linked to
executive functions and the attentional system. Twenty-nine percent of the
ADHD samples under study have this repeat allele, double its rate in the general
population (Baird, Stevenson, and Williams, 2000). Both Ebstein (1996) and
Benjamin, Patterson, Greenberg, *et al.* (1996) reported an association of the 7-
repeat allele of DRD4 with novelty seeking. Persons high on this personality
trait are judged to be impulsive, exploratory, excitable, and quick-tempered,
features frequently seen in patients diagnosed with ADHD. And although their
findings were not replicated in a subsequent study of psychiatrically screened
normal controls and a group of alcoholic offenders (Malhotra, Virrkunen,
Rooney, *et al.*, 1996), they were validated by the work of LaHoste, Swanson,
Wigal, *et al.* (1996), Sunohara, Barr, Jain, *et al.* (1997) and Swanson, Sunohara,
Kennedy, *et al.* (1998).

Biederman and Spencer (1999) continue, "Despite these encouraging DRD4
data, it would be premature to consider DRD4 to simply be an ADHD gene
because the positive association findings could be due to an unknown gene in
linkage dysequilibrium with DRD4" (p. 1235). Just so, researchers such as
Comings, Wu, Chiu, *et al.* (1996) followed receptor DRD2, enzyme dopamine-
b-hydroxylase, and transporter DAT1 gene polymorphisms in Tourette probands
and their relatives. They found significant associations between variations of
the three genes and those diagnosed with Tourette's, ADHD, stuttering,

oppositional defiant behavior, alcohol abuse, mania, and general anxiety. According to Baird *et al.* (2000), "(T)hese studies confirm what must be intuitively obvious: that these conditions have genetic underpinnings, are polygenic, and likely form a continuum that manifests itself in a variety of observed conditions, all interrelated" (p. 7).

Prenatal and Perinatal Factors

As ADHD was initially conceptualized as a result of minimal brain damage caused primarily by infection, trauma, or complications during pregnancy or at the time of delivery (Cruickshank, Eliason, and Merrifield, 1988), both prenatal and perinatal factors have been implicated in the etiology of ADHD. However, studies have been equivocal, and routine neurological examinations, clinical evaluation with CT scans, MRIs, and EEG studies typically have not revealed specific lesions or abnormalities in children with ADHD (Voeller, 1991; Shaywitz, Shaywitz, Byrne, *et al.,* 1993). However, more refined advances in electrophysiological methods have resulted in some evidence for structural/morphological differences in the brains of children with ADHD as a group (Voeller, 1991).

Nichols (1980) in a review of the findings of the Collaborative Perinatal Project, which followed 60,000 infants from birth to age seven, found hyperactivity to be associated with maternal smoking and birth complications. His findings are consistent with those reported by Chandola, Robling, Peters, *et al.* (1992) and Biederman, Milberger, Faraone, *et al.* (1995). On the other hand, Taylor, Sandberg, Thorley, and Giles (1991) did not find perinatal complications and toxin exposure to be associated with hyperactivity later in childhood. Sprich-Buckminster, Biederman, Milberger, *et al.* (1993) noted that studies they reviewed to that point in time had used heterogeneous groups of children with ADHD. In their study, they found evidence to suggest that the association between ADHD and the complications of pregnancy, delivery, and infancy was much stronger in the group with comorbidity (anxiety, major depression, conduct disorder) as compared to the group without comorbidity.

In addition to prenatal and perinatal factors, issues surrounding food additives, refined sugar, allergies and atopic disorders, and thyroid have been put forward as causative with respect to ADHD in children. To date, data to substantiate a causal relationships between any of these factors and ADHD have not been forth coming (Riccio, Hynd, and Cohen, 1997).

And, while researchers have consistently found a relationship between ADHD and certain psychosocial factors (Barkley, 1990), the issue remains one of the chicken or the egg, at best. Biederman and his colleagues (1995), following the classic studies of Rutter and his colleagues on the Isle of Wright, found more chronic family conflict, decreased family cohesion, and parental pathology, especially in the mother, in the families of children with ADHD than

anterior executive system (prefrontal cortex [PFC] and anterior cingulate gyrus), where the responsiveness of the PFC and anterior cingulate to incoming signals is modulated primarily by dopaminergic (DA) input from the ventral tegmental area of the midbrain. Ascending DA fibers stimulate postsynaptic D1 receptors on pyramidal neurons in the PFC and anterior cingulate, which in turn facilitate excitatory NMDA receptor inputs from the posterior attention system. DA selectively gates excitatory inputs to both the PFC and the cingulate which then effectively reduces irrelevant neuronal activity during the performance of executive functions. "According to Pliszka *et al* (1996), the inability of NE to prime the posterior attention system could account for the problems with inattention seen in children with ADHD, and the loss of DA's ability to gate inputs to the anterior executive system may be linked to the deficit in executive functions characteristic of ADHD" (Himelstein, Schulz, Newcorn, and Halperin, 2000, p. 463).

Hunt (1997) has proposed a neurobiological model of ADHD in which he attempts to link the particular brain systems involved with information processing, arousal, behavioral inhibition, and the limbic system, disturbances in their neurotransmitter pathways (DA, NE, 5-HT, and neuropeptides and endorphins), and the symptoms manifest in ADHD as a means to form the basis for pharmacological interventions. "The neurotransmitters and neuropeptides bridge information between neurons and are key to perception, cognitive processing, arousal, inhibition, and reward....Medications mitigate the neurobehavioral dysfunctions in ADHD by modulating the neurotransmitter mechanisms at the synapse" (p. 579).

According to Hunt's schema, a defect in the cognitive-processing system, primarily a disorder of selective attention and information processing and possibly related to hypoactivity of the dopamine system, is hypothesized to involve the gating capacity of the nucleus accumbens, cortical sensory integration centers, the ability of the hippocampus to identify change in the environment, and response selection capacities of the prefrontal cortex. Symptoms of excessive arousal (aggression, impulsivity, increased motor activity and comorbid mania and/or conduct disorder) are thought to relate to hyperactivity of noradrenergic circuitry involving the locus coerulus and the reticular activating system. Impaired behavioral inhibition results from the combined dysfunction of serotonergic and dopaminergic circuits in the prefrontal cortex and in the caudate nucleus and thalamus. Deficits in the reward system are thought to arise from affect regulation defects in limbic circuitry, which then impact responsivity to reward and punishment and faulty cognitive analysis and integration of information arising from defects in prefrontal and associative cortex. Both dopamine and the neuropeptides and endorphins are hypothesized to be dysregulated.

Taken as a whole, research devoted to the neurochemical aspects of ADHD does appear to give evidence of dysfunction in multiple neurotransmitter systems (Hornig, 1998; Zametkin and Liotta, 1998; Himelstein, Schulz, Newcorn, and Halperin, 2000). Although there are inconsistencies in the various findings, given the heterogeneity of individual symptom manifestations across groups, it is not surprising that a uniform deficiency in one neurotransmitter system may not be found across the varied presentations of the disorder. While the neuropsychological, neurochemical, genetic, and neuroanatomical literature gives partial support for the models of ADHD suggested by Pliszka *et al.,(1996)*, Arnsten *et al.*, (1996), Barkley (1997), and Hunt (1997), the inconsistencies in the research do not allow unqualified support for any single model of ADHD. "A most promising direction for future research in the neural substrates of ADHD appears to be in the continued efforts to find meaningful subgroups...within the disorder which yield more uniform neurobiological profiles" (Himelstein *et al.*, 2000, p.474).

COMPONENTS OF THE DIAGNOSTIC PROCESS

Triolo (1999) has set forth six sequential components for the diagnostic process with adults:
* Rule out medical problems that may mimic ADHD symptoms
* Conduct a clinical interview incorporating a retrospective history and observations as well as DSM-IV criteria as appropriate
* Conduct an independent collateral interview
* Quantify subjective reports of ADHD symptoms with standardized measures (Inventories)
* Conduct a brief analysis of personality traits and emotional dispositions
* When warranted, neuropsychological testing

In his text Triolo spends an entire chapter on the diagnostic process which is complete and readily accessible by the clinician. Thus, we will not review in detail all of the six components which he describes, but rather focus on the last three, namely, the use of self-report inventories, personality assessment, and the use of neuropsychological testing, as these are more typically included in evaluations conducted by psychologists and neuropsychologists in addition to the other three information sources.

Self-Report Inventories

While there are numerous checklists available for use with adults (Weiss, 1992; Hallowell and Ratey, 1994; Murphy and LeVert, 1995, Amen, 1997)), they are not standardized and at times the cutoff points are arbitrary at best. In addition, many checklists included in the lay literature and on the Internet are so inclusive that no one would escape identification as having ADHD. Triolo (1999) points out also that some checklists and questionnaires can appear to be statistically developed with normative parameters but are not. Here, he cites the Owens and Owens (1993) Adult Attention Deficit Disorder Behavior Rating Scales. That having been said, there are at least four published instruments which are normed through the entire age range for adults, the Adult Attention Deficit Evaluation Scale, A-ADDES (McCarney and Anderson, 1996), the Brown Attention Deficit Disorder Scales (Brown, 1996), the Attention Deficit Scales for Adults (ADSA) (Triolo and Murphy, 1997), and newest, the Conners' Adult ADHD Rating Scales (CAARS) (Conners, Erhardt, and Sparrow, 1999). The ones we have found most useful are the Brown ADD Scales, one for adolescents and one for adults.

Impetus for the Brown ADD Scales, according to the developer (Brown, 1996), came from clinical conversations with students who suffered from "chronic underachievement despite high IQ and apparently strong wishes to do well in school" (p. 4). The Scales cover the age ranges of 12 through 18 years and 18 years and older, and the 40 self report items are grouped into five clusters of "conceptually related symptoms" (Brown, 1996) of attention deficit disorders (ADDs). These are organizing and activating to work, sustaining attention and concentration, sustaining energy and effort, managing affective interference, and utilizing working memory and accessing recall. While the items assess symptoms included in the DSM-IV criteria, they also incorporate symptoms taken from clinical studies. Brown goes on to say that certain assumptions underlie the nature of the ADDs and thus the construction of the test items. These are listed below.

- ADDs are dimensional disorders.
- ADD symptoms may vary according to tasks and context.
- Difficulty with activating and getting started is often an important element of ADD impairment.
- Chronic impairments in working memory and in recall of learned information are often important in ADDs.
- Hyperactivity/Impulsivity is not an essential element in ADDs.
- ADDs often include aspects of other psychological disorders and frequently overlap with other emotional or behavioral disorders in comorbid combinations.
- ADDs are not impairments of attention only; they are disorders affecting many aspects of cognitive functioning.

Thus, Brown's definition of ADHD with adolescents and adults takes into account the frequency and intensity of symptoms, the stimulus bound nature of sustained attention, problems with activation of behavior in addition to insufficient inhibition, and impairments in active working memory (Baddeley, 1986; Goldman-Rakic, 1987, 1994) and its "file manager" (p. 8) function in accessing recall. The central impairment of ADHD is not viewed as disruptive behavior or failure of inhibition or of inattention only, but rather as impairments in a broad range of cognitive functions, and that a significant overlap of symptoms between ADD and other disorders is a given. The Scales also include a diagnostic form for the clinical history interview and the opportunity for multi-rater capacity on the Scales themselves.

There is one caveat that Triolo (1999) discusses with respect to the IQ levels of the groups on which the Brown Scales were normed. Of the 142 clinical subjects, 52 had an IQ within the average range and 90 had an IQ of 110 or greater. However, one must keep in mind that the nonclinical group used in the discriminant validity study were matched for age and socioeconomic status but not on IQ. That the IQ level of the majority of the clinical group is above average is not surprising given the fact that Brown's initial work with high school and college level students led to the development of the Scales.

Should IQ level be a concern for the practitioner, perhaps the items elicited by the ADSA (Triolo and Murphy, 1996) or those elicited by the CAARS (Conners, Erhardt, and Sparrow, 1999) might be more useful. The ADSA was initially normed on a community sample of 306 adults with no childhood history of problems with attention or hyperactivity, estimated IQs of 80 or above, no reported history of drug or alcohol abuse or felony convictions, and age 17 or older. Data were later collected on 97 clinical subjects, age 17 years or older, who were diagnosed with ADHD prior to involvement in the validity study of the ADSA (Triolo, 1999). Conners et al.(1999) report age and gender based norms from a sample of 2000 nonclinical community adults as well. The CAARS has a both a self-report and an observer rating format as well as long, short, and screening versions.

Triolo's (1999) other concern was that the Brown Scales overemphasized the core symptom of inattention. In this regard, the reader is referred to a study by Millstein, Wilen, Biederman, and Spencer (1997) in which they evaluated the clinical presentation of ADHD in adults. Their results indicated that inattentive symptoms were most frequently endorsed in over 90% of their adult sample. Fifty-six percent of the group met criteria for ADHD, Combined Type, 37% Inattentive Type, and 2% Hyperactive/Impulsive Type. Also, psychiatric comorbidity with ADHD was more prominent in adults with hyperactivity-impulsivity as part of their clinical picture. They concluded, "Given that ADHD adults are presenting from multiple domains, clinicians should carefully query for the inattentive aspects of ADHD when evaluating these individuals" (p. 159).

In summary, behavior rating scales have been the mainstay in the clinical assessment of children with ADHD for more than 20 years (Halperin, Newcorn, and Sharma, 1991). However, even with children, teacher ratings suffer from halo effects (Schachar et al., 1986), and parent ratings have been found to have poor reliability (Rapoport et al., 1986). With adults, in a study by Klee, Garfinkel and Beauchesne (1986), while the index group (diagnosed with ADHD) rated themselves as having more problems with concentration, lower frustration tolerance, impulsivity, and restlessness as children than did the control group, there was greater similarity between the two groups on current behavior rating as the index group rated themselves as much improved when compared to their childhood ratings. These findings suggest real limitations in relying on rating scales solely to identify symptoms in adults, when in fact, the nature of symptomatology in adults may well be altered. In addition, with the exception of the Brown Scales, behavior rating scales have generally not been particularly helpful in the diagnosis of ADHD, Inattentive Type, which has been documented to be more common in adults and in women (NIH Consensus Statement, 1998). Given these concerns, the use of self-rating scales should be considered as one among a number of measures used in the diagnosis of adults

Personality Measures

While the assessment of personality and emotional dispositions will tend to reflect the preferences of the clinician and an established comfort level with either objective or projective measures, we will present a selection of objective measures that we utilize on a regular basis with either adolescents or adults. These measures assist with rule outs regarding major psychiatric disorders or long standing personality traits, that may affect either the quality of performance on other cognitive measures or provide support for comorbidity.

With adolescents a clinically useful battery may consist of either the Beck Depression Inventory-II (BDI-II) (Beck, Steer, and Brown, 1996) or the Reynolds Adolescent Depression Scale (RADS) (Reynolds, 1987), the SCL-90-R (Derogatis, 1994), and the Adolescent Psychopathology Scale (APS) (Reynolds, 1998). Useful also, again depending upon the clinician's preference, are the Millon Adolescent Personality Inventory (MAPI) (Millon, Green, and Meagher, 1982) and the Millon Adolescent Clinical Inventory (MACI) (Millon, Millon, and Davis, 1993). While available as hand-scored measures, they are most efficiently scored and profiled using the NCS Microtest Q Software. The APS is also available in a software program with uses purchased in units of 25 through a Key Disk, much less expensively than the Microtest Q Software package, which requires an annual licensing fee in addition to a set fee per test use. In either case, having access to self-report data can be extremely useful in augmenting the clinical interview, and the redundancy of the measures to some extent has been valuable in counteracting the tendency of some adolescents to access the "zero" or "false" category as a default response pattern. The SCL-90-R and APS response format are most helpful in this regard.

With adults, use of the Beck, the SCL-90-R, and the MCMI-III (Millon, Davis, and Millon, 1997) is a standard part of the comprehensive evaluation process. The three measures give a good picture of the quality of depressive symptoms (neurovegetative vs. reactive), the current severity of psychological and/or somatic stressors, and long-standing behavioral patterns and personality traits.

Having said that, there are certain cautions that must be taken into consideration during the interpretation process, as with the exception of the APS, none of the other measures have necessarily included individuals with ADHD in their clinical norms. It is our experience, as has been reported elsewhere in the literature, that the Obsessive-Compulsive Scale on the SCL-90-R is generally elevated in adults and adolescents with ADHD because the items included in this scale deal with worrying excessively, ruminating thoughts, difficulty with decision making and concentration, and memory problems. With the BDI-II, items involving past failure, self-disappointment, agitation, and concentration difficulty are most often rated as problematic. These items on the BDI-II illustrate to some degree the reactive nature of the depressed feelings particularly when the individual has experienced failure in the school setting or on the job. With the MCMI-III, the scales tend to take on a spurious nature with individuals who have lived with their ADHD over the years particularly if they have a childhood history of hyperactivity and/or impulsivity. Resultant profiles often tend to reflect a pre-occupation with self and the lack of awareness or reported concern for others, which may or may not be totally accurate. As a result, the validity of personality measurement given the instruments available at this time should be viewed with caution and always in light of information derived from a comprehensive history and access to corroborating data whenever possible.

Neuropsychological Assessment

Barkley's (1991; 1994a) analysis of the utility of neurospychological tests in distinguishing children with ADHD and those without found them to be of little merit for the most part with the exception perhaps of continuous performance measures. At the same time he wrote a critical review on the assessment of attention in children (Barkley, 1994b) using Mirsky et al.'s (1991) model of human attention and the possible measures for evaluating its components: focus-execute, sustained, shift, and encode. In that chapter Barkley attempts to equate various attention measures with these components and then critiques their ecological validity as well. Some of the measures included were the Stroop Color-Word Interference Test (Stroop, 1935), the Trail Making Test (Parts A & B; Reitan and Wolfson, 1985); various Digit Symbol or Coding tests, the Wisconsin Card Sort Test (WCST) (Heaton, 1981) and the Categories Test from the Halstead-Reitan Battery (Reitan and Wolfson, 1985). Overall, his critiques can be summarized as "more research is needed on the ecological validity of this test as a measure of attention in children" (p.85), in reference to the Stroop, the Trail Making Test, the Digit Symbol and Coding subtests of the WAIS-R and WISC-R, and the Children's Embedded Figures Test (Witkin, Oltman, Raskin, and Karp, 1971) and "the ecological validity of this measure deserves further study" (p. 87) (in reference to the WCST). With respect to continuous performance tests (CPT), Barkley (1994b) concludes that while children having ADHD often make more errors as a group than do groups of children without such disorders, they have not been particularly effective in differentiating between children with ADHD and "other clinical groups presumed not to have sustained attention problems" (p. 80).

On the other hand studies utilizing neuropsychological measures have demonstrated deficits in adults consistent with those found in children (Matochik, Rumsey, and Zametkin, 1996; Downey, Stelson, Pomerleau, and Giordani, 1997; Jenkins, Cohen, and Malloy, 1998; Seidman, Biederman, and Weber, et al., 1998; Corbett and Stanczak, 1999; Lovejoy, Ball, and Keats, 1999). Further, work by Seidman et al. (1998), suggests that because the diagnosis of ADHD in adults is controversial to the degree that it is dependent on a retrospective diagnosis, external validation of cognitive-neuropsychological functions, particularly attentional and executive processes, which have been found to be frequently impaired in children with ADHD, "would help to clarify the validity of the adult diagnosis and supplement the clinical picture" (p. 260). In addition, cognitive performance measures are useful validating criteria because they do not share method variance with other measures and by their very nature allow direct assessment of performance. "Identification of core neuropsychological deficits in adults with ADHD is also important both as an empirical study of performance relevant to adaptive functioning and as a window into hypothesized alterations in brain functioning in frontostriatal systems (Grodzinsky and Diamond, 1992)" (Seidman et al., 1998, p. 260).

In the study involving unmedicated adults with ADHD and controls reported by Seidman et al. (1998), the neuropsychological battery utilized included an estimated Full Scale IQ from the WAIS-R (Wechsler, 1981), using the Vocabulary and Block Design subtests. The Digit Symbol, Digit Span, and Arithmetic subtests were used to compute a Freedom-from–Distractibility IQ as well. In addition, the Wide Range Achievement Test-Revised (WRAT-R) (Jastak and Jastak, 1985), Rey-Osterrieth Complex Figure (ROCF) (Rey, 1941), the California Verbal Learning Test (CVLT) (Delis et al., 1987), the Wisconsin Card Sorting Test (WCST) (Heaton et al., 1993), the Stroop Test (Golden, 1978), the scattered letters version of visual cancellations (Weintraub and Mesulam, 1985), and an auditory CPT (Zametkin et al., 1990) were administered. Overall, the adults with ADHD demonstrated milder neuropsychological impairments than had been previously reported with children and adolescents using an identical battery (Seidman, Biederman, Faraone, et. al, 1997). The adults assessed were not impaired on the Stroop, the WCST, or the ROCF as the children had been, nor did they show significant impairment on the Freedom-from-Distractibility Index. However, they were significantly more impaired than controls on the CVLT for words learned on trials 1-5, on semantic clustering, and on the number of words recalled after long delay; the auditory CPT; and on the arithmetic subtest of the WRAT-R. These results were similar to those reported by Holdnack *et al.* (1995).

In recognition of the high degree of comorbidity between ADHD and depression, which has been documented from both epidemiologic (Anderson *et al*, 1987; Bird *et al.*, 1988) and clinical studies (Jensen *et al.*, 1988; Woolston *et al*, 1989; Biederman *et al.*, 1990), we (Katz, Wood, Goldstein, *et al.*, 1998) investigated the potential of various neuropsychological measures to discriminate between groups of adults with ADHD comorbid with depression and those with a diagnosis of ADHD without depression. Variables derived from the CVLT, the Paced Auditory Serial Addition Test (PASAT) (Gronwall, 1977), and the Stroop Test were found to discriminate between the groups at a level significantly exceeding chance. But while the neuropsychological tests used appeared to be quite sensitive to ADHD, they were also sensitive to depression in some cases. Results suggested that the differential diagnosis of ADHD and depression in adults may be complicated to some extent because of the shared characteristics of the disorders in adults.

Suggested Neuropsychological Testing Protocol for Adolescents and Adults

Given that no standard battery of neuropsychological tests exists specifically for the identification of ADHD, the clinician is left with a variety of instruments that may be quite useful in identifying specific cognitive or processing deficits and in demonstrating the impact of the underlying ADHD on cognitive performance. From a neuropsychological perspective, an understanding of (1) how the brain processes information and novel stimuli, (2) the differential access to visual or auditory modalities on learning and memory, (3) the impact of working memory's encoding function on storage and retrieval, (4) the ability to sustain attention and vigilance to task, (5) the level of initial sensory arousal, and (6) the limitations imposed on reading comprehension and/or written language output can be helpful not only in validating the diagnosis of ADHD in adolescents and adults but also in facilitating their understanding of how the disorder impacts their learning or vocational endeavors.

Based upon assessments conducted with hundreds of adolescents and adults, we offer the following annotated testing protocol which we have found useful in addressing the cognitive variables listed above from a neuropsychological framework concerned with functional systems, impairment, and the possible limitations imposed on behavior/performance. The reader will also notice that the protocol contains a strong psychoeducational component. As well documented in the literature, comorbidity rates of from 40 to 60% for a learning disability have been reported (Cantwell and Baker, 1991).

- Wechsler Adult Intelligence Scale-III (WAIS-III) (Wechsler, 1997). It is our experience that the WAIS-III is an improvement over the WAIS-R in general because it allows for greater qualitative interpretation of test performance and error analysis. Specifically, having access to the Letter-Number Sequencing subtest allows for comparison with Digit Span. With individuals who are capable of hyperfocus when stimulus material is highly challenging, performance can be greatly enhanced. Thus, often the measured performance on the Letter-Number Sequencing Task is better than on the Digit Span subtest. One can examine also the requirement for repetition of auditory input to evoke initial sensory arousal on the Arithmetic subtest, which again enhances working memory, an opportunity not provided with Digit Span. The WAIS-III provides the opportunity to assess the impact of untimed performance on cognitive, nonverbal tasks via the Matrix Reasoning subtest in particular vs. the Block Design subtest. Also, access to cued and free recall for the Digit Symbol subtest gives additional evidence regarding the impact of repetition and practice on working memory. Difficulties with the Information subtest give some initial indication of the impact of a possible ADHD on the early learning environment. Finally, Verbal, Performance and Full Scale IQs give us a self-referent base for comparison purposes.

- Wide Range Achievement Test-III (Wilkinson, 1993). With adolescents and adults the WRAT-III provides a screening tool to establish the possible co-existence of a specific learning disorder, whose co-morbidity with ADHD has been well established and was reviewed under the co-morbidy section of this chapter. With the Spelling and Reading Recognition subtests, an analysis of error patterns enables the evaluator to determine whether to proceed with a more in-depth evaluation of language functions. Also, since two forms are available, math operations skills can be assessed with and without access to a calculator, and again error analysis can help pin-point errors resulting from inattention to detail (misaligning numbers, misreading "+" and "- " signs, etc.).

- Comprehensive Test of Phonological Processing (CTOPP) (Wagner, Torgesen, and Rashotte, 1999) or the Woodcock Language Proficiency Battery-Revised (Woodcock, 1991). Because research has demonstrated the necessity to evaluate for a phonological processing deficit highly specific to the majority of reading disorders, components of each or both of these measures are extremely useful and both provide norms for adults through the age of 24. However, it should be pointed out that there are differences more often than not between the core and alternative subtests with the CTOPP, and it has been our experience that it is necessary to administer the entire test in order to obtain a more accurate assessment of rapid naming, for example. This is further discussed in the chapter on disorders of reading and written language.

- Test of Mathematical Abilities-2 (TOMA-2) (Brown, Cronin, and McEntire, 1994). The TOMA-2 often provides additional information on math functions and operations should the need to rule out a specific mathematics disorder seem appropriate. The TOMA-2 provides subtests dealing not only with computation but also with story problems, math vocabulary, general concepts, and attitude toward math. As it is normed on individuals between the ages of 8 an 18-11, its use may be restricted more appropriately to young adults unless it is used primarily for providing qualitative information. Alternatively, the several math measures (calculation and applied problems) from the Woodcock-Johnson Tests of Achievement-Revised (Woodcock and Johnson, 1989) provide a more in-depth view of math skills for the college population in particular.

- Woodcock Language Proficiency Battery-Revised (WLPB-R) (Woodcock, 1991). The Woodcock provides several measures for assessing written language skills including punctuation, spelling, and grammar (usage). There is also a measure of writing fluency under constraints of timed performance. As with the Woodcock-Johnson Tests of Cognition and Achievement (WJ-R) (Woodcock and Johnson, 1989), norms are provided for adult subjects.

- Test of Written Language–3 (TOWL-3) (Hammill and Larssen, 1996). Should a spontaneous writing sample be required to further assess written language output, the TOWL-3 may be utilized, as long as one takes into account a degree of score inflation as the referent group is high school seniors. However, despite that issue, a qualitative analysis of theme development, logical thought progression, and efficient production of written language under timed and extended time conditions can be made.

- Nelson-Denny Reading Test (Brown, Fishco, and Hanna, 1993) and the Gray Oral Reading Test (GORT-3) (Wiederholt and Bryant, 1992). We routinely administer the Nelson-Denny, a silent reading comprehension measure, which also allows for measurement of reading rate, in addition to the GORT-3. Invariably, unless a reading disorder is present, the individual with ADHD will improve his or her comprehension and reading rate scores under conditions of oral reading. We suggest that these measures help to demonstrate the impact of multi-modal sensory input on working memory. Again, the norms are restricted to college graduates on the Nelson-Denny and ages 18-11 on the GORT-3. However, these measures much more closely resemble the kinds of reading materials and multiple-choice exam questions an individual is likely to experience in the later secondary and postsecondary years. Also, it is our experience that while the Woodcock-Johnson Tests of Achievement (Woodcock and Johnson, 1989) are normed on an adult population as well as children, the subtest assessing passage comprehension overestimates reading comprehension skills in individuals with above average measured IQ and fails to uncover the problems made manifest when individuals are faced with decoding extensive reading passages over a period of time similar to those found in college and/or post baccalaureate texts.

- Wechsler Memory Scale-III (WMS-III) (Wechsler, 1997). While we utilize this measure on a routine basis, we have found the results to be somewhat equivocal with respect to the Working Memory Index when evaluating adults. Based upon numerous clinical observations of test results, we hypothesize that because the Index is based solely on the performance scores from two measures, Letter-Number Sequencing and Spatial Span, that more often than not we are measuring the individual's ability to "hyperfocus" (as mentioned previously) and the impact of multi-modal sensory input (both tactile and visual for the Spatial Span subtest) vs. working memory per se.

- California Verbal Learning Test (CVLT) (Delis et al., 1987). On the other hand, if the individual manifests significant difficulty with the Paired Verbal Association subtest (performance is significantly below an expected level given his IQ), we will then administer the (CVLT) to help in understanding the differential in auditory processing, encoding, and retrieval. The CVLT also gives the opportunity to assess semantic learning strategies and the effects of cued recall and a condition of recognition recall.

- Routinely, we will include the Stroop Color and Word Test (Golden, 1978), the Paced Auditory Serial Addition Test (PASAT) (Gronwall, 1977), the Trail Making Test (Reitan and Wolfson, 1993), and the Smith's Symbol Digit Modalities Test (SSDMT) (Smith, 1982). The use of the Stroop and the PASAT further substantiates the ability to hyperfocus on discrete auditory or visual input and/ or demonstrates significant problems with selective attention and response inhibition. Thus, both factors must be taken into consideration when interpreting results. The SSDMT gives us another measure of psychomotor speed and working memory should we need to give certain measures under conditions of medication and without medication. With the Trail Making Test, it is our experience that one may often find a discrepancy between Trails A and Trails B performance scores, favoring one or the other, again dependent on how challenging the task is of the examinee's visual attention, that is, does it capture attention or it is perceived of as too simple and simply not worth the effort.

- Category Test (Reitan and Wolfson, 1993) or the Wisconsin Card Sorting Test (WCST) (Heaton, 1993). It is our experience that the brighter the subject the less challenging the WCST is. However, it is our choice with adolescents in particular. Although with both the Category Test and the WCST performance is somewhat variable, what concerns us most is whether there is a substantial impact on frontal lobe mediated executive functions as purportedly measured by either of these instruments.

Use of such a comprehensive battery in combination with an extensive clinical interview, access to collateral data (previous evaluations and/or interview with parent or significant other), and the use of self-report behavior and personality inventories have become the routine rather than the exception in our clinical practice. It is in keeping with the Educational Testing Service (ETS) policy statement and standards with respect to the documentation of ADHD in adolescents and adults (1998) and with those documentation standards imposed by professional organizations and licensing bodies such as the National Board of Medical Examiners and the various state law boards (Richard, Finkel, and Cohen, 1998).

TREATMENT AND INTERVENTIONS

Pharmacotherapy

Psychostimulants

Psychostimulants, first-line medications for treating the Combined and Inattentive Types of ADHD both in children and adults include the following: methylphenidate (MPH) (generic) Ritalin and Ritalin SR, and Concerta (brand names); dextroamphetamine (DEX) (generic), Dexedrine, Dexedrine Spansule, and Adderal (brand names); and pemoline (Cylert). Both MPH and DEX are thought to promote the release of dopamine and norepinephrine in the brain. They are taken orally and are absorbed within 30-45 minutes. While robust response rates have typically been reported in close to 70% of children (Barkley, 1977; Wilens and Biederman, 1992), studies with adults have shown much more equivocal results with response rates ranging from 25% to 73% in controlled studies (Spencer, Biederman, Wilens, Harding, *et al.* (1996).

Concerta (methylphenidate HCl) was just released in the summer of 2000. Concerta uses an osmotic system of delivery in a pulsed pattern, allowing a 12-hour response from a single daily dose. Several double-blind crossover studies with children between the ages of 6 and 12 have been conducted comparing once a day dosing to three times daily dosing with immediate release methylphenidate or placebo. Results supporting the efficacy of the medication were reported at the 46th Annual Meeting of the American Academy of Child and Adolescent Psychiatry in Chicago, Il (Pelham and Swanson, 1999).

Spencer, Biederman, Wilens, Harding, *et al.* (1996) reported that in contrast to the 155 controlled studies on the use of stimulants with children, there were fewer than ten in the adult literature. However, these studies do support the efficacy of stimulant medication with adults (Wood, Reimherr, Wender, and Johnson, 1976; Wender, Reimherr, and Wood, 1981; Yellin, Hopwood, and Greenberg, 1982; Mattes, Boswell, and Oliver, 1984; Gualtieri, Ondrusek, and Finley, 1985; Wender, Reimherr, Wood, and Ward, 1985; Wilens and Biederman, 1992; Matochik, Liebenauer, King, *et al.*, 1994; Spencer, Wilens, Biederman, *et al.*, 1995), the most recent of which has used a double-blind, placebo, controlled crossover design.

In a seven week study of 23 adults with ADHD, Spencer, *et al.*(1995) reported a 78% response rate for methylphenidate (MPH, Ritalin) treatment vs. a 4% response rate for placebo. The response rate was independent of gender, psychiatric morbidity, or family history of psychiatric disorders. They also reported a more robust improvement in symptoms with a 60-80 mg. daily dosage vs. a modest improvement with 30-40 mg. daily dosage.

In terms of clinical management of ADHD in adults with psychostimulants, Spencer, *et al.* (1995) suggest that treatment should be initiated with short-acting preparations at the lowest possible dose (5mg. of either MPH or DEX) once-daily in the morning, to 2 to 4 daily doses until an acceptable response is noted (average adult doses range from 20-80 mgs). In a study by Rush, Kollins, and Pazzaglia (1998) across an eightfold range of doses, methylphenidate produced discriminative-stimulus and participant rated effects that were essentially indistinguishable from those observed with *d*-amphetamine.

Side effects of the stimulants are generally considered mild and managed with adjustment of timing of administration or dose (i.e., insomnia, edginess, diminished appetite, weight loss, dysphoria, and headaches). In terms of adverse or serious toxicity, Diener (1991) reports, "Over a period of more than 30 years of worldwide clinical experience with MPH, remarkably few reports of adverse reactions or serious toxicity have been recorded and/or published in the medical literature. Even reports of adverse effects due to intentional overdosage or drug abuse are relatively rare" (p. 42). Diener adds that only a very few reports were cited by Baselt (1982) about the related hazard of intravenous MPH abuse and the development of talc granulomatosis resulting from the attempted solubilizing and injection of the contents from tablets intended for oral use.

Pemoline, because of its long half-life is given once or twice a day, usually in a 37.5 mg dose, and may take up to six weeks until it reaches efficacy. However, more recent concerns about toxic effects on liver functions have seen its use diminish in clinical practice (Jaffe, 1989; Fargason and Ford, 1994; Amen and Johnson, 1996; Wender, 1998).

Nonstimulant Medications

Despite the use of stimulant medication with adults diagnosed with ADHD, some 30% to 50% do not respond positively to the medication, experience unpleasant or untoward side effects, or have comorbid depressive or anxiety disorders. As a result, nonstimulant medications are used with adolescents and adults including various antidepressant medications, antihypertensive agents, and amino acids (Wender, Wood, Reimherr, and Ward, 1983; Wood, Reimherr, and Wender, 1983; Hunt, Capper, and O'Connell, 1990; Wender and Reimherr, 1990; Hunt, Arnsten, and Asbell, 1995; Wilens, Spencer, and Biederman, 1995a;Wilens, Spencer, and Biederman (1995b).

Wilens, Biederman, Mick, and Spencer (1995) reported positive responses to desipramine and nortriptyline; 52% of 37 adult subjects with a mean age of 41 years reported marked improvement in symptoms. In addition, Wender and Reimherr (1990) reported the atypical antidepressant, Wellbutrin (bupropion) to be helpful in reducing ADHD symptoms in a group of 19 adults treated with an average of 360 mg for a period of six to eight weeks (74% reported moderate to marked response). Gelenberg, Bassuk, and Schoonover (1991) suggested that bupropion might be most helpful for adults with ADHD who also have cardiac abnormalities (in contrast to the tricyclics) and/or comorbid mood instability. In the study by Rush, Kollins, and Pazzaglia (1998), bupropion produced some *d*-amphetamine-like, participant-rated drug effects but did not occasion significant levels of *d*-amphetamine-appropriate responding (Drug A or not Drug A) in an experiment involving *d*-amphetamine trained humans. They reported that their findings were congruent with previous studies of a dissociation between the discriminative-stimulus and participant-rated effects of drugs.

According to Ratey, Hallowell, and Leveroni (1993) the challenge to treating ADHD in adults is finding the medication or combination of medications that work for the individual. In prescribing tricyclics, they report positive effects experienced particularly at a very low dose range that is often lost as the dose is increased. Norpramin is prescribed initially at 10mg once daily for a period of one week to ten days and then raised to 20 to 30mg/day if needed. Ratey, Greenberg, and Lindem (1991) also reported the use of a combination psychostimulant and nadolol (a peripherally acting beta-adrenergic blocker). The medications were used in a group of adults with ADHD for whom the tricyclics were unsuccessful and methylphenidate alone did not help with symptoms of anxiety and impulsiveness. In treating adults, Ratey, *et al.*(1991) write that in their clinical experience the "persistent somatic anxiety created by the attention deficit itself...while sometimes fully treated in children and adolescents with methylphenidate alone...often remains a problem and requires dosage adjustment or adjuncts such as clonidine" (p. 700), [another noradrenergic agonist]. Williams, Mehl, Yudofsky, *et al.* (1982) had earlier hypothesized that propranolol's mechanism of action in modifying behavior might be in part secondary to beta adrenergic blockade "which breaks a vicious cycle of interaction between anxiety and adrenergically mediated physical sensations (Easton and Sherman, 1976)" (p. 134).

Amen and Goldman (1998) present a medication decision tree for the primary care physician listing clusters of symptoms, e.g., inattention, distractibility;

disorganization; hyperactivity and impulsivity, and ADD/overfocus symptoms (cognitive inflexibility, worrying, trouble shifting attention, etc.). Attached to each symptom cluster are first-line and seond-line medications. In the case of attention/focus symptoms and hyperactivity/impulsivity, the first line medications are the various psychostimulants; second line include tricyclics, bupropion, guanfacine (Tenex), and clonidine. For the ADD/overfocus symptoms, Amen and Goldman suggest the SSRIs (venlafaxine, sertraline, paroxetine, and fluoxetine) as first-line medications and fluvoxamine, clomipramine, and nefazodone as second-line medications.

Finally, a pilot study reported in the *American Journal of Psychiatry* (Wilens, Biederman, Spencer, *et al.*, 1999) held that a nicotine-like drug provisionally named ABT-418, might hold some promise for adults with ADHD. The drug is a prototype of a new class of compounds called *selective cholinergic channel activators*. Previous research has suggested that nicotine patches might be useful for some adults with ADHD (Conners, Levin, Sparrow, *et al.*, 1996). Conners *et al.* comment: "The high prevalence of smoking among adolescents and adults with ADHD and the stimulant-like properties of nicotine suggest that ADHD patients may smoke as a form of self-treatment for their symptoms" (p. 67). For a thorough discussion of medications and their use in ADHD the reader is referred also to the text by Copeland and Copps (1995), *Medications and Attention Disorders and Related Medical Problems.*

Alternative Medicines

Arnold (1999) presented the results from a meta-analysis of 23 alternative treatment approaches to ADHD other than psychoactive medication and behavioral/psychosocial interventions. The treatments included such interventions as oligoantigenic or few-foods diet, relaxation/EMG biofeedback, deleading, Chinese herbals, EEG biofeedback, meditation, channel-specific perceptual training, single-vitamin megadosage, laser acupuncture, and essential fatty acid supplementation, among others. Some of the procedures were conducted under controlled conditions, others were present in the literature as pilot or case studies. Arnold concludes his review with the comment that "the most basic recommendation for future research on treatment alternatives for ADHD is that there should be more....most...have been relatively neglected by... mainstream investigators and by peer-reviewed funding" (p.42). For those interested, suggested effects from various antioxidant, vitamin and mineral preparations, and herbal extracts are discussed in a paper by Ludwikowski and DeValk, (1998). Their clinical work is specifically with children, however, they are using some of these substances for medication-naïve patients and for others whose psychostimulant medication needs have been able to be reduced as a result.

Young Adults: College Students and Medications

With respect to individuals in postsecondary settings, the issue of whether or not medication is an efficacious treatment strategy to counteract the effects of inattention and distractibility on academic performance and /or interpersonal interactions has been well documented (Nadeau, 1995). What is at stake is the young adult's mind-set regarding the use of medication. Noncompliance becomes a serious issue in medication management for a number of reasons. First, with individuals diagnosed at an earlier age, medication management has become equated with behavior control or a form of discipline either at home or in the classroom. When the individual moves from mid-adolescence into young adulthood, discontinuance of medication heralds a breaking away from parental control, tangible evidence of independence and self-management.

At the same time, peer-pressure is still strong, and peer-endorsed drug and alcohol experimentation adds to the illusion of being in control of one's fate, engaging in independent judgments, and dealing effectively with consequences of those judgments. The very students who argue that prescribed "drugs" are changing their personalities, restricting their usual levels of high energy and enthusiasm, and altering their creativity and spontaneity, find themselves self-medicating with nicotine, caffeine, marijuana, LSD, and alcohol (Henningfield, Clayton, and Pollin, 1990; Lambert and Hartsough, 1998). This is particularly troublesome as there is an emerging literature showing that the persistence of ADHD into adulthood may be a risk factor for a pychoactive substance use disorder (Blouin, Bornstein, and Trites, 1978; Mannuzza, Kein, and Bessler, 1993; Wilens, Biederman, Spencer, *et al.,* 1994; Biederman, Wilens, Mick, *et al.,* 1995; Tzelepis, Schubiner, and Warbasse, 1995; Wilens, Biederman, Mick, *et al.,* 1997). It is has been reported as well that ADHD is associated with a longer duration of a psychoactive substance use disorder and a significantly slower remission rate (Wilens, Biederman, and Mick, 1998).

Third, college age young adults often have never been given the responsibility to understand the consequences of the disorder on their lives by treating clinicians. Medications are prescribed with little education for the prescribee; at other times dosages are not titrated with enough attention given to target behaviors. If they have been medicated as children, it is their parents, more often than not, who read up on the medications, ask questions, and observe behaviors. It is their parents who opt for medication holidays and summers without medication; it is their parents who reluctantly agree to the use of medication as a last resort. Young adults are left with no real understanding of what prescribed medications are intended to do. When a fellow student asks to use the prescribed medication or to offer to demonstrate how to "snort" Ritalin for a quick high, there is no internalized behavioral repertoire from which to draw. When the popular press demonizes the use of Ritalin (Gibbs, 1998), both the parents' guilt and the young person's reluctance are greatly reinforced.

Malcom Gladwell (1999) in critiquing the impact of the popular press on individuals with ADHD writes, "Only by a strange inversion of moral responsibility do books like *Ritalin Nation* and *Running on Ritalin* seek to make those parents and physicians trying to help children with ADHD feel guilty for doing so" (p. 84). He then opines that the rise of ADHD is a consequence of what might otherwise be considered a good thing. "...The world we live in increasingly values intellectual consideration and rationality—increasingly demands that we stop and focus. Modernity didn't create ADHD. It revealed it" (p. 84).

EDUCATIONAL, BEHAVIORAL, AND PSYCHOSOCIAL INTERVENTIONS

Strategies in the Postsecondary Education Environment

In addition to the use of medication, the single most important intervention for adults dealing with ADHD is education, whether in the academic arena, the world of work, or in the context of personal and social relations. Hallowell (1995) writes that the comprehensive treatment of ADHD begins with diagnosis followed by education, structure, psychotherapy, and medication. "The first two" (diagnosis and education) "are invariably essential; the third, almost always; each of the final two may or may not be necessary" (p. 147).

Self-education and self-awareness are keys to well-informed decision making and to understanding the expectations and roles that derive from being a student in a post-secondary college or university setting. Without them, the student is confronted with a myriad of pitfalls that mitigate the chance for success. Despite a reliance on external structures that were in place in the earlier years or self-devised compensatory strategies that might have proved more than adequate for the demands posed by earlier educational experiences, once faced with the complexity of demands on the person in this unstructured, self-directed, highly diverse environment, the old approaches are no longer functional. Lack of well-integrated and self-regulated time management, organization, and planning skills coupled with the inability to cope with an inertia that feeds upon itself and culminates in excessive procrastination, [that reacts only to intense pressure], leaves the young adult student vulnerable to failure, low-esteem, and depression. Self-evaluation becomes laden with self-criticism, negative projections, and self-anger if the individual does not understand the role that ADHD plays in his or her academic life.

Direct, explicit instruction in how to set priorities, how to manage the demands on one's time while at the same time planning for down-time, and how to replace the unincorporated "parent monitor" with strategies and devices that are one's own, either internal or external, are critical. The instructor or counselor cannot assume that once the individual has a day-planner or palm pilot, for example, that he or she will be able to follow a schedule, get to class on time, hand in reports on time, or establish a sense of priorities. The key will be in connecting relevance to behavior by establishing a direct link between desired outcome and steps to achieve that outcome and positively reinforcing behaviors that reflect cognitive and metacognitive understanding in their enactment. Knowing "what works" and why and then being willing to give up ineffective learning strategies that have been intermittently and successfully reinforced in the past are examples of both cognitive and metacognitive understanding.

Reasonable Accommodations in Postsecondary Settings

In addition to self-education and self-awareness, the university or advanced degree student is also eligible for reasonable and appropriate accommodations. In 1991, the U.S. Department of Education issued a memorandum clarifying the status of ADD, recognizing that ADD can result in significant learning problems, and confirming that children with ADD may be eligible for services under the Disabilities Education Act (IDEA), passed in 1975 as The Education for All Handicapped Children Act, and under the Rehabilitation Act of 1973 (29 U.S.C. 701). The rights of postsecondary students with ADHD stem primarily from three sources, the Constitution, statutes and regulations prohibiting discrimination, and cases decided by courts, departments, and agencies (Latham, 1995).

The two principal laws giving rise to the legal rights of postsecondary students are the Rehabilitation Act of 1973 and the Americans with Disabilities Act of 1990 (ADA). Section 504 of the Rehab Act applies to postsecondary institutions that receive federal funds; Title II of the ADA applies to public postsecondary institutions, and Title III of the ADA applies to private postsecondary institutions. (Latham, 1995). Eligibility under these statutes is individually determined (ADD is a disability when it substantially limits a major life activity) (Latham and Latham, 1993), and not all students with ADHD benefit from identical modifications and accommodations, nor do they use them in the same way or to the same degree (Richard, 1995).

Postsecondary students with ADHD, who provide documentation of their disabilities in a timely manner and are qualified for the program, are entitled to appropriate academic adjustments and auxiliary aids and services. Standard criteria for documenting attention deficit disorders have been developed by the Consortium on ADHD Documentation (1998) and are available for use by "postsecondary personnel, examining, certifying, and licensing agencies, and consumers who require documentation to determine reasonable and appropriate accommodation (s)…"(p.4).These accommodations must be provided at no additional expense to the student, unless such provision would pose an undue hardship (Southwestern Community College v. Davis, 1979).

Life-Management Skills

When working with the young adult as therapist, counselor, or coach, the roles outlined by Nadeau (1995) are highly appropriate in this regard. Nadeau writes that the clinician working with adults with ADHD needs to take into consideration all of the aspects of daily functioning that are affected by the cognitive skills deficits associated with ADHD. Citing the work of Zametkin, Nadeau states that as the frontal lobes are one of the major neurological structures involved in attention deficit, the executive functions they control are the "oversight or managerial functions so often affected in adults with ADD" (p.191). She lists various executive functions that include attention, memory, organization, planning, initiation, self-inhibition (self-discipline), ability to change set, strategic behavior, and self-monitoring in relation to time. Her chapter is then devoted to the effect of executive functions on practical life management skills.

Next, Nadeau (1995) sets forth roles for the therapist. She writes that an essential role is to educate and thereby enable the individual to better understand the neurological basis for the ADHD symptoms. The process of education is supported through reading, participation in support groups, and ongoing therapy in some cases. The therapist is also a supporter, moving the individual from "victimization to empowerment in relation to the ADD symptoms" (p. 193). The therapist is an interpreter, validating the disabling effect of ADHD on the individual's life whether to a spouse or employer. Finally, the therapist is a structurer and a rehabilitation counselor, providing guidelines, homework assignments, and information and strategies for both accommodations and environmental restructuring. She goes on to detail strategies focused on attention-enhancing techniques; on the avoidance of prolonged under or over stimulation, everyday, semantic and prospective memory problems, and the use of compensatory strategies; building problem-solving skills; time management issues including chronic lateness; and stress management and the reduction of distractions. Her model, which is based on an assessment of executive functions in daily living, relies in part on the work of Sohlberg and Geyer (1986) and Pollens, McBratnie, and Burton (1988).

Coaching

Hallowell (1995) writes that in psychotherapy with patients who have ADHD it is useful to be overtly encouraging rather than emotionally neutral and to be directive rather than withholding of advice. "In this posture the therapist becomes like a coach: that individual standing on the sidelines with a whistle around his or her neck, barking out encouragement, directions, and reminders to the player in the game" (p. 148). According to Nancy Ratey (1997) "coaching is about a partnership ...it's about helping the person learn how to manage their brain" (p.8).   Coaching is also an example of a point of performance intervention (Barkley, 1997).   Barkley sees the problems experienced by individuals with ADHD not as skill deficits but rather problems with behavioral execution.   Because of the difficulties encountered in executive functions, successful performance is impaired despite the individual's existing knowledge of effective coping strategies.

Consistent with Barkley's theory, Turnock (1998) reported the results of a survey conducted at Colorado State University involving students with ADHD. Results suggested that students within the high-symptom group used significantly fewer coping behaviors than their low-symptom peers.   They approached studying in a less organized, less methodical way, procrastinated more, and employed fewer self-control/self-disciplinary behaviors. Academic success in the high-symptom group was related primarily to their level of intelligence, but significantly lower grades and high drop-out rates were greater among this group than among their low-symptom peers.   In the words of Hallowell again, "This approach (coaching) takes into account the neurological inability of the ADD mind to focus and organize as efficiently as other minds" (p. 149).

In like manner, Ratey, Hallowell, and Miller (1997) define coaching as an action oriented rather than insight oriented process. They suggest that while the coach may be a partner or friend, retaining a professional coach may be the most productive arrangement. The interaction between the coach and the adult with ADHD may be face-to-face meetings, phone calls, faxes, or e-mails, and in this relationship the coach acts as a kind of "neurocognitive prosthetic device" (p. 586). As such, the coach assists the individual to compensate for deficiencies in his or her executive functions that impede the ability to plan, organize, and monitor behavior.

Coleman and Sussman (Unpublished manuscript) suggest that a comprehensive approach towards coaching individuals with ADHD can be summarized in four words: structure, support, skills, and strategies. Structure is operationalized as (1) clearly defined vision, goals and values that are clarified in the early phases of coaching; (2) systems for managing daily life (e.g., shopping, bill paying, handling mail); (3) a time management system that enables the individual to identify priorities, break them into manageable steps, and schedule them into a calendar; (4) a single action taken every day to reinforce a sense of accomplishment; and (6) daily habits that are small, constructive actions done on a routine basis.

Support is provided through a variety of means. In this regard the coach serves a variety of roles that include witness, empathizer, provider of feedback, and a personal advocate, among others.   Hallowell (1995) organizes these functions with the acronym H-O-P-E (Help, Obligations, Plans, Encouragement). Skill building focuses on consistency of application most generally in the areas of time management, goal setting, setting boundaries, and dealing with transitions. Strategies are those creative and highly individualized tools developed in partnership to deal with every day life management tasks and for achieving personal goals. Hallowell would liken these strategies to external structure such as lists, notes to self, color coding, rituals, reminders, files, and choosing healthy addictions, O.H.I.O. (with paperwork, only handle it once). He offers "50 Tips on the Management of Adult Attention Deficit Disorder" (p. 157). These are a series of directive suggestions/ behavioral prescriptions that can be given to patients to help them in their day-to-day lives, and that he hands out to his patients at the beginning of treatment.

Two other strategies that Coleman and Sussman (Unpublished manuscript) suggest are visualization and verbalization. Mind mapping is particularly useful for students who tend to get overwhelmed because they see the whole picture but cannot pick out the details. The technique can be used also with detail-intensive texts where the student is trying to put a complex of ideas into order or into perspective. The software, *Inspiration*, can be useful to the college or university student who experiences a mental block when faced with a writing project because there is no way to express or contain the flood of ideas that are present simultaneously in their brains. Visualization can also be used to deal with time, for example. Here the mental image involves size and shape vs. a linear construct.

Verbalization is a means for individuals to "down load" extraneous thoughts so that they can focus on the task at hand. The coach sets aside a specified amount of time either by phone or in person during which the individual can verbalize the myriad of thoughts and ideas, which are racing unproductively and getting in the way of directed performance. Peterson (Unpublished manuscript) suggests that students write down their creative ideas or distracting thoughts at the point at which they occur rather than allowing them intrude when a significant amount of attention to task is required. Peterson calls this creating a home for thoughts, a parking lot of sorts. Use of this strategy may enable the individual to gain more control over his or her creative ideas while at the same time modifying the dysfunctional nature of impulsivity and/or obsessive ruminations.

Finally, there is a program known as "Work Flow Coaching" based on the model developed by David Allen & Co. (www.davidco.com) that is applicable to persons with ADHD in the work place. In the words of Allen, "Our trainers and coaches deliver well-defined and proven methods that help individuals manage the intensity and volume of 'knowledge work'—a meta-skill set encompassing time and project stress management, team building, and communication issues" (www.davidco.com). The program was developed for implementation in the individual's physical work environment with subsequent telephone reinforcements. Phase one of the program, Installation Intensive, is done in two consecutive days, on site at the individual's place of work followed up with a telecoaching session one to two weeks afterward. The second phase, Building Consistency Telecoaching Program, consists of telephone calls over an extended period of time, usually structured as four end-of-week one-hour private telephone sessions scheduled at the individual's convenience.

THE WORKPLACE AND REASONABLE ACCOMMODATIONS

Developmental Issues

Although anecdotal and clinical reports are available that may be useful in understanding the employment issues faced by individuals with ADHD (Weiss, 1992; 1994; Hallowell and Ratey, 1994; Latham and Latham, 1994; Kelly and Ramundo, 1995; Levine, 1995; Nadeau, 1995), there is no empirical documentation to support the use of any particular strategy (Carroll and Ponterotto, 1998). Thus, we are left with relying on the clinical experiences of these individuals for the most part. Further, Nadeau (1995) writes that career counseling with adults who have ADHD is a complex process that requires knowledge of career issues, neurodevelopmental issues as they affect workplace performance, psychological disorders that may be related to ADHD, and personality factors that interact with attentional difficulties. "There is no single course of training that can provide this level of expertise in such a broad range of disciplines" (p.326).

Moore (1997) writes that making the transition from student to worker is a difficult process for most individuals, but the individual with ADHD may face some significant obstacles from the start. In addition to possible issues surrounding emotional maturity, the tendency toward impulsive responding may be problematic from the perspectives of both interpersonal relationships (e.g., impulsive comments that interrupt coworkers or meetings) and overcommitments, taking on projects that cannot be handled successfully by one person. In addition, the "flush of enthusiasm" (p. 3) often gives way to boredom when the task requires follow-through and attention to details that are perceived to be tedious. Other obstacles involve frustrations by coworkers on account of the problems with clutter, confusion, lack of time management, and idiosyncratic "piling systems" that person with ADHD often evidence. Lastly, according to Moore, the most difficult job relationship for many to handle may be the crucial connection between the employee and the supervisor, because of the tendency to display independent attitudes vs. a teamwork approach, chafing at traditional procedures and rules, and a distaste for authority figures. She then goes on to write about the work of Brainworks in Carrollton, Texas, where both individual and common problems for individuals with ADHD in the workplace and in their personal relationships are the focus of treatment.

In an effort to assist school counselors with decisions regarding postsecondary preparation or direct job placement, Levine (1995) investigated "ADHD-friendly" occupations using three criteria: 1) does a given occupation facilitate autonomy; 2) does it provide for active engagement and movement rather than staying in one place all day; and 3) does it provide a variety of duties, that allow creative contributions in some form. She investigated 30 job areas including computer technology, consulting, engineering, education, nursing, technical, legal, medical, managerial, laborer, construction, and scientific. As an example in the technical area, some of the representative jobs that allowed for autonomy, variety, and multiple settings were those involving biomedical equipment technician, sound effects technician, field engineer, and electronics mechanic. Interestingly, in the area of law, while the nature of the work of trial attorneys and litigators was judged to be "ADHD-friendly," insurance or corporate law, requiring constant attention to detail, made it an "ADHD-unfriendly" occupation. Her work has been cited by several authors working in the area of employment counseling (Carroll and Ponterotto, 1998; Schwiebert, Sealander, and Bradshaw, 1998).

Reasonable Accommodations and Personal Accommodations

In her chapter on *ADD in the Workplace* Nadeau (1995) provides a list of reasonable accommodations to be provided by employers of adults with ADHD, which were gleaned from a variety of sources. Among these are suggestions for the provision of a nondistracting work space, flextime, more structure and immediate deadlines, assistance with a filing system, and the use of memos and e-mail in addition to verbal directions. In one of the few studies investigating accommodations that have proven useful for adults with ADHD in the workplace, the Job Accommodation Network (JAN), a service of the President's Committee on Employment of People with Disabilities, conducted a follow up survey of accommodation outcomes (Means, Stewart, and Dowler, 1997). Respondents to the survey were from 25 states, the District of Columbia, and one Canadian province, and included employers, persons with disabilities, and others (rehabilitation professionals, parents). ADD was reported as the only disability in 41% of the 61 participants. The accommodations were categorized as environmental changes, policy changes, assistive devices, training/retraining, or medical. In contrast to the ADD/LD group, those in the ADD only group were more likely to incorporate assistive devices and environmental changes as a means of accommodation and twice as likely to self-accommodate. The authors commented that environmental changes that reduce or eliminate distractions aid in task organization, and while these are low cost or no cost, they can dramatically impact a worker's performance.

Nadeau (1995) also lists numerous practical and direct symptom management techniques and strategies that the adult with ADHD might employ in the workplace. These strategies are clustered around problems with hyperactivity/motor restlessness, distractibility, organization, time management, procrastination, interpersonal conflicts on the job, prioritization, and memory. The recommendations offered would be highly beneficial for any clinician, coach, or educator to share with adults entering or already in the workplace, both young and older, who are diagnosed with ADHD. Their relevance is even more critical given the results from the JAN study (Means, Stewart, and Dowler, 1997), that found individuals with ADHD more likely to self-accommodate than workers with learning disabilities or psychiatric disorders.

FOLLOW-UP AND OUTCOME STUDIES

Limitations

In reviewing nearly all follow-up and outcome studies involving adults with ADHD, certain methodological concerns must be taken into account that suggest that interpretations drawn from these studies must be narrowly defined. First and foremost, nearly every major study (Hechtman, Weiss, Perlman, Hopkins, and Wener, 1981; Weiss, Hechtman, Milroy, and Perlman, 1985; Mannuzza, Klein, Bessler, 1993; 1998; Hansen, Weiss, and Last, 1999) has involved males who were diagnosed as children and in DSM-IV terminology would meet criteria for ADHD, Hyperactive/Impulsive Type. Data that address outcomes in ADHD, Inattentive Type with adults are largely nonexistent (Schwean, 1999). Second, the samples were all clinically drawn and thus, by their very nature, reflect concern for behaviors that were judged to be highly indicative of pathology in the first place, often times conduct disorder. And third, the loss of one-third of the sample in the 15 year follow-up study reported by Weiss *et al.* (1985) gives reason for pause in terms of generalization of results, although the researchers speculated that those subjects lost might have represented a worst outcome subgroup, coloring to some degree their outcome findings. They concluded, however, that "There was evidence that the hyperactives had more overall psychopathology and functioned generally less well than did normal controls" (p.211).

Results reported by Biederman, Wilens, Mick, et al. (1995), Mannuzza et al (1998), and Hansen, Weiss, and Last (1999) concur, suggesting that children with ADHD are at significantly higher risk for a specific negative course marked by antisocial and substance-related disorders, are more likely to have dropped out of high school, and more likely than controls to report problems in psychological functioning. Again, the samples were drawn primarily from Caucasian (The Mannuzza study in particular, as the others do not specify race.)

males diagnosed as children as hyperactive. Findings were similar in the study reported by Barkley, Murphy, and Kwasnik (1996), although their sample contained both males and females. Adults with ADHD were found to have shorter durations of employment in their full time jobs than adults in the control group, as well as greater psychological distress and maladjustment on all scales of the SCL-90-R. They also reported committing more antisocial acts, particularly involving thefts and disorderly conduct.

While studies exploring the mental health of parents of children with ADHD report a higher prevalence of mental disorder as well as ADHD (Biederman, Faraone, Keenan, Knee, and Tsuang, 1990; Biederman, Faraone, Keenan, et al., 1992; Biederman, Farone, Spencer et al, 1993), much research underscores the protective role that families play in successful adjustment of children and adults. In a recent study by Gardiner and Schwean (1998), one of the most powerful protective factors associated with resilient adults with ADHD was the family. "Those adults who grew up in families who were warm and affectionate and where there were clear and fair parameters for behavior expressed significantly greater happiness and satisfaction with their lives as adults" (p. 601). In addition, greater life satisfaction was expressed by those adults who had a strong, close relationship with at least one grandparent as they were growing up.

Finally, in the few studies that look at college students, with a childhood history of ADHD (Dooling-Litfin and Rosen, 1997), self-esteem was positively correlated with greater social skills and negatively correlated with current symptoms. On the other hand, achievement/talent, having had a mentor or special person, and treatment history were not associated with self-esteem in college students with an ADHD history.

Hechtman (1989) summarized the then available literature on the adult adjustment of children previously diagnosed with ADHD and identified three possible outcomes: Adults who function fairly normally compared to matched controls; adults who continue to have significant difficulties with work, interpersonal relations, poor self-esteem, irritability, impulsivity, anxiety, and emotional lability to varying degrees; and adults who have significant psychiatric and antisocial pathology. Given the nature of the study samples previously discussed, one is struck that two out of the three possible outcomes are relatively positive. Outcome three more than likely represents individuals having comorbid psychiatric disorders as has been well documented in the literature reviewed. In addition, 50% of the time ADHD symptoms do not continue into adulthood, requiring no particular treatment or intervention. Aggregate findings would suggest, finally, that particular adult outcomes are not associated with any one specific or initial variable but with the additive interaction of personality characteristics and social and familial parameters (Schwean, 1999).

SUMMARY

Throughout this chapter we have made an effort to highlight the many problems associated with the diagnosis of adults with ADHD as well as the presentation and ramification of the disorder in their lives, with a particular focus on young adults in postsecondary educational settings. In addition, we have reviewed a number of significant studies in the fields of genetics, neurobiology, neurochemistry, and neuropsychology in an attempt to capture data that are relevant to our understanding of ADHD in an adult population. Strategies including pharmacotherapy, psychosocial interventions, and current intervention practices have been detailed, again with a focus on adults, recognizing that much of the knowledge is based on clinical rather than empirical validation. [In light of the existing limitations on research involving adults and the outcome studies currently in the literature, in the future, we will be most anxious to see research that includes both men and women, differentiates between Inattentive, Hyperactive/Impulsive, and Combined Types in the subjects drawn for study, begins to address the subtypes suggested by Amen and others for purposes of treatment interventions. Investigations of treatment strategies such as coaching, support groups, and directive psychotherapy as they may impact on the lives of adults with ADHD, whether diagnosed as children or adults will be critical as well].

5

HIGH FUNCTIONING AUTISM

INTRODUCTION

Autism is a developmental mental disorder that we usually associate with childhood. We hear the phrase "autistic children" so commonly that it is easy to forget that autism is a life-span illness that begins in early childhood, but is an incurable disease that persists throughout life. Autism is also a disorder with extremely varying severity. Some individuals with the disorder are mute and severely retarded, while others have fluent speech and levels of intellectual function that may range to superior. The research evidence clearly supports the view that it is all the same disorder in which intellectual level will vary substantially. As a widely accepted convention, first suggested by Michael Rutter, IQ is considered to be a reasonable index of the severity of autism (Rutter and Schopler, 1987). An IQ of 70 has usually been adopted as the cut-off point separating high functioning from low functioning autism.

In this chapter, we will only discuss high functioning autism for several reasons. Since the book is about learning disabilities, individuals with IQs in the retarded range would typically not have learning disabilities as they are currently diagnosed, and it is more likely that any academic difficulties they may have are more likely to be attributable to mental retardation than to a specific learning disability. There is also the practical matter that low-functioning individuals with autism are generally not good candidates for the psychometric and neuropsychological testing that provide the basis for much of the learning disability literature. It is now widely accepted that the information gained from such assessments is pertinent to the entire ability spectrum of autism, but is only obtainable from higher functioning individuals. In high functioning individuals, it is also possible to separate what is attributable to the autism from the frequently confounding influences of mental retardation. Finally, autistic individuals with mental retardation frequently have other disorders as well, and their influences would have to be determined in each case. Higher functioning individuals often find their ways into regular schools and special education classes, but that is rarely the case for lower-functioning individuals. When these high functioning individuals enter school, they typically demonstrate forms of learning disorder that appear to be relatively unique, and are, in any event, quite different from what characterizes dyslexia and other academic skill disorders.

DIAGNOSIS

In contemporary practice, autism is diagnosed quite precisely. There are other disorders that share some of the features of autism, and there are autism-like syndromes associated with identifiable diseases, but these conditions are currently not diagnosed as autism. Some of the diseases that can produce autistic like syndromes are Fragile-X syndrome, tuberous sclerosis, and other genetic and infectious disorders. One also encounters the term "autistic behaviors" or behaviors that characterize autism without the full syndrome being present, as in the DSM IV diagnosis of Pervasive Developmental Disorder Not Otherwise Specified (APA, 1994). The DSM system classifies autism as a pervasive developmental disorder within a category of diagnoses described as "Disorders Usually First Diagnosed in Infancy, Childhood, or Adolescence." These disorders are associated with deficits in multiple areas of development, and typically involve impairment in social relations, communication, and range of interests and activities. DSM-IV diagnostic criteria for Autistic Disorder are divided into three sections, the first of which includes behaviors that characterize the disorder with regard to impairment in social interaction, communication, and the presence of restrictive, repetitive, and stereotyped patterns of interest. Examples of impaired social relations would be failure to develop peer relationships appropriate to developmental level and lack of social or emotional reciprocity. Communication deficits are manifested as impairment of language development, lack of ability to sustain a conversation, stereotyped or idiosyncratic language, and lack of spontaneous or imitative play. There may be an encompassing preoccupation with stereotyped and restricted patterns of interest, inflexible adherence to routines and rituals, stereotyped, repetitive movements, or persistent preoccupation with parts of objects. The second section of the criteria requires delays in social, language, or play development with onset before age 3 years. Finally, the disturbance cannot be better described as one of the other pervasive disorders.

The criteria are somewhat child-oriented, but they appear to work well with adults. They do so because the diagnosis is of necessity based in part on an adequate developmental history and cannot be made from current clinical phenomenology. For that reason, a structured diagnostic interview has been developed for autism, the Autism Diagnostic Interview (ADI) (LeCouteur *et al.*, 1989; Lord, Rutter and LeCouteur, 1994). It is administered to a parent or caregiver who has knowledge of the individual's early history. It is particularly important to document the existence of a developmental delay before age 3 years, because the diagnosis cannot be made without such evidence. Administration of the ADI is often accompanied by use of the Autism Diagnostic Observation Schedule (ADOS) (Lord, Rutter, and Goode, 1989), a structured role-playing procedure that allows for direct observation of the patient. The ADI and ADOS were designed to facilitate making of a reliable DSM diagnosis.

HIGH FUNCTIONING AUTISM

The group of older children or adults with high functioning autism constitutes about 20 - 25% of the cases. The remaining cases have varying degrees of mental retardation or are mute. The conclusion reached by most experts is that autism is the same disorder regardless of level of intelligence and communicative ability. These latter factors are indicators of severity, and do not define the disorder itself. Autism is thought to be present if DSM-IV criteria are met, and if further clinical and laboratory examination does not rule it out.

The high functioning individuals, despite the early developmental delays, go on to develop adequate language and often enter special education programs or regular schools. As noted earlier, they often have academic difficulties, but they are quite different from the learning problems typically experienced by children with dyslexia or other forms of academic skill disorder. For this reason, special attention needs to be paid to the educational needs of children with autism, since the more traditional remedial methods do not appear to be applicable (Siegel, Goldstein, and Minshew, 1996). We will elaborate on this point extensively as we proceed. These differences appear not to be directly related to the social skill impairment or clinical phenomenology of the autism, but to major differences in cognitive function among autism, the specific academic skill disorders, and normal function. Indeed, some authorities hold the view that the clinical phenomenology of autism is founded in the way in which individuals with autism think. There is a very large literature on cognitive function in autism that we will briefly summarize before dealing more directly with the matter of learning disability.

COGNITIVE FUNCTION IN AUTISM

The core cognitive deficit in autism has been sought for many years, and there is no consensus in the field at present. Domains of function implicated have included attention, memory, language, conceptual reasoning, and executive function. More specifically, impairments of working memory and selective attention have been viewed as areas of particular involvement. Autism has been characterized in terms of comprehensive conceptualizations describing it as a disorder of memory, executive function, or complex information processing. While the neurobiology of autism is essentially unknown, these theoretical formulations have suggested various localizations of the disorder including the temporal-limbic system, the frontal lobes, the amygdala, and the cerebellum. A wealth of formal experiments comparing individuals with autism with appropriate control and comparison groups has been accomplished in efforts to document these theories. Early work in this area is difficult to interpret because of the lack of agreed upon diagnostic criteria, but since the appearance of DSM-III, the diagnostic problem has been largely resolved.

We will briefly review the general theories of cognitive function in autism, and attempt to make an evaluation and synthesis. Originally, autism was thought by Kanner and his co-workers (Kanner, 1943; Kanner, 1977; Kanner, Rodriguez, and Ashenden, 1972) to be an environmentally acquired disorder produced by obsessive, distant parents; so-called "refrigerator parents." Since these early observations, it has become increasingly apparent that autism is a neurodevelopmental disorder, and that while Kanner's description of its phenomenology was quite astute, his assumptions about its cause were essentially incorrect. Most modern theories of autism are variants of the general concept of a neurodevelopmental disorder, although the neuropathology is not yet understood. There is also a, at least implicit, widely held view that autism is fundamentally a cognitive disorder, despite the fact that the clinical phenomenology most apparently involves social function and communicative behavior. It could be said that autism is now thought to be a neuropsychological disorder, and a great deal of the research done in recent years involves experimental neuropsychology. There have been numerous studies of the major domains of neuropsychological function, which include attention, memory, language, spatial abilities, perceptual and motor skills, and conceptual abilities or executive function.

Memory

Historically, the memory theory was the first of the neurocognitive theories extensively considered. Some time ago, we had the so-called "amnesic theory" of autism that asserted that memory is a cardinal deficit in autism, particularly since post-mortem studies have identified abnormalities in the hippocampus

(Bauman and Kemper, 1985), and animal model studies have proposed a resemblance between autistic behavior and that observed in monkeys with medial temporal structure ablations (Bachevalier, 1991). Boucher and Warrington (1976) found resemblances between the pattern of memory found in individuals with autism and those with amnesic disorders. These resemblances were impaired free recall, a reduced primacy effect with a normal recency effect on list learning, and improvement with external cuing but not through use of internally produced cues. That is, they shared the pattern of intact and impaired memory function found among individuals with an amnesic syndrome. Numerous studies confirmed the existence of a reduced primacy effect, and the apparent lack of ability of individuals with autism to produce internal cues that aided new learning. Subsequent studies supported the view that failure to produce organizational strategies was the key to the memory difficulty in autism, and further, when demands on such cuing was minimal, as in the cases of simple associative learning or short-term memory, the memory of individuals with autism was as good as that of appropriate normal controls.

To confirm this view a study of memory involving a detailed investigation of the California Verbal Learning Test was done by Minshew and Goldstein (1993). Comparing high functioning subjects with autism with matched controls. They looked for differences on the many scores that can be derived from this procedure. Very few significant differences were found. Of the 33 measures compared, significant differences were obtained for number correct on Trial 5 for List A, List A Total Intrusions, List B - Number Correct, Semantic-Cluster Ratio and Global Cluster Ratio, and List A Short Delay - Total Intrusions. The major findings therefore were that the subjects with autism produced more intrusions than controls, and they did less semantic clustering than controls. They were also more susceptible than controls to proactive interference. We should add the cautionary note that when a Bonferroni correction for multiple comparisons was made, all significant differences disappeared. An additional analysis determined for each measure whether the mean score for the autistic sample was better, worse, or tied with the control sample. Of the 33 scores, there were only 3 on which the subjects with autism did better than the controls. Using a sign test, it was determined that this result far exceeded chance. It was also found that the learning curves for the 5 A List trials had similar shapes in both groups, but the score was lower for each of the trials in the case of the autism group. It was concluded that memory in autism is less efficient than normal as indicated by analysis of the direction of the differences between autistics and controls.

In subsequent research in the area of memory, differences from controls were found on delayed recall tasks but not on associative memory tasks (Minshew, Goldstein, and Siegel, 1997). Increasing difficulty with memory as task complexity increased was also found in autism. For example, on a stylus maze task, the impairment of a sample of individuals with autism relative to controls significantly increased as the number of elements in the stimulus increased. Furthermore, while it was originally thought that nonverbal memory was relatively spared in autism, more recent evidence suggests that task complexity is the crucial element rather than stimulus modality. Of particular interest to the area of education is a study by Boucher (1981) in which it was shown that individuals with high functioning autism remembered less about activities they recently engaged in than did controls. In summary, while memory difficulties are typically present, high functioning autism is not an amnesic syndrome. That is, while individuals with high functioning autism are not severely forgetful or disoriented, they do have difficulties in learning and retaining new information that has important implications for education.

Deficits of Attention

Attention dysfunction also has a long history in the study of autism. It became a matter of particular interest when attentional difficulties were associated with recent findings concerning abnormalities in the cerebellum of at least some individuals with autism (Courchesne *et al.*, 1995). Numerous models of attentional dysfunction have emerged in the autism literature and may be divided into those proposing that the origin of the dysfunction is at the sensory-perceptual level and those supporting the view that the dysfunction is at the conceptual level (Burack, Enns, and Johannes, 1997). More recent theories have generally taken the latter view. Early models generally understood attention deficit in autism to exist at the sensory-perceptual level. For example, one theory attempted to explain the propensity to engage in repetitive, stereotypical movements, respond in an atypical manner to the environment, and the failure to develop socially, as a deficit in the modulation of arousal (Dawson and Levy, 1989; Hutt, Hutt, Lee, and Ounsted, 1964; Ornitz and Ritvo, 1968). Another early but still widely cited attentional model attributed the autistic individuals' intense focus on detail and failure to interpret multiple social cues in the environment to overselective attention (Lovaas, Koegel, and Schriebman, 1979; Pierce, Glad, Schriebman, 1997). Rincover and Ducharme (1987) contended this overselectivity of attention was due to "tunnel vision" or an overly selective attentional gaze.

In contrast, other studies have explored the possibility of deficits in the ability to filter out irrelevant stimuli in autism (Bryson, Wainwright, and Smith, 1990; Burack, 1994). Deficits in reflexive orienting have also been reported in individuals with autism (Casey, Gordon, Mannheim, and Rumsey, 1993). Many of these theories were later disconfirmed or reformulated, although there are limited data to suggest that individuals with autism are slower in processing the demand characteristics of more complex tasks (Burack and Iarocci, 1995; Wainwright and Bryson, 1996; Wainwright-Sharp and Bryson, 1993).

Another much researched attentional model hypothesized that the lack of interest in people was due to an inability to direct attention to extrapersonal space or from one stimulus to the next (Ornitz, 1988; Townsend and Courchesne, 1994). This proposed deficit in the ability to direct attention to extrapersonal space has been implicated as a core symptom underlying the clinical manifestations of autism (Ornitz, 1988; Townsend and Courchesne, 1994). The dysfunction in directing attention to extrapersonal space was attributed to parietal lobe dysfunction. Courchesne and colleagues have also hypothesized that individuals with autism are deficient in the ability to shift their attention between modalities and to disengage their attention (Courchesne et al., 1994). Support for this hypothesis was derived from modality shift and reaction time tasks (Courchesne et al., 1993; Courchesne, Akshoomoff, Townsend, and Saitoh, 1995; Courchesne et al., 1994), and was attributed to cerebellar abnormalities by Akshoomoff and Courchesne, (1992). As these investigators put it, the difficulty is in rapidly and accurately moving the "spotlight of attention." Taken together, the above models and investigations imply that the attention problem in autism is a perceptual one.

Difficulty in shifting attention has also been extensively explored with cognitive measures, notably the Wisconsin Card Sorting Test (WCST) (Ozonoff, 1995a, Ozonoff, Pennington, and Rogers, 1991; Prior and Hoffmann, 1990). These studies concluded that the difficulty in shifting of attention was the result of a primary deficit in executive function in autism. Numerous investigations have eventuated in a well-developed model proposing that individuals with autism perform poorly on tasks that involve executive function, such as joint attention, inhibition of responses, difficulty shifting cognitive sets, and working memory tasks (Hughes and Russell, 1993; McEvoy, Rogers, and Pennington, 1993; Ozonoff, Pennington, and Rogers, 1991; Ozonoff Strayer, McMahon, and Filloux; 1994; Pennington, Rogers, Bennetto, et al, in press). Yet another recent model described attention deficits in autism as associated with an inability to coordinate and modulate attentional resources, and not a deficit in shifting attention (Pascualvaca, Fantie, Papageoriou, and Mirsky, 1998).

In summary, apparent behavioral deficits in autism have been attributed to varying components of the general theoretical construct of attention. Theoretical models generated from extensive research efforts have differed in their views of whether attentional problems in autism are at the perceptual, reflexive, conceptual, or executive control level. Strong evidence has been generated from more recent, well-controlled studies to indicate abnormalities in attention in autism are related to the information processing aspects of tasks and the voluntary or executive control of attention, and not to deficits in reflexive, orienting abilities (Burack, Enns and Johannes, 1997).

In order to provide a comprehensive assessment of attention and to clearly define the components of attention evaluated, an empirically derived four factor neuropsychological model was applied (Mirsky, Anthony, Duncan, et al.,

1991). This model was based upon a series of distinctions among types of attention originally formulated by Zubin (1975). In this model, attention is divided into the ability to 1) focus on a target object and perform a task in the presence of distracting objects, 2) maintain vigilance over a sustained time period, 3) adaptively shift focus of attention, and 4) efficiently receive and interpret incoming information. The factors derived from this model were termed focus-execute, sustain, shift, and encode. The model was applied in the Mirsky *et al.*, study in order to clarify what components of attention might be intact and impaired in autism.

In many tests of attention, speed of performance is used as the response measure. Such tests load in the Mirsky group factor analysis on the Focus-Execute factor. Indeed Mirsky *et al.*, (1991) characterized that factor as reflecting perceptual-motor speed. It has been well established that individuals with autism commonly have psychomotor deficits in the form of slowness, awkwardness, or poor coordination (Bauman, 1992; Gillberg and Coleman, 1992; Hughes, 1996, Smith and Bryson, 1994; Rapin, 1997). Thus, the direct interpretation of tests involving speed scores as measures of attention is confounded in autism by psychomotor impairment, and it is necessary to account for the influence of that impairment on performance outcome.

This comprehensive analysis of attentional functioning in individuals with carefully diagnosed high functioning autism demonstrated that the major dysfunctions relative to normal controls are on those measures of attention that utilize psychomotor speed, as opposed to accuracy or span of apprehension, as a dependent measure, or that require cognitive flexibility. That is, differences were noted only on the Focus-Execute and Shift factors of the Mirsky group model, and not the Vigilance and Encode factors. Correspondingly, the Mirsky group was unable to confirm the view that individuals with autism have difficulties in encoding information and sustaining attention over time. This finding is well supported by other studies in which subjects with autism performed normally at repeating digits and calculating (Minshew, Goldstein, Muenz, and Payton, 1992; Minshew, Goldstein, and Siegel, 1997). The sustained attention or vigilance data indicate that when a challenging attentional task does not have a conceptual or psychomotor component, the autism group does not differ from controls.

The data would suggest that in the case of autism, unequivocal evaluation of attention cannot be accomplished using dependent measures based on speed of movement. We would offer the proposal that significant differences between individuals with autism and controls may be found on experimental measures of attention that actually assess such processes as conceptual reasoning, executive function, rapid decision making, problem solving, and working memory; abilities that are widely believed to be impaired in autism (McEvoy, Rogers, and Pennington, 1993; Minshew, Goldstein, and Siegel, 1997; Ozonoff, 1995b; Ozonoff *et al.*, 1994, Ozonoff, Pennington, and Rogers, 1991). With regard to the Mirsky model shift factor, there is evidence from other research indicating that individuals with autism do not have difficulty with elementary perceptual shift tasks, but do have difficulty when shifting must be accomplished at a conceptual level. In a study of saccadic eye movements, subjects with autism performed normally on visually guided saccade tasks involving shifting of focus of attention. However, they performed abnormally on a volitional saccade task in which the eyes must accurately move to the point at which the target stimulus was previously present, but had disappeared. This latter task has a substantial working memory component (Minshew, Luna, and Sweeney, 1999). Furthermore, numerous other studies involving the WCST have produced equivocal results, with several reports of normal functioning by autism samples on several of the measures derived from this test (Minshew, Goldstein, and Siegel, 1997, Ozonoff, 1995a). In the Mirsky group study, the autism group did not differ from controls on a relatively simple perceptual shifting task, but made significantly more perseverative errors on the WCST than controls. The Mirsky group's subjects averaged 9 years of age, and had a mean WISC-III Full-scale IQ score of 78. The group studied by Minshew *et al.*, (1992) with the WCST averaged 21 years of age, and had a mean WAIS-R Full Scale IQ score of 96. This group of individuals with autism made considerably fewer perseverative errors on the WCST (M = 18.3) than the Mirsky group's autism sample (M = 60.7) Considering the literature as a whole, including these results, differences in various scores from the WCST between individuals with autism and normal controls may be a matter of the presence of autism in combination with developmental considerations and general ability level. Thus, evidence for impaired shifting of attention in autism appears to be associated with working memory and other aspects of complex information processing, and not with perceptual shifting of focus of the type that may be mediated by cerebellar function. Furthermore, this deficit, at least when measured by such procedures as the WCST, may not appear in higher functioning individuals with autism. These findings make it appear likely that the well established cognitive deficits and their associated abnormal behaviors associated with autism are not the result of a failure to incorporate information, or to sustain concentration, or to resist distraction. Such considerations as working memory, the ability to organize information, and the capacity to monitor ongoing events and make rapid adjustments are likely to be relevant considerations.

Language and Communication Skills

Language and communication in autism have been extensively studied. The high functioning individual with autism who is not mute or retarded may nevertheless have significant language problems, some of which involve academic skills. Studies of academic abilities in autism were originally stimulated by reports of autistic-savants who did remarkably well at calculation or related specific skills, and by a literature suggesting that high functioning individuals with autism may master the mechanical aspects of reading, but may not comprehend affective, metaphorical, or inferential aspects of text. Their reading is sometimes characterized as hyperlexic, connoting excellent command of phonetics, but limited comprehension of what is read. Much of the language research in autism contrasts procedural and mechanical academic skills with skills requiring comprehension and interpretation. Three test batteries that allow for such comparisons are the Revised Woodcock Reading Mastery Tests (Woodcock, 1987), the Kaufman Test of Educational Achievement (Kaufman and Kaufman, 1985), and portions of the Detroit Tests of Learning Aptitude (Hammill, 1985). In a series of studies (Goldstein, Minshew, and Siegel, 1994; Minshew, Siegel, Goldstein, and Weldy, 1994) it was found that, comparing high functioning subjects with autism with well-matched controls on these batteries, the autism group did not differ from controls on mechanical tasks such as those assessing spelling ability or phonetic analysis, but did differ on the Passage Comprehension subtest of the Woodcock Reading Mastery Test and the Reading Comprehension subtest of the Kaufman Test of Educational Achievement.   Thus, individuals with autism are not dyslexic, nor do they exhibit the academic deficits found in individuals with verbal learning disability. The difficulty appears to be at the level of comprehension and interpretation. A surprising finding occurred in the case of the Detroit Tests.   Significant differences were found for the Oral Directions, Word Sequences, and Letter Sequences subtests, with Oral Directions producing the greatest difference. These tests do not require judgment or inference making, but the sequence strings are relatively long and complex, and therefore may have required formation of organizing strategies to promote accurate recall.   We have considered the possibility that a specific deficit in working memory is involved here.

While DSM-IV does not specifically require delay in language development to make the diagnosis of autism, in neuropsychological assessment it is desirable to require it to make a specific diagnosis in order to avoid inclusion of individuals with Asperger's disorder. To diagnose Asperger's disorder, which has many resemblances to autism, there must be no clinically significant delay in language development. Therefore, language development may be a crucial consideration in differential diagnosis and possible associated neurobiological differences among developmental disorders.

In an autism vs. control developmental study of a series of psychoeducational tests (Goldstein, Minshew, and Siegel, 1994) subjects were divided into age groups ranging from less than 8 to over 18. A cross-sectional analysis was accomplished. Two tests were of particular interest, one assessing a procedural skill and the other an interpretive skill. The Word Attack (procedural skill) and the Passage Comprehension (interpretive skill) subtests from the Revised Woodcock Reading Mastery Test with age adjusted standard scores were used as the measures. On Word Attack, the subjects with autism were actually a little better than the controls, and this relationship persisted into the 18 years and older group. The picture for Passage Comprehension was quite different. The younger subjects with autism did better than or as well as controls up until the 10-11 year old group, after which the controls did consistently better, and dramatically so in the 18 and older group. It would therefore appear that individuals with high functioning autism might keep up with their peers indefinitely with regard to mechanical or procedural linguistic tasks, but lose ground as the cognitive demands of tasks increase as appropriate for normal language development.

Upon combining formal language and psychoeducational tests in studies of autism there appears to be a consistent pattern of absence of significant differences on the simple tests including measures of verbal fluency, phonetic analysis, word knowledge, and calculation, as contrasted with significant differences on measures of language comprehension, pragmatic language, and comprehension of complex grammatical structures. The role of working memory may be important in conceptualizing these results, but the deficits noted on several of the complex tests suggested a more pervasive impairment of language comprehension than could be explained solely on the basis of a deficit in working memory.

Abstract Reasoning and Problem Solving

Going on to abstract reasoning and problem solving, many autism scholars were clearly struck by the failure to obtain significant differences between subjects with autism and controls on the "gold standard" measures; the WCST, the Halstead Category Test, and Part B of the Trail Making Test. Minshew, Goldstein, Muenz, and Payton (1992) made the observation that subjects with autism failed to shift from one basis of sorting to another on the Goldstein-Scheerer Object Sorting Test, often remarking that the way they placed the objects was the way they belonged or there was no way of sorting them differently. We therefore felt that they had identified a deficit in cognitive flexibility that was not sufficiently challenged by the WCST. A method used in a later study (Minshew, Siegel, Goldstein, and Weldy, 1994) was a Twenty Questions procedure used some time ago by Nelson Butters (Laine and Butters, 1982) to study problem solving in chronic alcoholic patients, and by Mosher and Ornsby (1966) to study the cognitive development of children. The results were quite striking. The subjects with autism did exceptionally poorly on this task. The important variable was the constraint seeking score that indicates the percentage of times the subject asks a question that constrains the number of possibly correct answers. This is the classic "Is it animal, mineral or vegetable?" question. Rather than ask such questions, the participants with autism were more inclined to ask hypothesis-scanning questions, which amounts to guessing.

Thus, if one divides abstraction, as the literature suggests, into rule learning, attribute identification, and hypothesis testing or true concept formation rather than identification, then subjects with autism in the non-retarded range appear to have their major difficulty in the hypothesis-testing component. Another way of putting it is that they can identify concepts, but have difficulty in forming them.

A Summary of Cognitive Findings

It appears that individuals with high functioning autism have cognitive deficits in various domains at the complex, but not at the simple skill level. That conclusion applies to memory, attention, language, and abstraction and problem-solving domains. Recent investigations suggest there does not appear to be modality specificity. That is, vision or hearing is not specifically involved in the cognitive function of individuals with autism. However, visuospatial abilities appear to remain intact, for unknown reasons, and individuals with autism may do exceptionally well on spatial and constructional tasks that do not use social stimuli.

In order to suggest that this cognitive profile has some biological significance, we can briefly mention a portion of a study in which cognitive test results were correlated with Phosphorous Magnetic Resonance Spectroscopy (MRS) data (Minshew, Rogers, and Pennington, 1993). We will only comment on the correlational data for phosphomonoesters (PME) and phosphodiesters (PDE), both of which reflect phospholipid metabolism. The conclusion reached was that phospholipid findings in autism reflect under synthesis and enhanced degradation of brain membranes. There were very robust correlations between cognitive test scores and PME and PDE levels. PDE goes up and PME goes down as scores get worse. These high correlations were not seen in the normal controls, nor were they seen in the subjects with autism for such basic skill tasks as the Reading Decoding and Spelling subtests of the Kaufman Test of Educational Achievement. Correlations with low information processing load tasks of this type were non-significant in both autism and control groups. While this study was very preliminary, there is nevertheless the suggestion that there is an association between cognitive function and metabolic energy state of phospholipids involved in high functioning autism.

Based on these results and a review of the now extensive literature on high functioning autism, we would like to propose the following conclusions.
1. Autism represents a deficit state in complex information processing with sparing of basic, simple cognitive processes.
2. The underlying cognitive deficits for autism are not specific to any particular domain of cognitive function or to any particular modality. Autism is not primarily a deficit in attention, memory, language, or executive function, but involves all of these cognitive domains.

3. The most likely neurobiological basis for autism is in the form of a network of numerous subcortical and cortical structures. The actual pathology may be at the cellular level, reflecting some variation in dendritic architecture. The preliminary magnetic resonance spectroscopy findings would support this view.

4. Correspondingly, autism is not a localized or lateralized disorder. It is a disorder at the system level. While frontal, temporal-limbic, and subcortical localizations have been suggested, none of these views has shown a consistent relationship between the hypothesized localizations and the clinical phenomenology of the disorder.

5. The specifics of the network remain unknown, but would appear to be ultimately discoverable with more research and emerging technologies.

In autism, the brain has invented a disorder that does not have a neat, discrete neurocognitive space. It doesn't seem to live anywhere. It isn't like ideational apraxia or the WCST or other entities that appear to have found homes in the frontal lobes or elsewhere. What this appears to suggest is that the brain can code complexity. If it couldn't, it couldn't produce a disorder in which complexity appears to be selectively impaired. Furthermore, in autism, complexity is selectively impaired regardless of domain or modality. The impetus to localize autism in the frontal lobes, or cerebellum, or hippocampus appears to be based upon traditional views arising from modularity or localization concepts. However, it is a disorder that can be more economically explained in what have been described in the past as mass action, equipotentiality, or holistic concepts. These early conceptualizations have evolved into system or network theories in which localized functions are integrated in the manner of Luria's functional systems. Since the brain can produce a disorder like autism, it would appear to be able to process information at a system level just as if it can produce a disorder like alexia without agraphia, it can process information in a highly discrete, circumscribed way. It is not necessary to return to the days when there was some belief that the brain always functions as a unified whole. On the other hand, autism helps teach us that it is not always necessary to understand cognitive function as representing some specific domain or modality, or even some combination of them. There appears to be the implicit belief that complex activities are based on the interaction of localized structures that work together in a seamless way, giving rise to the illusion of unified behavior. When a link in the system is disrupted, the behavior becomes impaired. The problem in autism is that we have not been able to find the disrupted link. It is not in attention, or memory, or language, or executive function, but is in all of them. It therefore appears more like the mischief is in the system itself, and not in some particular component. Perhaps we need to know more about the emergent properties of systems as they apply to brain function.

NEUROPSYCHOLOGICAL ASSESSMENT

Neuropsychological assessment of individuals with high functioning autism is typically highly feasible utilizing standard tests and batteries. We have found these individuals to be quite cooperative, and fully capable of providing valid and reliable test data. They usually tolerate extensive testing quite well, and the more lengthy standard batteries can be administered in a manner that is routine for most clinical settings. The extensive neuropsychological research done provides extensive information regarding selection of tests. Much work has been done with experimental procedures designed for particular studies, but much of the research has been done with standard clinical tests including the various Wechsler intelligence scales (WAIS; WAIS-R; WAIS-III) (Wechsler, 1955; 1981; 1997), the Revised Wechsler Memory Scale (Wechsler, 1987), portions of the Halstead-Reitan Battery (Reitan and Wolfson, 1993), the Luria-Nebraska Battery (Golden, Purisch, and Hammeke, 1985), the WCST (Heaton, Chelune, Talley, et al., 1993), the California Verbal Learning Test (Delis, Kramer, Kaplan, and Ober, 1987), the Rey-Osterrieth Complex Figure (Osterrieth, 1944) and numerous psychoeducational tests and batteries.

In the following, we will outline a model for assessment that will hopefully characterize the major features of high functioning autism, and provide useful recommendations. Consistent with recent thinking about psychiatric diagnosis, neuropsychological assessment should not be used to diagnose autism. That matter is better left to other established procedures, notably the ADI and ADOS. However, neuropsychological and psychoeducational tests have been found to be quite useful in characterizing autism, and may reveal core deficits that underlie the clinical phenomenology.

As is the case for all neuropsychological assessment, the assessment of autism should generate data from the major cognitive domains; abstract reasoning and problem solving, memory, attention, language, spatial abilities, and perceptual and motor skills. There should also be an evaluation of general intelligence and academic achievement. Personality evaluations, such as the MMPI, are not typically done for individuals with autism, for reasons that are unclear. Perhaps the disorder is so blatant, and the ADI, ADOS, and other scales, notably the Childhood Autism Rating Scale (CARS) (Schopler, Reichler, and Rochen-Renner, 1980) serve that purpose so well, particularly in mentally retarded individuals, that tests of the MMPI type add little unique information. Based on the literature, it is also important to include in the battery both simple and complex tests within the same domain, and to place some stress on areas likely to be dysfunctional including concept formation, metaphoric language, skilled motor activity, reading comprehension, and delayed recall of material that is verbally or geometrically complex, such as stories or the Rey-Osterrieth Figure. Since spatial-constructional abilities are typically good or better in autism, it is valuable to assess this area for its compensatory potential. Because of varying reports of discriminative validity concerning the same tests, it has become critically important to carefully evaluate the samples upon which the studies were based. As indicated, autism is an extremely variable disorder from the standpoint of general ability level and what discriminates between individuals with autism and controls in one IQ range may not discriminate in another range. Thus, while the domains mentioned here should ideally all be assessed, the particular tests chosen may vary with regard to sensitivity and specificity across ranges. Particularly in the case of those tests that tend to be highly correlated with IQ, relatively small differences in IQ level can be associated with presence or absence of abnormal scores. The clinician should therefore have available a repertoire of tests in each of the domains that vary in level of difficulty.

The Wechsler Scales

The Wechsler intelligence scales have proven to be of particular value in autism because of the large number of studies done, and the clinically useful results (Siegel *et al.*, 1996). There is a reasonably good prototypic profile characterized by a high point on Block Design and a low point on Comprehension. It is not unusual for the Block Design score to be in the 12-13 range, even when the rest of the profile does not attain that level. From the standpoint of differential diagnosis, individuals with high functioning autism have a dramatically different WAIS-R profile from what is seen in adult learning disability, as illustrated in Figure 1. These profiles were derived from samples of 102 adults with learning disability (McCue and Goldstein, 1991) and 35 individuals with high functioning autism. While the Performance subtests are reasonably comparable, the Verbal subtests have very different patterns, with the LD group showing an elevation on Comprehension and Similarities and a depression on Information, Arithmetic, and Digit Span. Essentially the case is reversed in the autism group. The WAIS-R profile characterizes the autism group nicely, as having relatively normal development of semantic knowledge relative to poor development of both linguistic and social comprehension, as well as particularly good spatial-constructional ability when the task does not have a social component. This dissociation between social and non-social performance tasks is not seen in the LD group. It has the anticipated evidence of poor development of semantic knowledge and calculation skills. There is, in fact, preliminary evidence that the WAIS-R has a different factor structure in autism from what is found in normal individuals and people with adult LD, reflecting differences largely with regard to social content of the test material (Lincoln *et al.*, 1988). The Wechsler intelligence scales therefore can be recommended as a good assessment procedure for autism and for discriminating between autism and adult LD.

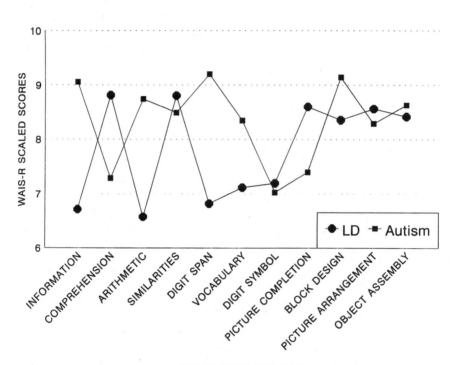

WAIS-R SUBTEST

Figure 1. WAIS-R profiles comparing samples of individuals with high-functioning autism and learning disabilities.

Abstract Reasoning

The assessment of abstract reasoning and concept formation in autism requires a rather sophisticated approach. It has been noted that the WCST, taken to be the "gold standard" for conceptual reasoning tests, did not discriminate between autism and control groups in several studies, despite the heavy emphasis placed by some authorities on perseverative thinking and executive dysfunction in autism. Review of several studies suggests that the absence or presence of a significant difference is a matter of general level of ability, or IQ. This absence of significance has also been noted for the Halstead Category Test and Part B of the Trail Making Test, both of which are widely accepted measures of conceptual reasoning ability. In ongoing unpublished work done in collaboration with Dr. Nancy Minshew, one of the authors (GG) noted a distinction in autism between two classes of conceptual reasoning tests, one evaluating rule learning or attribute identification, and the other, concept formation. A concept formation test is different from rule-learning and attribute identification tests in that in the latter tests, the concept is predetermined and the test-taker has to identify it, or learn what it is. In concept formation, the test-taker has to generate hypotheses in an open-field situation. The classic concept formation task is the sorting test in which an array of material is placed before the test-taker, who is asked to group those together that belong together. An increased challenge is presented by having the test-taker group the material in ways different from what was done on the initial sort. The Goldstein-Scheerer Object Sorting and Color Sorting tests (Goldstein and Scheerer, 1941) and the Hanfman-Kasanin Concept Formation Test have this characteristic (1936). The 20 Questions task used in our own work also has it. Clinically, we have seen patients with autism who did well on the WCST and Category Test but who could not form a consistent organization of questions that corresponded with formation of hypotheses that would constrain the number of possible correct answers. In the case of tests of this type, consistently robust significant differences between subjects with autism and controls have been found (Minshew *et al.*, 1994).

The general principle here seems to be that the rule learning and attribute identification tests may be done at an impaired level by individuals with autism in the lower end of the high functioning range. However, individuals with higher IQs often need to be more challenged with concept formation tasks. It would therefore be wise to have in one's assessment repertoire tests of the free sorting or 20 questions type. The discriminative validities of these kinds of tests appear to be better across a broader range of high functioning autism.

Memory

The evaluation of memory is probably best accomplished with tests of the Wechsler Memory Scale type that contain both simple and complex material. One can generally anticipate normal or near normal performance on simple material such as repeating digits or paired-associate learning, and abnormal performance on story recall or recall of complex material, particularly under delayed memory conditions. More elegant analyses of simple material such as analyzing for a primacy-recency effect or for semantic clustering of the items may also reveal areas of impairment. The research suggests that the general principle is that individuals with autism do not benefit from contextual cues that support memory. Theoretically, they may do no better at remembering a story than a random list of words of the same length. Several studies have shown that they do not show the anticipated improvement in learning from organized material compared with unorganized material. Simple associative learning and short-term memory tests may be administered for contrast purposes, but they are likely to produce normal results.

Attention

The clinical assessment of attention in autism is a complex matter. The standard measures of simple attention such as repeating digits are typically non-revelatory, and tests for which psychomotor speed variables are used as the score (e.g., reaction time, cancellation tasks) are confounded because of the well-established reduction in psychomotor function often found in individuals with autism. Spatial attentional deficits, such as unilateral neglect, are not a part of autism. Probably the most sensitive tests of attention for autism are measures of working memory in which ongoing activity is monitored. In particular, span tasks that contain multiple components appear to be particularly sensitive. For example, the Word Span and Oral Directions subtests from the Detroit Tests of Learning Aptitude (Hammill, 1985) or the Daneman and Carpenter (1980) Reading Memory Test may be quite sensitive. Apparently more complex tests of attention such as Part B of the Trail Making Test are less suitable because of confounding with psychomotor speed, as well as the existence of data from several studies indicating that this test does not discriminate between individuals with high functioning autism and controls (Minshew et al., 1992).

Language and Academic Skills

While individuals with low-functioning autism may be mute, individuals with high functioning autism are not aphasic. Therefore, the language difficulties they evolve are not generally captured by the standard aphasia examinations, with few exceptions. Specifically, these individuals do not have difficulties with word finding, repetition, enunciation, oral reading, spelling, handwriting, simple calculation, and basic auditory analysis. Their language difficulties lie mainly in the areas of prosody, reading comprehension, understanding of metaphor and figurative speech, and analysis of complex grammatical structures. Thus, the only aphasia tests that may show some sensitivity to the disorder are instruments of the Token Test type. This sensitivity is found particularly for instructions that have complex grammatical structures. The language tests that are most sensitive are generally from intelligence tests and psychoeducational batteries, notably tests like the Comprehension subtest of the Wechsler series, and the various standard reading comprehension tests. Research supporting this conclusion has been done with the reading comprehension sections of the Woodcock Reading Mastery Test and the Kaufman Test of Educational Achievement. The Test of Language Competence (TOLC) (Wiig and Secord, 1989) has also been shown to be very sensitive to high functioning autism, particularly the Metaphoric Expression subtest.

The clinical phenomenology of the language dysfunction involves fluent speech with limited intonation and a variety of comprehension deficits such that spoken or written prose are often, at best, only partially understood. The severity of the comprehension loss increases with the complexity or the metaphoric content of the language used. There is often a failure to respond to humor. Discourse is typically not bizarre or incoherent, as in the case of schizophrenia, but may reflect the individual's narrow range of interests. This narrowness sometimes has "idiot-savant" characteristics such that there is remarkable expertise regarding one topic, but little breadth of information. The man with autism in the movie "The Rain Man" is a good example of this phenomenon, as illustrated by his fear of flying in combination with his extremely detailed knowledge of accident statistics.

The evaluation of academic skills is of particular importance for autism, even in adults who have completed their educations, because the tests most sensitive to communicative dysfunction associated with the disorder are found in psychoeducational tests, clearly to a greater extent than is the case for the traditional neuropsychological tests of language. Also quite important are the tests of verbal reasoning and comprehension contained in intelligence tests, and tests of the 20 Questions type. We have referred to WAIS-R Comprehension, but such tests as the Verbal Absurdities, Picture Absurdities, and Plan of Search from the Binet scales are relevant also to the language dysfunction of high functioning autism. As indicated above, the TOLC, which deals with issues of metaphor, ambiguity, and inference making, seems to be exceptionally sensitive to the language deficit in autism. In the following section we will deal more specifically with learning disability aspects of autism and their management, but here we wish to point out that the psychoeducational tests contain what are perhaps the most important parts of the language evaluation for high functioning autism.

Spatial Abilities and Perceptual-Motor Skills

Perhaps one of the most widely observed but puzzling aspects of cognition in high functioning autism is the intact, and often better than intact, spatial abilities found in individuals with autism. They are good at building things, analyzing visual material, and solving pictorial puzzles, and seem to enjoy doing those things. The exception seems to be the task that has a social content, such as the Picture Arrangement subtest of the Wechsler intelligence scales, where comprehension of the social situation contributes to the solution. As indicated previously, Block Design is typically the high score on the Wechsler scales, and other constructional and copying tasks are usually done in a comparably normal manner. However, when a spatial task is combined with a delayed recall task mild impairment may be found, particularly if the spatial task is complex. For example, a study has shown that individuals with high functioning autism do less well than controls on delayed recall of the Rey-Osterrieth Complex Figure. It has been suggested that the network dysfunction that underlies autism is not of the type that is thought to mediate spatial abilities, such as the pattern of cerebral organization found primarily in the right cerebral hemisphere. Largely because of the apparent communicative problems seen in autism, it was suggested in the past that it was primarily a disorder of the left cerebral hemisphere (Hoffman and Prior, 1982), but that view is not widely supported at present.

With regard to perceptual and motor skills, autism does not involve any apparent physical disability with regard to any of the senses or the motor system. However, there is a commonly observed motor awkwardness or dyskinesia often documented by neuropsychological tests of dexterity. The typical pattern is normal simple motor skill, such as finger tapping, with impaired dexterity as assessed with psychomotor speed or pegboard tasks. A similar pattern exists for perception such that basic sensory-perceptual skills are usually intact, but there may be impairment at a more complex level as is assessed by such procedures as fingertip number writing from the Halstead-Reitan Battery.

It has been reported that relatively pure tests of psychomotor speed can discriminate better between individuals with autism and normal controls than can tests in which the psychomotor component of the task is combined with a challenging cognitive component. Thus, individuals with autism may do significantly worse than controls on Part A of the Trail Making Test, which has minimal cognitive demands, but not on Part B, which requires substantial cognitive resources (Minshew et al., 1994). The documentation of impairments of skilled planned action in autism is provided by an extensive experimental literature (Smith and Bryson, 1994).

The Neuropsychological Profile and Its Implications

The profile we have been describing contains a combination of some rather distinct, straightforward dissociations and some more subtle distinctions. There is an apparent dissociation between simple and complex abilities across domains, with intact basic skills and often significantly impaired complex skills. There is also an apparent intactness of spatial-constructional skills, except in those cases in which the stimulus material has social content. Even with social content, however, spatial tasks are done better than linguistic tasks with social content. For example, on the WAIS-R, Picture Arrangement is typically done better than Comprehension. In language and memory, a key factor appears to involve voluntary utilization of contextual cues. While basic linguistic and associative skills appear to be intact, the application of strategies that utilize contextual cues or that provide them appear to be impaired in autism. For example, individuals with autism do not tend to organize words into semantic categories when learning a list, nor do they utilize contextual cues in stories in promoting recall. Since they do not organize material effectively, comprehension may be substantially compromised. The classic situation is the individual with autism who reads a passage aloud without error, but has little understanding of what was read.

With regard to abstract reasoning, there is a dissociation between the ability to identify relevant attributes of a stimulus array and to learn rules regarding them, and an impairment in concept formation, which involves voluntary initiation of alternative hypotheses. Thus, individuals may perform normally on rule-learning and attribute identification tasks such as the Wisconsin Card Sorting Test, but poorly on sorting tasks that require initiation of hypotheses.

There is often a dissociation between normal performance on basic perceptual and motor tasks and at least mildly impaired performance on tasks that require integration of sensory input, such as identifying numbers on the fingertips, or that require dexterity and speed, such as pegboard tasks. We would add here that seizures occur in individuals with autism more frequently than they do in the general population (Minshew, Sweeney, and Bauman, 1997). Thus, neurological dysfunction may occur in association with the seizures or the medications used to treat them.

This profile is probably most consistent with the theory of autism that characterizes it as a disorder of complex information processing. It is apparently not a domain specific disorder of language or memory, because impairments have been identified across several domains. Characterization of autism as a disorder of executive function has much to be said for it, except for two considerations. First, individuals with high functioning autism often perform normally on the WCST, the test that most authorities use as the "gold standard" measure of executive function. Second, the deficits noted in reading comprehension, understanding of metaphor, and perceptual integration go beyond the usual definition of executive function involving maintenance of goal-directed behavior, adapting to changes, and planning abilities. It is not being suggested that individuals with autism do not often have executive function deficits. Rather, it is being suggested that the core deficit appears to go beyond that particular construct.

INTERVENTIONS

Preliminary Remarks

In order to provide a basis for what we will describe as "Interventions" it seems advisable to point out that autism is a life-long incurable disorder, and while there may be some developmental changes in symptom severity, the disease process does not remit spontaneously or in response to any known biological or psychological treatment. In essence, there is no cure for autism. We therefore will limit the use of such terms as treatment, therapy, and rehabilitation in describing interventions accomplished with individuals with autism. However, there is substantial evidence that individuals with autism can learn, and may alter their behavior as a result of behavior modification efforts (Schriebman, Koegel, Charlop, and Egel, 1982). It is also the case that individuals with autism are entitled to an education, and it is proper to use the best educational methodologies and strategies that show promise of being effective with the disorder. We will not be discussing the behavior therapy work here, but rather, will focus on the design of instruction and educational environment. This section is based largely on a paper by Minshew, Goldstein, and Siegel (1996), to which the reader is referred for more detailed information. We would note that the paper is largely devoted to providing ideas based upon what is known about cognitive function in autism and how certain available educational programs and strategies may be productively applied. There is little if any published research establishing the empirical basis for efficacy of these methods as applied to individuals with autism. This information may also help to distinguish between instruction appropriate for individuals with autism and other disabled learners, such as individuals with dyslexia and other specific academic skill disorders (Rumsey and Hamburger, 1990; Shea and Mesibov, 1985; Bartak and Rutter, 1976; Lincoln *et al.*, 1988). While individuals with high functioning autism have educational difficulties that may be characterized as learning disability, they typically do not have dyslexia, or the specific academic skill disorders.

Reading

Neuropsychological study of high functioning individuals with autism has demonstrated a psychoeducational profile distinct from dyslexia (Rumsey and Hamburger, 1990; Shea and Mesibov, 1985) and characterized by intact encoding and declarative skills with impaired comprehension and interpretative skills (Goldstein, Minshew, and Siegel, 1994; Minshew, Goldstein, Taylor, and Siegel, 1994). There is a dissociation between mechanical reading ability and acquiring meaning from printed text (Frith and Snowling, 1983 Minshew *et al.*, 1994). The phenomenon of excellence in oral reading may be seen as a savant skill in the hyperlexic autistic individual who in the absence of any formal instruction demonstrates an advanced ability to read single words (Goldberg, 1987; Whitehouse and Harris, 1984). Deficits in comprehending text are evident, however, despite adequate word knowledge and general fund of information, and this often excellent oral reading fluency.

Considering an intact ability to employ phonetic analysis rules to read fluently, with deficient comprehension of reading material, certain implications emerge for teaching. Unlike instruction designed for the dyslexic individual, there does not need to be training for phonological deficits such as sound-symbol relationships, remediation of phonetic or structural analysis skills, or teaching the orthographic features of words, syllabication, or blending. Rather, the emphasis needs to be on understanding what was read, something that is often quite deficient even in high functioning individuals with autism. Numerous methods of specific strategy training for reading comprehension are reviewed in Siegel, Goldstein, and Minshew (1996). They all involve previewing the passage, outlining the main ideas, re-reading it in greater detail, asking questions about it, and reviewing the passage again if necessary. Appropriate interventions would also be the use of vocabulary material that develops knowledge of secondary meanings of words, use of organizers that represent story events in a temporal sequence with pictures, or instruction in interpreting cause and effect and other logical relationships, and developing hypotheses about intervening events. Practice in answering *Who, What, Where, Why, When* questions about a reading selection can function as an aid for organizing story details.

Compensatory approaches to reading instruction might include the use of high interest reading material, perhaps involving the student's special interest, and using text that is grammatically simple. During class discussion of reading material, if there is a relative emphasis on recalling facts and details rather than on understanding the motivation of characters or formulating inferences about story events, the student with autism might be relatively successful. Capitalizing on the strength in mechanical reading ability, individuals with autism can participate in classroom activities by reading instructions or class announcements, thereby possibly gaining positive peer recognition. The focus, however, should be directed toward comprehension, and development of organizing skills that become increasingly self-initiated. There is some evidence that oral reading improves comprehension when well-organized text is used (Hinchley and Levy, 1988), opening the possibility that the systematic use of an intact ability may support learning of an impaired ability.

Mathematics

Arithmetic calculation is an automatic, procedural skill that is not typically deficient in high functioning autism (Minshew *et al.*, 1994). Indeed there are case reports of individuals with autism who are lightning calculators (Steel, Gorman, and Flexman, 1984). In contrast to intact computational abilities, there is often a deficit in understanding mathematical concepts as applied to everyday applications, and mathematical reasoning and problem solving such as are required in arithmetic story problems (Minshew *et al.*, 1994). These deficits may be attributable to several factors including the complex language embedded in the wording of the problems, the need to generate hypotheses and strategies to solve the problem, and the ability to proceed toward a solution by flexibly testing hypotheses.   Thus, in autism, there may be dissociation between mechanical arithmetic skills and mathematical reasoning, a somewhat different situation from what is the case in other individuals with mathematical learning disabilities (Rourke, 1993).

If this situation is the case, then instruction may deal mainly with mathematical problem solving rather than the more traditional areas of number concept and calculation skills.   Mathematical language may be emphasized such that the student may become familiar with the mathematical terminology in story problems that indicate the process required to solve the problem.   For example, key words such as *both, combined,* and *more* indicate that the operation of addition is required, while *part, equal,* and *half,* convey that division should be performed.   The student underlines such words in the problem statements, as an aid in comprehending the question.   Story problems can also be organized into component parts by separating the information given from the question to be answered.   Problem statements can be represented pictorially to illustrate the processes necessary for obtaining a solution.

Communication and Language

The high functioning individual with autism possesses basic communicative competence but demonstrates selective linguistic deficits (Minshew *et al.*, 1994). In high functioning autism there is fluent narrative discourse and intact word knowledge, with specific linguistic impairment in semantic and pragmatic aspects of language (Baltaxe and Simmons, 1992; Brook and Bowler, 1992). In particular, the comprehension of metaphorical or figurative aspects of language are deficient in high functioning individuals with autism. There is a disability in understanding figures of speech or ambiguous statements. Complex relational terms may also be poorly understood (Goldstein *et al.*, 1994). Reciprocal communication is impaired by a limited capacity to adopt another's perspective, accurately interpret affective meanings, understand cause and effect or temporal relationships, develop inferences about intervening events, or to alternately exchange speaker-listener roles (Baltaxe, 1977). Comprehension of humor is likely to be deficient (Van Bourgondien and Mesibov, 1987). Limited use of inflection, prosody, eye contact, and recognition of gestural cues are present and impact adversely on social functioning (Yirmiya and Sigman, 1991).

Considering these deficits, the student with autism will experience difficulty learning in educational settings where there is a preference for oral presentation, reliance on verbal instructions and lecture, use of figurative expressions in conversational speech, and reference to meaning by way of analogy, metaphor, or humor. The social deficits persist throughout life, and relationships will always be difficult to develop. The individual with autism may be perceived by others as odd, and thus, difficult to relate to in both work and play situations. These deficits are part of the autism and cannot be reversed except in the sense that specific target behaviors such as eye contact or abnormal posturing may be altered through behavior modification procedures. However, it is possible to capitalize on assets and to provide various accommodations.

The relative strength in fluency and verbal production can be used as an asset since it is possible to request the student to make oral presentations containing factual information, describe special interests, or recite poems, or share story details or current events. Clinically, we have heard high functioning individuals with autism make relatively eloquent presentations of their special interests. Due to the deficit commonly found in the auditory or visual comprehension of language, instructors can provide accommodation by communicating in short, syntactically simple sentences that contain one idea per utterance. Oral directions, particularly those containing multiple sequences or complex phrasing should not be used, while lengthy discourse should be generally avoided. Directions may need to be repeated by the teacher and then spoken aloud by the student to insure commands have been understood. It has been demonstrated that individuals with autism while impaired in their ability to respond immediately to spoken communications, are as capable as normal controls when written information is present (Boucher and Lewis, 1989). Therefore, printed instructions should always be available on assignment sheets and displayed in the room for ready reference by the student with autism, or instructions may be provided both orally and in writing. The difference between oral and written instruction may relate to processing time. Once an oral instruction is given it is gone, but written instructions are more amenable to being reviewed over a lengthy time span. Thus, accommodation may be provided by allowing more time for receiving instructions, with the opportunity for repeating the instructions in the case of oral presentation.

Teachers should be sensitive to the inability of individuals with autism to misunderstand or not comprehend slang, jokes, pop culture jargon, and nonverbal communication through gesture or expression. It is generally desirable to explain social conventions, rules, and standards in concrete terms. It is always necessary to consider that a message may not have been understood, and may require repetition, rephrasing, or concretization. Sarcasm and non-verbal communication to praise, kid, or reprimand through tone of voice, facial expression, or physical posture may well not be understood by the high functioning individual with autism. Active, declarative, and affirmative speech without use of transformations or complex phrasing is preferred. Alternatively, the student with autism should not be expected to deliver complex messages to others.

Reasoning and Problem Solving

Deficits in verbal reasoning, concept formation, and in generating strategies for problem solving have been documented by autism research (Minshew, *et al.*, 1992; Rumsey and Hamburger, 1988; Tager-Flusberg, 1985). These difficulties are made evident in perseverative efforts at problem solving with an inability to shift and develop strategies that are heuristic (Minshew *et al.*, 1994; Prior and Hoffman, 1990; Rumsey, 1985). Nevertheless, as indicated above, rule-learning and attribute identification aspects of abstraction have been reported to be intact in at least some high functioning individuals with autism (Minshew *et al.*, 1992). Those that possess these abilities, however, may still require instruction in concept formation, development of self-initiated strategies, and conceptual flexibility. The issues here revolve around how one forms hypotheses, drops prepotent tendencies when they don't work, and develops alternatives. Appropriate methods for teaching conceptual skills to mentally ill patients have been developed outside of the area of autism, and, in particular, there have been extensive efforts to teach patients with schizophrenia to improve their performance on the WCST (e.g., Green, Satz, Ganzell, and Vaclav, 1992). The results have been mixed, but some success has been obtained either by using monetary reinforcement or simplifying the task. One simplification method is providing in advance the relevant categories, such as form, color, and number, and requiring the student only to identify the appropriate one. Concept development can be taught in general through teaching recognition of relevant, salient features of a stimulus array, suppressing prepotent responses, and identifying principles such as similarity and difference, part-to-whole relationships, and causality. Abstract ideas and concepts are often introduced to children through concrete representations. Ongoing monitoring of behavior through such means as self-questioning may aid in breaking down rigidity and perseveration. For example, after a response the student may be encouraged to ask, "Is this right?" "Why did I get this wrong?" "Can it be done some other way?" A clinical observation made in a study of an object sorting test was that when asked to shift sorts, almost all of the participants with autism indicated that there was no other way possible to sort the objects. The initial sorts were generally quite plausible, but there was little capacity to formulate other bases for sorting (e.g., going from color to function) (Minshew *et al.*, 1994). Presenting alternatives may be helpful in breaking down this severe rigidity along with stopping perseverative behavior when it occurs.

Memory

Early clinical accounts of autism noted an excellent memory for remote events, often phenomenal rote memory for poems and names, and the precise recollection of complex patterns and sequences (Kanner, 1943). As part of the observation of preoccupation with sameness, clinicians noted the remarkable capacity of individuals with autism to detect the slightest change in a familiar environment, such as a room. Memory ability in autism is quite different from that of individuals with learning disabilities. For example, in a study comparing members of the two groups, the participants with autism demonstrated intact performance on an auditory rote memory task while demographically matched dyslexics demonstrated deficient rote memory (Rumsey and Hamburger, 1990).

Considering intact rote memory processes involving visual and verbal modalities, the capacity for high functioning individuals with autism to benefit from the use of semantic information to encode information, and the difficulty using strategies to organize new information, several implications emerge for instruction that would make such instruction different from what would be appropriate for dyslexia. A strength-matched approach could exploit the intact ability to form verbal associations, as demonstrated by good performance on paired-associate learning tasks. This method of developing recall can be adapted to curriculum content. For example, this procedure might work in geography by associating the names, locations, natural resources, and capitals of states; in history for learning the names of explorers and their discoveries, and in science when learning equations for velocity and acceleration. It is therefore possible that intact associative learning can be utilized through providing students with autism with organized lists of materials rather than expecting them to generate meaningfully related content and categories from text.

Ecological and Other Considerations

Clinical reports of individuals with autism describe such characteristic behavioral features as resistance to change and an insistence on sameness (Kanner, 1943; 1971). Processing of sensory information is also often deficient and may be evident in a heightened sensitivity to noise or physical contact, an apparent insensitivity to pain, a fascination with certain sensory input such as textures or smell, or diminished performance in settings where stimuli are inconstant. Abnormal motor behavior involving odd body posture, poor coordination, or stereotypies, and hyperactivity may also be observed (Minshew and Payton, 1988). This cluster of behaviors can be accommodated for in school by providing considerable structure (Volkmar, Hoder, and Cohen, 1985). Consistent and predictable behavior by the teacher in the delivery of consequences and reinforcement with the use of established routines will provide security and comfort. Daily schedules can be reviewed upon entering the classroom in the morning or posted. Work periods should be brief, structured, with tasks organized into small units that can be completed within reasonable time periods. This is especially important when new skills are introduced. Any change in location or content of activities should be planned in advance and supported. Alertness to special events as they occur in the course of the year is important (e.g., assembly programs, a class party or trip, teacher absence) in order to assist the student in anticipating these changes in advance. If repetitive statements, conversation only about the student's restricted range of interest, or arguments persist, it may be helpful to rephrase directions, require that the individual prepare a list of concerns that can be examined at another time, or firmly redirect the conversation.

It has been demonstrated that small group arrangements in the classroom is effective in increasing the amount of interaction time for students with autism (Kamps, Walter, Maher, and Rotholz, 1992). If collaborative projects or structured recreational activities (e.g., playing table games) are provided, conversation may more likely be appropriately related in content to performing the common activity. Pursuit of the object of the game or completion of the task can also serve as intrinsic mechanisms for turn-taking in communications. While individuals with autism may be able to participate in simple table games, adaptations to the physical education program may be necessary to provide success and avoid social censure due to their poor motor coordination skills. High functioning individuals with autism seem to share with individuals with attention-deficit hyperactivity disorder (ADHD) executive function deficits involving the ability to initiate, sustain, inhibit, and shift mental activity (Denckla, 1989). Differences between these disorders in other aspects, however, are greater than their similarities. For example anything novel, challenging, and varied may enhance the performance of individuals with ADHD while individuals with autism encounter considerable difficulty tolerating change in the environment.

Considering the heightened activity level and inattentiveness described for some individuals with autism, distractions and disruptions need to be minimized with extraneous classroom stimuli eliminated. Seating assignments need to consider proximity to the teacher, egress to the room, high-activity areas, and the behavior of other students which may overload thresholds for stimulation. Brief time-out periods may be beneficial in enabling the student to become comfortable subsequent to excessive stimulation. These considerations extend to adults not in school but who are with other people at work or in social situations. A low-key, stable, small group environment seems to be preferable.

Educating high functioning individuals with autism poses unique challenges. Knowledge of the neuropsychological profile is valuable in this effort because it contributes to understanding aptitude and educational interactions specific to the disorder. We have presented some suggestions for educational intervention consistent with the neuropsychological findings. It was not intended to evaluate the use of specific teaching methodologies developed for students with autism such as auditory training or facilitated communication, special curriculum such as TEACCH (Reichler and Schopler, 1976), or technology and materials such as computers. Some of these interventions remain controversial and are often only appropriate for severely impaired students, while some may be considered for use with high functioning students with autism. It should also be noted that while the strategies developed for instruction and the classroom environment emerge from research on neuropsychological functioning in autism, they are presented only as possible interventions.

SUMMARY

Based on extensive research, it has been suggested that the particular educational needs of individuals with high functioning autism are in relatively delimited areas. These include (1) instruction in organization and planning to promote improved comprehension and recall of complex material, such as text. (2) Teaching skills in initiation of hypotheses during problem solution that consider alternatives and that discourage perseverative behavior. (3) Providing accommodation through limiting use of figures of speech, metaphors, and extended, grammatically convoluted language in communicating information. (4) Providing accommodation for the social deficit that is a part of autism through various means including maintenance of a relatively subdued and stable environment, adequate preparation for and gradual introduction of change, and behavioral management of self-destructive and socially inappropriate actions.

This field does not have a set of established, empirically based treatments, and it is only possible at this point to provide a tentative blueprint of educational needs based upon a large amount of cognitive research. Actual validation of the effectiveness of these strategies will need to be obtained from systematic and controlled studies, but hopefully the available research may guide us away from inappropriate but firmly entrenched methods such as phonics training. Clearly, the specific educational needs of a high functioning individual with autism cannot be based only on group results, as the individual may depart from the performance of the group by a considerable degree.

As a final comment on intervention, possibly the optimal treatment program for high functioning autism involves a multidimensional approach coordinated by a case manager who has particular expertise in the area. The case manager can coordinate medical intervention activities, particularly if there is an associated illness such as epilepsy, teachers, parents, and clinicians who provide specialized procedures, notably behavior therapy. Very often, the case manager is the individual who is most prepared to deal with the frequent life crises commonly occurring with individuals with autism because of episodes of inappropriate behavior or exposure to an unanticipated stressor. Behavioral management techniques in combination with instructional strategies may provide an ideal program for maximizing learning for the high functioning student with autism.

6

CONCLUDING THOUGHTS

We have addressed a group of learning disabilities in young adults from a neuropsychological perspective with the intent that such a perspective would indeed have clinical utility. In doing so we have discovered that while the knowledge base in each of the disorders reviewed in the previous chapters has been enlarged considerably within the past decade, much remains to be understood. In many cases, research is lacking and clinical practice reflects the biases of the practitioner's specific discipline. For example, when we look at those disorders most reflective of academic pursuits, reading, written expression, and math, there is little crossover between the fields of special education, cognitive psychology, neurology, or neuropsychology. Hiscock and Hiscock (1991) go so far as to challenge the educational utility of neuropsychological data in relation to academic problems, opining that the "disease model" gathers extraneous information with little utility (see a discussion of this issue in the chapter on Nonverbal Learning Disability). Medical research in the area of "dyslexia" has confined itself to neuroanatomical case studies and/or genetic transmission and twin studies. And while the Shaywitz group, which does in contrast involve pediatrics, neurology, and educational psychology, has one of the most comprehensive of the follow up studies ever conducted, not all researchers agree with their basic assumptions regarding the etiology and definition of reading disorders. Further, in their work and that of others, while the basis for deficits in reading with young children has certainly been addressed in terms of early acquisition of phonological skills, at times the focus on such a highly specific deficit has prevented the inclusion of constructs such as temporal processing and orthographic processing in the research design. This "one size-fits-all" paradigm is particularly distressing to those of us who work with adolescents and adults and certainly should be distressing to those who work with children, each of whom has a unique learning style.

When we then look at continued problems with efficient reading and/or comprehension in the young adult population, interventions based upon strategies developed with young children tend to remain in practice in many literacy programs, although work on metacognitive strategies has produced curricular offerings at the high school level (e.g., the work coming out of Deshler's group at the University of Kansas). Other investigators continue to focus on the non-utility of intelligence measures in the assessment of reading disorders in children and adults, and in their singular focus on this issue, fail to appreciate the cognitive processing information that such instruments provide to the trained clinician that consequently contribute to treatment plans involving remediation and/or appropriate accommodations for young adults in academic or vocational settings.

Even more discipline-specific is work in the areas of written language and math disorders in adults. Neuropsychology has tended to focus on acquired disorders affecting language or math calculations following some sort of brain trauma, while special educators are still not of one mind with respect to the existence of these disorders as stand alone conditions. Other educational researchers focus entirely on spelling as the single manifestation of written language production again in terms of early acquisition of skills. While the use of manipulatives has been demonstrated to enhance the acquisition of basic mathematical operations, there is little if any empirical research on effective methods for teaching higher-level math functions even though these skill subjects remain especially difficult for many college level students. However, more recent work by investigators such as Geary (2000) give us hope that studies incorporating neuroimaging and work done on semantic and phonological memory systems may shed light on the cognitive underpinnings of mathematical disorders, which have been postulated in the literature (Nolting, 1988), and ultimately on intervention strategies.

In contrast to the predominant discipline-specific nature of research in the academically based disorders, work done in the areas of autism and attention deficit disorder illustrate what can be accomplished when research and practice are multidisciplinary in nature. The work of all of the major researchers in both fields utilizes data coming from the areas of educational psychology, neuropsychology, psychopharmacology, and neurology. The work of Minshew's group at the University of Pittsburgh and the Biederman group at the University of Massachusetts illustrate the rich knowledge base that can be made available to the clinician who works with adults, although work with high functioning autistic adults in still in the infancy stage. Particularly rich is the more recent focus on psychopharmacology with the ADHD population including adults as the disorder has come to be recognized as a life-long condition much in the same way that "LD" was acknowledged to affect the lives of adults twenty years ago. That research taps behaviors in a variety of settings and has included measures specific to academic performance as well as working memory.

As with the reading and written language disorders literature, the issue of sub-typing remains dominant in the ADHD diagnostic literature. Subtyping studies with reading disorders in children have produced numerous subclassifications, but their utility in the classroom setting has never been demonstrated. Studies involving subtyping in adults with have been rather simplistic and thus have not proved to be particularly useful to clinicians. On the other hand, subtyping classifications such as those postulated in studies with individuals, adults and children alike, with ADHD would appear to be more useful to the clinician as well as fruitful areas of investigation (see the neurochemical mechanisms section of the ADHD chapter).

The new kid on the block, NLD, suffers from neglect to some degree. While the Rourke group has done seminal work in the field in terms of identification, there is little empirical research involving a cross-disciplinary approach perhaps as a consequence of the controversy that surrounds the diagnosis of a specific right-hemisphere disorder. Work such as that on the neuroanatomical underpinnings of dyslexia or on neuroimaging studies including *f*MRIs are surprisingly absent in the literature. Studies involving the adjustment of adults with NLD, academically, or vocationally, would seem to be lumped together with LD outcome studies in general, and thus we can say little about outcome. Future studies including the spectrum of NLDs (e.g., Asperger's) may shed light on appropriate interventions in much the same way that the early work on high-functioning autism is now doing. The work of Klin *et. al* (1995) with respect to the similarities in neuropsychological functions between NLD and Asperger Syndrome give us strong hints that interventions for the two groups may well be compatible.

Several other concerns need to be raised in our overall understanding of the spectrum of learning disorders in young adults. The first of these involves how these young adults or their parents can afford to access the extensive battery that we have advocated with respect to the diagnosis of ADHD in particular. Insurance companies routinely deny the need for an evaluation process that includes psychological or educational testing even though we know that the comorbidity for learning disabilities in the population of individuals with ADHD is 60% or more and the comorbidity for other psychiatric disorders including major depression, anxiety disorders, or Obsessive Compulsive Disorder has a prevalence rate of between 15% and 20%. Organizations such as C.H.A.D.D. have been working for some time with other mental health organizations to achieve parity, but until researchers and clinicians across a variety of disciplines acknowledge the need for such evaluations, the consumer will be forced to bear the expense of the labor-intensive process. If the young adult is still within a secondary school system, some of the psychoeducational components of the evaluation may be accessed through the school district as covered by special education law or Section 504 of the Rehabilitation Act. With adults facing major academic or vocational failures and who have financial need, partial support for an evaluation to

establish eligibility status might be available through the state vocational rehabilitation agency. And while paying for a comprehensive evaluation is costly,
that fact alone does not diminish its clinical validity or utility in much the same
way that an MRI is costly but critical to clinical care for certain conditions in
medical practice.

Second, there is a real necessity for work directed at the psychological sequelae of these various disorders of learning on adults. While follow-up studies
report a series of negative outcomes in terms of psychosocial functioning for
heterogeneous groups of individuals diagnosed with learning disabilities and/or
ADHD during childhood, the clinical utility of these studies is questionable, as
we have discussed previously throughout these chapters, because the target
population is never clearly defined and what constitutes positive or negative
outcomes is often narrowly defined. Gerber's (1992) work on reframing and the
ethnographic research reported by him and his colleagues come closest to providing therapists and counselors with some understanding of the synergistic effect of the learning disabilities and their implications for adult functioning. The
effectiveness of interventions such as coaching and directive therapy have yet to
be addressed in any comparative studies, and yet they are in the mainline of approaches used with adults who have ADHD. This is not surprising, however, as
it has only been within the very recent past that behavior modification approaches have been compared with psychopharmacological therapies in any
systematic way in the case of children with ADHD, although their use was discussed extensively in the child ADHD literature as a substitute for medication.

Third, it is critical for persons with learning disorders that the incorporation
of assistive technology into the academic arena and work place be given the
highest priority by clinicians and researchers. It is our strong belief that assistive technology has the potential to transform human cognitive potential in ways
that were previously unimaginable. We have seen just the tip of the iceberg as
voice recognition, for example, has many bugs still to be worked out. Thus, it is
imperative that practitioners and others with particular knowledge about neuropsychological functioning and learning have input into the development of assistive technology devices to assure their efficacy for persons with learning disabilities.

Finally, it is our contention that processes to foster cross-professional collaboration are needed in terms of both research and clinical practice. This can certainly be accomplished by organizations sponsoring national meetings and
workshops and by organizations collaborating at the national level to influence
policies that affect their constituent members across diagnostic categories. The
recent efforts at collaboration between C.H.A.D.D. and the national organization
of Community Mental Health Centers is an example of efforts to reach out for
mutual benefit and with a stronger voice to federal agencies and policy makers,
as is C.H.A.D.D.'s effort to engage and utilize a multidisciplinary professional
advisory board. The various professional journals might also reach out in spe-

cial issues to bring a multidisciplinary focus to a topic with researchers and practitioners exchanging perspectives in a real effort to learn from each other vs. advocating a singular point of view. The field of learning disabilities in general has suffered to some degree from an adherence to narrowly prescribed theories, supporting research studies that reflect that narrow focus, and at times a lack of openness by some practitioners to a research and knowledge base outside of their respective domains of expertise. This remains a danger always in fields of study where passions run high. And in the words of Alexander Pope, "What reason weaves, by passion is undone" (*An Essay on Man II*). Let this be a caution for all of us, clinician and researcher alike. We would like to believe that this is some of what we have come to understand in producing this work.

REFERENCES

Aaron, P. G., Malatesha, J., & Williams, K. (1999). Not all reading disabilities are alike. *Journal of Learning Disabilities, 32*(2), 120-137.

Abbott, J. (1987). *Accessing vocational education and vocational rehabilitation training and employment programs.* Paper presented at the ACLD International Conference, San Antonio, TX.

Abbott, R., & Berninger, V. (1993). Structural equation modeling of relationships among developmental skills and writing skills in primary and intermediate grade writers. *Journal of Educational Psychology, 85*, 478-508.

Achenbach, T. M. (1991). *Manual for the child behavior checklist/4-18 and 1991 profile.* Burlington, VT: University of Vermont Department of Psychiatry.

Achenbach, T. M., & Edelbrock, C. S. (1981). Behavioral problems and competencies reported by parents of normal and disturbed children aged 4 through 16. *Monographs of the Society for Research and Child Development, 46*, 1-82.

Ackerman, P. T., Anhalt, J. M., Dykman, R. A., & Holcomb, P. J. (1986). Effortful processing deficits in children with reading and/or attention disorders. *Brain and Cognition, 5*, 22-40.

Ackerman, P. T., Anhalt, J. M., & Dykman, R. A. (1986). Arithmetic automatization failure in children with attention and reading disorders: Associations and sequilae. *Journal of Learning Disabilities, 19*, 222-232.

Adams, M. J. (1990). *Beginning to read: Thinking and learning about print.* Cambridge, MA: MIT Press.

Adelman, H. S., & Taylor, L. (1986). The problems of definition and differentiation and the need for a classification schema. *Journal of Learning Disabilities, 19*(9), 514-520.

Akshoomoff, N. S., & Courchesne, E. (1992). A new role for the cerebellum in cognitive operations. *Behavioral Neuroscience, 43*, 613-622.

Alexander, G. E., DeLong, M. R., & Strick, P. (1986). Parallel organization of functionally segrated circuits linking basal ganglia and cortex. *Annual Review of Neuroscience, 9*, 357-381.

Alster, E. H. (1997). The effects of extended time on algebra test scores for college students with and without learning disabilities. *Journal of Learning Disabilities, 30*, 222-227.

Amen, A. J., Johnson, S., & Amen, D. G. (1996). *A teenager's guide to ADD.* Fairfield, CA: MindWorks Press.

Amen, D. G. (1997). *Windows into the A.D.D. mind: Understanding and treating attention deficit disorders in the everyday lives of children, adolescents and adults.* Fairfield, CA: MindWorks Press.

Amen, D. G., & Goldman, B. (1998). Attention-Deficit Disorder: A guide for primary care physicians. *Primary Psychiatry, July.*

Amen, D. G., Paldi, J. H., & Thisted, R. A. (1993). Brain SPECT imaging. *Journal of the American Academy of Child and Adolescent Psychiatry, 32*, 1080-1081.

American Psychiatric Association. (1968). *Diagnostic and statistical manual of mental disorders* (2nd Ed.). Washington, DC: Author.

American Psychiatric Association. (1980). *Diagnostic and statistical manual of mental disorders* (3rd Ed.). Washington, DC: Author.

American Psychiatric Association. (1987). *Diagnostic and statistical manual of mental disorders* (3rd Ed., Rev.). Washington, DC: Author.

American Psychiatric Association. (1994). *Diagnostic and statistical manual of mental disorders* (4th Ed.). Washington, DC: Author.

Americans with Disabilities Act (ADA). (1990). P.L. 101-336, 42 U.S.C. 1201 et seq.

Anderson, J. C., Williams, S., McGee, R., & Silva, P. A. (1987). DSM-III disorders in preadolescent children: Prevalence in a large sample from the general population. *Arch General Psychiatry, 44,* 69-76.

Applegate, B., Lahey, B. B., Hart, E. L., Waldman, I., Biderman, J., Hynd, G. W., Barkley, R. A., Ollendick, T., Frick, P. J., Greenhill, L., McBurnett, K., Newcorn, J., Kerdyk, L., Garfinkel, B., & Shaffer, D. (1995). *The age of onset for DSM-IV attention-deficit-hyperactivity disorder: A report of the DSM-IV field trials. .*

Arnold, L. E. (1999). Treatment alternatives for attention-deficit/hyperactivity disorder (ADHD). *Journal of Attention Disorders, 3*(1), 30-48.

Arnsten, A. F. T., Steere, J. C., & Hunt, R. D. (1996). The contribution of alpha 2 noradrenergic mechanisms to prefrontal cortical cognitive functions: potential significance to Attention-Deficit Hyperactivity Disorder. *Archives of General Psychiatry, 53,* 448-455.

Asberger, H. (1979). Problems of infantile autism. *Communication, 13,* 45-52.

Auchenbach, T. M. (1991). *The Child Behavior Checklist - 1991.* Burlington, VT: Department of Psychiatry.

Bachevalier, J. (1991). Memory loss and socio-emotional disturbances following neonatal damage of the limbic system in monkeys: An animal model for childhood autism. In C. A. Tamminga & S. C. Schultz (Eds.), *Advances in psychiatry* (Vol. 1, pp. 129-140). New York: Raven Press.

Baddeley, A. D. (1986). *Working memory.* New York: Oxford University Press.

Badian, N., McAnulty, G. B., Duffy, F. H., & Als, H. (1990). Prediction of dyslexia in kindergarten boys. *Annals of Dyslexia, 40,* 159-169.

Baird, J., Stevenson, J. C., & Williams, D. C. (2000). The evolution of ADHD: A disorder of communication? *Quarterly Review of Biology, 75,* 1-21.

Bakwin, H. (1973). Reading disability in twins. *Developmental Medicine and Child Neurology, 15,* 184-187.

Baltaxe, C. A. M. (1977). Pragmatic deficits in the language of autistic adolescents. *Journal of Pediatric Psychology, 2,* 176-180.

Baltaxe, C. A. M., & Simmons, J. Q. (1975). Language in childhood psychosis: A review. *Journal of Speech and Hearing Disorders, 40,* 439-458.

Barkley, R. (1993). *Attention deficit hyperactivity disorder: Workshop manual.* Worcester, MA: Author.

Barkley, R. (1994). Impaired delayed responding: A unified theory of attention deficit hyperactivity disorder. In D. K. Routh (Ed.), *Disruptive behavior disorders in childhood* (pp. 11-57). New York: Plenum Press.

Barkley, R. A. (1977). A review of stimulant drug research with hyperactive children. *Journal of Child Psychology and Psychiatry, 18,* 137-165.

Barkley, R. A. (1981). *Hyperactive children: A handbook for diagnosis and treatment.* New York: Guilford Press.

Barkley, R. A. (1990). *Attention Deficit Hyperactivity Disorder: A Handbook for Diagnosis and Treatment.* New York: Guilford Press.

Barkley, R. A. (1991). The ecological validity of laboratory and analogue assessment methods of ADHD symptoms. *Journal of Abnormal Child Psychology, 19*(2), 149-178.

Barkley, R. A. (1994a). Can neuropsychological tests help diagnose ADD/ADHD? *The ADHD Report, 2*(1), 1-3.

Barkley, R. A. (1994b). The assessment of attention in children. In R. G. Lyon (Ed.), *Frames of reference for the assessment of learning disabilities* (pp. 69-102). Baltimore, MD: Paul H. Brookes.

Barkley, R. A. (1997). Behavioral inhibition, sustained attention, and executive functions: Constructing a unifying theory of ADHD. *Psychology Bulletin, 121,* 65-94.

Barkley, R. A. (1997a). *ADHD and the nature of self-control.* New York: Guilford Press.

Barkley, R. A. (1997b). Behavioral inhibition, sustained attention, and executive functions: Constructing a unifying theory of ADHD. *Psychological Bulletin, 121*(1), 65-94.

Barkley, R. A., Duple, G. J., & McMurray, M. B. (1990). Comprehensive evaluation of Attention Deficit Disorder with and without hyperactivity as defined by research criteria. *Journal of Consulting Clinical Psychology, 58,* 775-789.

Barkley, R. A., Fischer, M., Edelbrock, C. S., & Smallish, L. (1990). The adolescent outcome of hyperactive children diagnosed by research criteria: An 8 year prospective follow-up study. *Journal of the American Academy of Child and Adolescent Psychiatry, 29,* 546-557.

Barkley, R. A., Murphy, K., & Kwasnik, D. (1996). Psychological adjustment and adaptive impairments in young adults with ADHD. *Journal of Attention Disorders, 1,* 41-54.

Barrouillet, P., Fayol, M., & Lathuliere, E. (1997). Selecting between competitors in multiplication tasks: An explanation of the errors produced by adolescents with learning disabilities. *International Journal of Behavioral Development, 21,* 253-275.

Bartak, L., & Rutter, M. (1976). Differences between mentally retarded and normally intelligent autistic children. *Journal of Autism and Childhood Schizophrenia, 126,* 127-145.

Baselt, R. C. (1982). *Disposition of toxic drugs and chemicals in man.* (2nd ed.). Davis, CA: Biomedical Publications.

Bassett, D. S., Polloway, E. A., & Patton, J. R. (1993). Learning disabilities: Perspective on adulthood. In P. J. Gerber & H. B. Reiff (Eds.), *Learning disabilities in adulthood: Persisting problems and evolving issues .* Boston, MA: Andover Medical.

Basso, A., Taborelli, A. M., & Vignolo, L. A. (1978). Dissociated disorders of speaking and writing in aphasia. *Journal of Neurology, Neurosurgery, and Psychiatry, 41,* 556-563.

Bauermeister, J. (1992). Factor analyses of teacher ratings of attention-deficit hyperactivity and oppositional defiant symptoms in children aged four through thirteen years. *Journal of Clinical Child Psychology, 21,* 27-34.

Bauman, M. L. (1992). Motor dysfunction in autism. In A. B. Joseph & R. R. Young (Eds.), *Movement disorders in neurology and neuropsychiatry* (pp. 659-661). Boston, MA: Blackwell Scientific.

Bauman, M. L., & Kemper, T. L. (1985). Histoanatomic observations of the brain in early infantile autism. *Neurology, 35,* 866-874.

Beasley, G. F. (1996). Learning disabilities in the workplace. In S. C. Cramer & W. Ellis (Eds.), *Learning disabilities: Lifelong issues* (pp. 141-144). Baltimore, MD: Paul H. Brookes.

Beck, A. T., Steer, R. A., & Brown, G. K. (1996). *Beck depression inventory.* (2nd ed.). San Antonio, TX: Psychological Corporation.

Beers, S. R. (1993). Neuropsychological profiles of college students having learning problems: A comparison of students with a history of mild head injury and students with learning disabilities. *Dissertation Abstracts International, 53*(9-B), 4943-4944.

Beers, S. R. (1998). Rehabilitation assessment and planning for children and adults with learning disabilities. In G. Goldstein & S. Beers (Eds.), *Rehabilitation* (pp. 201-228). New York: Plenum Press.

Beers, S. R. (2000). Cognitive profiles of high and low functioning adults with learning disability. In R. L. Mapou (Ed.), *They don't go away: Research and perspectives* on *adult learning disabilities*. Denver, CO: International Neuropsychological Society.

Beers, S. R., Goldstein, G., & Katz, L. J. (1994). Neuropsychological differences between college students with learning disabilities and those with mild head injury. *Journal of Learning Disability, 27*, 315-324.

Beers, S. R., Goldstein, G., & Katz, L. J. (2000). Cognitive profiles of high and low functioning adults with learning disability (LD). *Journal of the International Neuropsychological Society, 6*, 210.

Beilke, J. R., & Yssel, N. (1999). The chilly climate for students with disabilities in higher education. *College Student Journal, 33*, 364-371.

Bellak, L., & Black, R. B. (1992). Attention deficit hyperactivity disorder in adults. *Clinical Therapeutics, 14*, 138-147.

Bender, W. N. (1997). *Understanding ADHD, A Practical Guide for Teachers and Parents*. Trenton, NJ:: Prentice-Hall.

Bender, W. N., Rosenkrans, C. B., & Crane, M. K. (1999). Stress, depression, and suicide among students with learning disabilities: Assessing the risks. *Learning Disability Quarterly, 22*, 143-156.

Benjamin, J., Patterson, C., Greenberg, B. D., Murphy, D. L., & Hamer, D. H. (1996). Population and familial association between the D4 dopamine receptor gene and measures of novelty seeking. *Nature Genet, 12*, 81-84.

Benson, D. F. (1991). The role of frontal dysfunction in attention deficit hyperactivity disorder. *Journal of Child Neurology, 6*(S), S9-S12.

Berger, H. (1926). Ueber rechenstoerungen bei herderkrankungen des grosshirns [On arithmetic problems of focal diseases of the cerebrum]. *Arch Fuer Psychiatrie, 78*, 238-263.

Berninger, V. (1994). *Reading and Writing Acquisition: A Developmental Neuropsychological Perspective*. Madison, WI: WCB Brown & Benchmark.

Berninger, V., & Hart, T. (1992). A developmental neuropsychological perspective for reading and writing acquisition. *Educational Psychologist, 27*, 415-434.

Berninger, V. W. (1994). Future directions for research on writing disabilities: Integrating endogenous and exogenous variables. In G. R. Lyon (Ed.), *Frames of reference for the assessment of learning disabilities: New views on measurement issues* (pp. 419-439). Baltimore, MD: Paul H. Brookes.

Berninger, V. W. (1996). Coordinating transcription and text generation in working memory during composing: Automatic and construction processes. *Learning Disability Quarterly, 22*, 99-112.

Berninger, V. W., & Abbott, R. D. (1994). Redefining learning disabilities: Moving beyond aptitude-achievement discrepancies to failure to respond to validated treatment protocols. In G. R. Lyon (Ed.), *Frames of reference for the assessment of learning disabilities: New views on measurement issues* (pp. 163-184). Baltimore, MD: Paul H. Brookes.

Berninger, V. W., & Fuller, F. (1992). Gender differences in orthographic verbal, and compositional fluency: Implications for assessing writing disabilities in primary grade children. *Journal of School Psychology, 30*, 363-382.

Berninger, V. W., Fuller, F., & Whitaker, D. (1996). A process approach to writing development across the life span. *Educational Psychology Review, 8*, 193-218.

Berninger, V. W., & Hart, T. (1993). From research to clinical assessment of reading and writing disorders: The unit of analysis problem. In R. M. Joshi & C. K. Leong (Eds.), *Reading disabilities: Diagnosis and component processes* (pp. 33-61). Amsterdam: Kluwer Academic Publishers.

Berninger, V. W., Mizokawa, D. T., & Bragg, R. (1991). Theory-based diagnosis and remediation of writing disabilities. *Journal of School Psychiatry, 29*, 257-280.

Berry, C. A., Shaywitz, S. E., & Shaywitz, B. A. (1985). Girls with attention deficit disorder: A silent majority? *Pediatrics, 76*, 801-809.

Biederman, J., Faraone, S., Milberger, S., Curtis, S., Chen, L., & et al. (1996). Predictors of persistence and remission of ADHD into adolescence: Results from a four-year prospective follow-up study. *Journal of the American Academy of Child and Adolescent Psychiatry, 35,* 343-351.

Biederman, J., Faraone, S. V., Keenan, K., Benjamin, J., Krifcher, B., & et al. (1992). Further evidence for family-genetic risk factors in attention deficit hyperactivity disorder. *Archives of General Psychiatry, 49,* 728-738.

Biederman, J., Faraone, S. V., Keenan, K., Knee, D., & Tsuang, M. T. (1990). Family-genetic and psychosocial risk factors in DSM-III attention deficit disorder. *Journal of American Academy of Child and Adolescent Psychiatry, 29,* 526-533.

Biederman, J., Faraone, S. V., Spencer, T., Wilens, T., Mick, E., & Lapey, K. S. (1994). Gender differences in a sample of adults with attention deficit hyperactivity disorder. *Psychiatry Research, 53,* 13-29.

Biederman, J., Faraone, S. V., Spencer, T., Wilens, T., Norman, D., Lapey, K. S., Mick, E., Krifcher Lehman, B., & Doyle, A. (1993). Patterns of psychiatric comorbidity, cognition, and psychosocial functioning in adults with attention deficit hyperactivity disorder. *American Journal of Psychiatry, 150*(12), 1792-1798.

Biederman, J., Milberger, S., Faraone, S. V., Kiely, K., & et al. (1995). Impact of adversity on functioning and comorbidity in children with attention-deficit hyperactivity disorder. *Journal of the American Academy of Child and Adolescent Psychiatry, 34,* 1495-1503.

Biederman, J., Newcorn, J., & Sprich, S. (1991). Comorbidity of attention deficit hyperactivity disorder with conduct, depressive anxiety, and other disorders. *American Journal of Psychiatry, 148,* 564-577.

Biederman, J., Russell, R., Soriano, J., Wozniak, J., & Faraone, S. V. (1998). Clinical features of children with both ADHD and mania: Does ascertainment source make a difference? *Journal of Affective Disorders, 51,* 101-112.

Biederman, J., & Spencer, T. (1999). Attention-deficit/hyperactivity disorder (ADHD) as a noradrenergic disorder. *Biological Psychiatry, 46,* 124-1242.

Biederman, J., Wilens, T., Mick, E., Milberger, S., Spencer, T. J., & Faraone, S. V. (1995). Psychoactive substance use disorders in adults with attention deficit hyperactivity disorder (ADHD): Effects of ADHD and psychiatric comorbidity. *American Journal of Psychiatry, 152,* 1652-1658.

Bigler, E. D. (1989). On the neuropsychology of suicide. *Journal of Learning Disabilities, 22,* 180-185.

Bigler, E. D. (1992). The neurobiology and neuropsychology of adult learning disorders. *Journal of Learning Disabilities, 25*(8), 488-506.

Bigler, E. D., Lajiness-O'Neill, R., & Howes, N. L. (1988). Technology in the assessment of learning disability. *Journal of Learning Disabilities, 31*(1), 67-82.

Bird, H. R., Canino, G., Rubio-Stipec, M., Gould, M. s., Ribera, J., Sesman, M., & et al. (1988). Estimates of the prevalence of childhood maladjustment in a community survey in Puerto Rico. *Archives of General Psychiatry, 45,* 1120-1126.

Bird, H. R., Gould, M. S., & Staghezza, B. M. (1993). Patterns of diagnostic comorbidity in a community sample of children aged 9 through 16 years. *Journal of the American Academy of Child and Adolescent Psychiatry, 32,* 361-368.

Bireley, M. (1995). *Crossover children.* Reston, VA: Council for Exceptional Children.

Blackorby, J., & Wagner, M. M. (1997). The employment of outcomes of youth with learning disabilities: A review of findings from the national longitudinal transition study of special education students. In P. J. Gerber & D. S. Brown (Eds.), *Learning Disabilities and Employment.* Austin, TX: Pro-Ed.

Blalock, J. (1981). Persistent problems and concerns of young adults with learning disabilities. In W. Cruickshank & A. Silver (Eds.), *Bridges to tomorrow: The best of ACLD* (Vol. 2, pp. 35-55). Syracuse, NY: Syracuse University Press.

Blalock, J. (1982). Persistent auditory language deficits in adults with learning disabilities. *Journal of Learning Disabilities, 15*(10), 604-609.

Blalock, J. W. (1987). Persistent problems and concerns of young adults with learning disabilities. In D. Johnson & J. W. Blalock (Eds.), *Adults with learning disability* (pp. 35-55). New York: Grune & Stratton.

Blouin, A., Bornstein, R., & Trites, R. (1978). Teenage alcohol use among hyperactive children: A five-year follow-up study. *Journal Pediatric Psychology, 3,* 188-194.

Boder, E. (1970). Developmental dyslexia: A new diagnostic approach based on the identification of three subtypes. *The Journal of School Health, 40,* 289-290.

Boder, E. (1973). Developmental dyslexia: A diagnostic approach based on three atypical reading-spelling patterns. *Developmental Medicine and Child Neurology, 15,* 663-687.

Boder, E., & Jarrico, S. (1982). The Boder Test of Reading-Spelling Patterns: A Diagnostic Screening Test for Subtypes of Reading Disability . New York: Grune and Stratton.

Bolden-Watson, C., & Richelson, E. (1993). Blockage by newly developed antidepressants of biogenic amine uptake into rat brain synaptosomes. *Life Science, 52,* 1023-1029.

Boreland, B. L., & Heckman, H. K. (1976). Hyperactive boys and their brothers. *Archives of General Psychiatry, 33,* 669-675.

Boucher, J. (1981). Memory for recent events in autistic children. *Journal of Autism and Developmental Disorders, 11,* 293-302.

Boucher, J., & Lewis, V. (1989). Memory impairments and communication in relatively stable autistic children. *Journal of Child Psychology and Psychiatry, 30,* 99-122.

Boucher, J., & Warrington, E. K. (1976). Memory deficits in early infantile autism: Some similarities to the amnesic syndrome. *British Journal of Psychology, 67,* 73-87.

Bourke, A. B., Strehorn, K. C., & Silver, P. (2000). Faculty members' provision of instructional accommodations to students with LD. *Journal of Learning Disabilities, 33,* 26-32.

Bradley, C. (1937). The behavior of children receiving Benzedrine. *American Journal of Psychiatry, 94,* 577-588.

Bradley, L., & Bryant, P. (1978). Difficulties in auditory organization as a possible cause of reading backwardness. *Nature, 271,* 746-747.

Bradley, L., & Bryant, P. (1983). Categorizing sounds and learning to read - a casual connection. *Nature, 310,* 419-421.

Brady, S., & Shankweiler, D. (Eds.). (1991). *Phonological Processes in Literacy: A Tribute to Isabelle Y. Liberman.* Hillsdale, NJ: Earlbaum.

Brandys, C. F., & Rourke, B. P. (1991). Differential memory abilities in reading- and arithmetic-disabled children. In B. P. Rourke (Ed.), *Neuropsychological validation of learning disability subtypes* (pp. 73-96). New York: Guilford Press.

Breen, M. J. (1989). Cognitive and behavioral differences in ADHD in boys and girls. *Journal of Child Psychology and Psychiatry, 30,* 711-716.

Brinckerhoff, L., Shaw, S., & McGuire, J. M. (1993). *Promoting postsecondary education for students with learning disabilities.* Austin, TX: Pro-Ed.

Brinckerhoff, L. C., Dempsesy, K. M., Jordan, C., Keiser, S. R., McGuire, J. M., Pompian, N. W., & Russell, L. H. (1998). *Guidelines for documentation of attention-deficit/hyperactivity disorder in adolescents and adults* : Consortium on ADHD Documentation.

Brinckerhoff, S. C., Shaw, S. F., & McGuire, J. M. (1996). Promoting access, accommodations, and independence for college students with learning disabilities. In J. R. Patton & E. A. Pollock (Eds.), *Learning disabilities: The challenge of adulthood.* Austin, TX: Pro-Ed.

Bronowski, J. (1967). *Human and animal languages. To Honor Roman Jakobson.* (Vol. 1). The Hague, Netherlands: Mouton & Cox.

Brook, S. L., & Bowler, D. M. (1992). Autism by another name? Semantic and pragmatic impairments in children. *Journal of Autism and Developmental Disorders, 22*, 61-81.

Brown, A. L. (1980). Metacognitive development and reading. In R. J. Spiro, B.Bruce, & W. E. Brewer (Eds.), *Theoretical issues in reading comprehension*. Hillsdale, NJ: Lawrence Earlbaum.

Brown, D. *Counseling and accommodating the student with learning disabilities*. Washington, DC: President's Committee on Employment of the Handicapped.

Brown, D., & Gerber, P. J. (1993). Employing people with learning disabilities. In P. J. Gerber & H. B. Reiff (Eds.), *Learning disabilities in adulthood: Persisting problems and evolving issues* (pp. 194-203). Boston, MA: Andover.

Brown, J. I., Fishco, V. V., & Hanna, G. (1993). *Nelson Denny Reading Test*. Chicago, IL: Riverside Publishing Company.

Brown, J. J., Bennett, J. M., & Hanna, G. (1981). The Nelson-Denny Reading Test . Chicago, IL: Riverside Publishing Company.

Brown, T. E. (1996). *Brown attention-deficit disorder scales*. San Antonio, TX: The Psychological Corporation.

Brown, V. L., Cronin, M. E., & McEntire, E. (1994). *Test of mathematical abilities*. Austin, TX: Pro-Ed.

Bruck, M. (1986). Social and emotional adjustments of learning disabled children. In S. Ceci (Ed.), *Handbook of cognitive social, neuropsychological aspects of learning disabilities* (Vol. 1, pp. 361-380). Hillsdale, NJ: Lawrence Earlbaum.

Bruck, M. (1987). The adult outcomes of children with learning disabilities. *Annals of Dyslexia, 37*, 252-263.

Bruck, M. (1990). Word recognition skills of adults with childhood diagnoses of dyslexia. *Developmental Psychology, 26*(439-454).

Bruck, M. (1992). Persistence of dyslexia's phonological awareness deficits. *Developmental Psychology, 28*(5), 874-886.

Bruck, M. (1993). Component spelling skills of college students with childhood diagnosis of dyslexia. *Learning Disability Quarterly, 26*, 171-184.

Bruck, M., & Waters, G. (1988). An analysis of the spelling errors of children who differ in their reading and spelling skills. *Applied Psycholinguistics, 9*, 77-92.

Bryson, S. E., Wainright-Sharp, J. A., & Smith, I. M. (1990). Autism: A developmental spatial neglect syndrome? In J. Enns (Ed.), *The development of attention: Research and theory* (pp. 405-427). Amsterdam: Elsevier.

Buchanan, M., & Wolf, J. S. (1986). A comprehensive study of learning disabled adults. *Journal of Learning Disabilities, 19*, 34-38.

Burack, J. A. (1994). Selective attention deficits in persons with autism: Preliminary evidence of an inefficient lens. *Journal of Abnormal Psychology, 103*, 535-543.

Burack, J. A., Enns, J. T., & Johannes, E. A. (1997). Attention and autism: Behavioral and Electrophysiological Evidence. In D. J. Cohen & F. R. Volkmar (Eds.), *Handbook of autism and pervasive developmental disorders* (2nd ed., pp. 226-247). New York: John Wiley and Sons, Inc.

Burack, J. A., & Iarocci, G. (1995). *Visual filtering and covert orienting in autism*. Paper presented at the Society for Research in Child Development, Indianapolis, IN.

Burenstein, B. (1995). *Giving voice to student writing: Exploring the uses of speech recognition and speech synthesis in a writing curriculum: Activities for word processing* (ERIC Document Reproduction Service No. ED395110).

Bursuck, W. D., Rose, E., Cowens, & Yamaya, M. A. (1989). Nationwide survey of postsecondary education services for students with learning disabilities. *Exceptional Children, 56*, 236-245.

Buschsbaum, M. S., Haler, R. J., Sostek, A. J., Weingertner, H., & et al. (1985). Attention dysfunction and psychopathology in college men. *Archives of General Psychiatry, 42*, 354-360.

Cantwell, D. P. (1975). Genetics of hyperactivity. *Journal of Child Psychology Psychiatry, 16*, 261-264.

Cantwell, D. P., & Baker, L. (1991). Association between Attention-Deficit-Hyperactivity Disorder and learning disorders. *Journal of Learning Disabilities, 24*(2), 88-95.

Carey, M. P., Diewald, L. M., Esposity, F. J., & et al. (1998). Differential distribution, affinity and plasticity of dopamine D-1 and D-2 receptors in the target sites of the mesolimbic system in an animal model of ADHD. *Behav Brain Res, 94*, 173-185.

Carlson, C. L., Lahey, B. B., & Neeper, R. (1986). Direct assessment of the cognitive correlates of attention deficit disorders with and without hyperactivity. *Journal of Psychopathology and Behavioral Assessment, 8*, 69-86.

Carroll, C. B., & Ponterotto, J. B. (1998). Employment counseling for adults with attention-deficit/hyperactivity disorder: Issues without answers. *Journal of Employment Counseling, 35*, 79-95.

Casey , J. E., Rourke, B. P., & Picard, E. M. (1991). Syndrome of nonverbal learning disabilities: Age differences in neuropsychological, academic, and socioemotional functioning. *Development and Psychopathology, 3*, 329-345.

Casey, B. J., Castellanos, F. X., Giedd, J. N., Marsh, W. L., & et al. (1997). Implication of right frontostriatal circuitry in response inhibition and attention-deficit/hyperactivity disorder. *Journal American Academy Child and Adolescent Psychiatry, 36*, 374-383.

Casey, B. J., Gordon, C. T., Mannheim, G. B., & Rumsey, J. M. (1993). Dysfunctional attention in autistic savants. *Journal of Clinical and Experimental Neuropsychology, 15*, 933-946.

Casstellanos, F. X., Giedd, J. N., March, W. L., & et al. (1996). Quantitative brain magnetic resonance imaging in attention-deficit hyperactivity disorder. *Archives of General Psychiatry, 53*, 607-616.

Castellanos, F. X. (1997). Toward a pathophysiology of attention-deficit/hyperactivity disorder. *Clinical Pediatrics, 36*, 381-393.

Castellanos, F. X., Giedd, J. N., Eckburg, P., March, W. L., & et al. (1994). Quantitative morphology of the caudate nucleus in attention deficit hyperactivity disorder. *American Journal of Psychiatry, 151*, 1791-1796.

Cawley, J. F., & Miller, J. H. (1989). Cross-sectional comparisons of the mathematical performance of children with learning disabilities: Are we on the right track toward comprehensive programming? *Journal of Learning Disabilities, 22*, 250-259.

Cazden, C. B. (1992). *Whole language plus: Essays on literacy in the United States and New Zealand*. New York: Teachers College Press.

Chandola, C. A., Robling, M. R., Peters, T. J., Melville-Thomas, G., & McGuffin, P. (1992). Pre- and perinatal factors and the risk of subsequent referral for hyperactivity. *Journal of Child Psychology and Psychiatry, 33*, 1077-1090.

Chase, C. H., & Tallal, P. (1991). Cognitive models of developmental reading disorders. In J. E. Obrzut & G. W. Hynd (Eds.), *Neuropsychological foundations of learning disabilities* (pp. 199-240). San Diego, CA: Academic Press.

Chruch, R. P., Fessler, M. A., & Bender, M. (1998). Diagnosis and remediation of dyslexia. In B. K. Shapiro, P. J. Accardo, & A. J. Capute (Eds.), *Specific Reading Disability: A View of the Spectrum*. Timonium, MD: York Press.

Clark, D. B., & Uhry, J. K. (1995). *Dyslexia: Theory and Practice of Remedial Instruction*. (2nd ed.). Baltimore, MD: York Press.

Clearinghouse on Adult Education and Literacy. (!989). *Instructional strategies for adults with learning disabilities*. Washington, DC: Division of Adult Education and Literacy, U. S. Department of Education.

Cleaver, R. L., & Whitman, R. D. (1998). Right hemisphere, white-matter learning disabilities associated with depression in adolescent and young adult psychiatric population. *Journal of Nervous and Mental Disease, 186*, 561-565.

Cohen, J. (1957). Factor analytically based rationale for Wechsler Adult Intelligence Scale. *Journal of Consulting Psychology, 21*, 451-457.

Cohen, R. M., Semple, W. E., Gross, M., & et al. (1988). Functional localization of sustained attention: Comparison to sensory stimulation in the absence of instruction. *Neuropsych Neuropsychol Behav Neurol, 1*, 3-20.

Coldman-Rakic, P. A. (1987). Circuitry of primate prefrontal cortex and regulation of behavior by representational memory. In F. Plum (Ed.), *handbook of physiology, the nervous system, higher functions of the brain* (pp. 373-417). Bethesda, MD: American Physiological Society.

Coleman, S., & Sussman, S. (1996). *The four S's: A comprehensive program for coaching people with ADD.* .

Coles, G. (1978). The learning-disabilities test battery: Empirical and social issues. *Harvard Educational Review, 48*, 313-340.

Coles, G. (1987). *The learning mystique.* New York: Pantheon Books.

Comings, D. E., & Comings, B. G. (1988). Tourette's syndrome and attention deficit disorder. In D. J. Cohen, R. D. Bruun, & J. F. Leckman (Eds.), *Tourette's syndrome and tic disorders: Clinical understanding and treatment* (pp. 120-135). New York: John Wiley and Sons.

Comings, D. E., & Comings, B. G. (1990). A controlled family history of Tourette's Syndrome, I: Attention-deficit hyperactivity disorder and learning disorders. *Journal of Clinical Psychiatry, 51*(7), 275-280.

Comings, D. E., Wu, S., Chiu, C., Ring, R. H., Gade, R., & et al. (1996). Polygenic inheritance of Tourette syndrome, stuttering, attention deficit hyperactivity, conduct and oppositional defiant disorder: the additive and subtractive effect of the three dopaminergic genes – DRD2, DbH, and DAT1. *American Journal of Medical Genetics, 67*, 264-288.

Connors, K. C., Erhrdt, D., & Sparrow, E. (1999). *Conners' adult ADHD rating scales (CAARS).* Odessa, FL: Psychological Assessment Resources, Inc.

Cook, E. H., Stein, M. A., Krasowski, M. D., Cox, N. J., Olkon, D. M., Kieffer, J. E., & Leventhal, B. L. (1995). Association of Attention-Deficit disorder and the dopamine transporter gene. *American Journal of Human Genetics, 56*, 993-998.

Copeland, E. D., & Copps, S. C. (1995). *Medications for attention disorders and related medical problems.* Plantation, FL: Specialty Press, Inc.

Corbett, B., & Stanczak, D. E. (1999). Neuropsychological performance of adults evidencing attention-deficit hyperactivity disorder. *Archives of Clinical Neuropsychology, 14*, 373-387.

Corcos, E., & Willows, D. M. (1993). The processing of orthographic information. In D. M. Willows, R. S. Kruk, & E. Corcos (Eds.), *Visual processes in reading and reading disabilities* (pp. 163-190). Hillsdale, NJ: Earlbaum Associates, Inc.

Courchesne, E., Akshoomoff, N. A., Townsend, J., & Saitoh, O. (1995). A model system for the study of attention and the cerebellum: Infantile autism. *Electroencephalography and Clinical Neurophysiology - Supplement, 44*, 315-352.

Courchesne, E., Townsend, J., Akshoomoff, N. A., Saitoh, O., Yeung-Courchesne, R., Lincoln, A. J., James, H. E., Haas, R. H., & Lau, L. (1994). Impairment in shifting attention in autistic and cerebellar patients. *Behavioral Neuroscience, 108*, 848-865.

Courchesne, E., Townsend, J. P., Akshoomoff, N. A., Yeung-Courchesne, R., Press, G. A., Murakmi, J. W., Lincoln, A. J., James, H. E., Saitoh, O., Egaas, B., Haas, R. H., & Schriebman, L. (1993). A new finding: Impairment in shifting of attention in autistic and cerebellar patients. In S. H. Broman & J. Grafman (Eds.), *Atypical deficits in developmental disorders: Implications for brain function.* New Jersey: Lawrence Earlbaum Associates.

Cox, B. A. (1985). Alphabetic phonics: An organization and expansion of Orton-Gillingham. *Annals of Dyslexia, 35*, 187-198.

Critchley, M. (1928). *Mirror-writing.* London: Paul Trench Trubner.

Critchley, M. (1964). *Developmental dyslexia.* Springfield, IL: Charles C. Thomas.

Critchley, M. (1970). *The dyslexic child.* (2nd ed.). London: William Heinemann.

Critchley, M. (1973). Some problems of the ex-dyslexic. *Bulletin of the Orton Society, 23*, 7-14.

Cruickshank, B. M., Eliason, M., & Merrifield, B. (1988). Long-term sequelae of cold water near-drowning. *Journal of Pediatric Psychology, 13*, 379-388.

Daneman, M., & Carpenter, P. A. (1980). Individual differences in working memory and reading. *Journal of Verbal Learning and Verbal Behavior, 19*, 450-466.

David Allen & Company. www.davidco.com

Dawson, G., & Lewy, A. (1989). Arousal, attention and the socioemotional impairments of individuals with autism. In G. Dawson (Ed.), *Autism: Nature, diagnosis, and treatment* (pp. 144-173). New York: Guilford Press.

De La Paz, S. (1999). Composing via dictation and speech recognition systems: Compensatory technology for students with learning disabilities. *Learning Disability Quarterly, 22*, 173-82.

De La Paz, S., & Graham, S. (1995). Dictation: Applications to writing for students with learning disabilities. In T. E. Scruggs & M. A. Mastropieri (Eds.), *Advances in learning and behavioral disabilities* (Vol. 9, pp. 227-247). Greenwich, CT: JAI Press.

DeFries, J. C., Olson, R. K., Pennington, B. F., & Smith, S. D. (1991). Colorado reading project: An update. In D. D. Duane & D. B. Gray (Eds.), *The Reading Program* (pp. 53-87). Parkton, MD: York Press.

DeFries, J. D., Stevenson, J., Gillis, J., & Wadsworth, S. J. (1991). Genetic etiology of spelling deficits in the Colorado and London twin studies of reading disabilities. *Reading and Writing, 3*, 271-283.

Delis, D. C., Kramer, J. H., Kaplan, E., & Ober, B. A. (1987). *California Verbal Learning Test: Adult Version.* San Antonio, TX: Psychological Corporation.

Denckla, M. A. (1974). Development of motor coordination in normal children. *Developmental Medicine and Child Neurology, 16*, 729-741.

Denckla, M. B. (1978). Minimal brain dysfunction. In J. S. Chall & A. F. Mirsky (Eds.), *Education and the brain* (pp. 223-268). Chicago, IL: University of Chicago Press.

Denckla, M. B. (1979). Childhood learning disabilities. In K. M. Heilman & E. Valenstein (Eds.), *Clinical neuropsychology* (pp. 535-573). New York: Oxford University Press.

Denckla, M. B. (1983). The neuropsychology of social-emotional learning disability. *Archives of Neurology, 40*, 461-462.

Denckla, M. B. (1989). Executive function, the overlap between attention deficit hyperactivity and learning disabilities. *International Pediatrics, 4*, 155-160.

Denckla, M. B. (1993). The child with developmental disabilities grown up: Adult residual of childhood disorders. *Neurologic Clinics: Behavioral Neurology, 11*, 105-125.

Derogatis, L. R. (1994). *SCL-90-R.* Minneapolis, MN: National Computer Systems, Inc.

Deshler, D. D., & Lenz, B. K. (1989). The strategies instructional approach. *International Journal of Disability Development and Education, 36*, 203-224.

Deshler, D. D., & Schumaker, J. B. (1986). Learning strategies: An instructional alternative for low-achieving adolescents. *Exceptional Children, 52*(6), 583-590.

Diener, R. M. (1991). Toxicology of Ritalin. In L. L. Greenhill & B. B. Osman (Eds.), *Ritalin theory and patient management* (pp. 35-43). Larchmont, NY: Mary Ann Liebert.

Dixon, B. (1994). Research guidelines for selecting mathematics curriculum. *Effective School Practices, 13*(2), 47-55.

Doehring, D. G., & Hoshko, I. M. (1977). Classification of reading problems by the technique of factor analysis. *Cortex, 13*, 281-294.

Dooling-Litfin, J. K., & Rosen, L. A. (1997). Self-esteem in college students with a childhood history of attention deficit hyperactivity disorder. *Journal of College Student Psychotherapy, 11,* 69-83.

Douglas, V. I. (1972). Stop, look, and listen: The problem of sustained attention and impulse control in hyperactive and normal children. *Canadian Journal of Behavioral Science, 4,* 259-282.

Douglas, V. I. (1983). Attention and cognitive problems. In M. Rutter (Ed.), *Developmental neuropsychiatry* (pp. 282-329). New York: Guilford Press.

Dowdy, C. A., Smith, T. E. C., & Noewll, C. H. (1996). Learning disabilities and vocational rehabilitation. In J. R. Patton & E. A. Pollock (Eds.), *Learning disabilities: The challenge of adulthood* (pp. 61-70). Austin, TX: Pro-Ed.

Dowdy, C. A., Smith, T. E. C., & Nowell, C. H. (1992). Learning disabilities and vocational rehabilitation. *Journal of Learning Disabilities, 25*(7), 442-447.

Downey, K. K., Stelson, F. W., Pomerleau, O. F., & Giordani, B. (1997). Adult attention deficit hyperactivity disorder: Psychological test profiles in a clinical population. *Journal Nerv. Ment. Dis., 185,* 32-38.

Drewe, E. A. (1975). Go-no learning after frontal lobe lesions in humans. *Cortex, 11,* 8-16.

Duane, D. D. (1983). Neurobiological correlates of reading disorders. *Journal of Educational Research, 77*(1), 6-15.

Duane, D. D. (1991). Biological foundations of learning disabilities. In J. E. Obrzut & G. W. Hynd (Eds.), *Neuropsychological foundations of learning disabilities* (pp. 7-27). San Diego, CA: Academic Press.

Dunham, M. D., Multon, K. D., & Koller, J. R. (1999). A comparison of adult learning disability subtypes in the vocational rehabilitation system. *Rehabilitation Psychology, 44,* 249-265.

Dykman, R. A., & Ackerman, P. T. (1993). Behavioral subtypes of attention deficit disorder. *Exceptional Children, 60*(2), 132-141.

Easton, J., & Sherman, D. (1976). Somatic anxiety attacks and propranolol. *Arch Neurol, 33,* 689-691.

Ebstein, R. P., Novick, O., Umansky, R., & et al. (1996). Dopamine D4 receptor (D4DR) exon III poly-morphism associated with the human personality trait of novelty seeking. *Nature Genet, 12,* 78-80.

Eden, G. F., VanMeter, J. W., Rumsey, J. M., Maisog, J. M., Woods, R. P., & Zeffiro, T. A. (1996). Abnormal processing of visual motion in dyslexia revealed by functional brain imaging. *Nature, 382,* 66-69.

Educational Training Service (ETS). (1998). Policy Statement for Documentation of Attention-Deficit/Hyperactivity Disorder in Adolescents and Adults. Office of Disability Policy Educational Testing Service. Princeton, NJ.

Ehri, L. C. (1980). The role of orthographic images in learning printed words. In J. F. Kavanagh & R. L. Venezky (Eds.), *Orthography, reading, and dyslexia* (pp. 155-170). Baltimore, MD: University Park Press.

Eicheler, A. J., & Antelman, S. M. (1979). Sensitization to amphetamine and stress may involve nucleus accumbens and medial frontal cortex. *Brain Research, 176,* 412-416.

Elbert, J. C., & Seale, T. W. (1988). Complexity of the cognitive phenotype of an inherited form of learning disability. *Developmental Medicine and Child Neurology, 30,* 181-189.

Elbro, C., Nielsen, I., & Petersen, D. K. (1994). Dyslexia in adults: Evidence for deficits in non-word reading and in the phonological representation of lexical items. *Annals of Dyslexia, 44,* 205-227.

Elkind, J. (1998). Computer reading machines for poor readers. *Perspectives, 24*(2), 2-7.

Eme, R. F. (1992). Selective female affliction in development of disorders of childhood: A literature review. *Journal of Clinical Child Psychology, 21,* 354-364.

Emily Hall Tremaine Foudation. (1995). *Learning disabilities and the American public: A look at Americans' awareness and knowledge*. Washington, DC: Author.

Englert, C. S., & Mariage, T. V. (1991). Shared understandings: Structuring the writing experience through dialogue. *Journal of Learning Disabilities, 24*(6), 330-342.

Enns, J. T., & Akhtar, N. (1989). A developmental study of filtering in visual attention. *Child Development, 60*, 319-337.

Eno, L., & Woehlke, P. (1980). Diagnostic differences between educationally handicapped and learning disabled students. *Psychology in the Schools, 17*, 469-473.

Ernst, M., Liebenauer, L. L., Jons, P. H., King, A. C., Cohen, M. D., & Zametkin, A. J. (1994, October). *Sexual maturation and brain metabolism in ADHD and brain metabolism in ADHD and normal girls*. Paper presented at the 41st Annual Meeting of the American Academy of Child & Adolescent Psychiatry, New York.

Ernst, M., Liebenauer, L. L., King, C., Fitzgerald, G. A., Cohen, R. M., & Zametkin, A. J. (1994). Reduced brain metabolism in hyperactive girls. *Journal American Academy of Child & Adolescent Psychiatry, 33*, 858-868.

Faas, L. A., & D'Alonzo, B. J. (1990). WAIS-R scores as predictors of employment success and failure among adults with learning disabilities. *Journal of Learning Disabilities, 23*, 311-316.

Faigel, H. C. (1998). Changes in services for students with learning disabilities in the U.S. and Canadian medical schools, 1991 to 1997. *Academic Medicine, 73*, 1290-1293.

Faraone, S., & Beiderman, J. (1946b). Is attention deficit hyperactivity disorder familial? *Harvard Review Psychiatry, 1*, 271-287.

Faraone, S., & Biederman, J. (1946a). Genetics of attention-deficit hyperactivity disorder. *Child Adoles Psychiatric Clin North America, 3*, 285-302.

Faraone, S. V., Beiderman, J., Lehman, B. K., Keenan, K., & et al. (1993). Evidence of the independent familial transmission of attention deficit hyperactivity disorder and learning disabilities: Results from a family genetic study. *American Journal of Psychiatry, 150*, 891-895.

Faraone, S. V., & Biederman, J. (1997). Do attention deficit hyperactivity disorder and major depression share familial risk factors? *Journal of Nervous and Mental Disease, 185*(9), 533-541.

Faraone, S. V., Biederman, J., Menin, D., Wozniak, J., & Spencer, T. (1997). Attention-Deficit Hyperactivity disorder with Bipolar disorder: A familial subtype? *Journal American Academy of Child and Adolescent Psychiatry, 36*(10), 1378-1387.

Faraone, S. V., Biederman, J., Mennin, D., & Russell, R. (1997). Bipolar and antisocial disorders among relatives of ADHD children: Parsing familial subtypes of illness. *American Journal of Medical Genetics (Neuropsychiatric Genetics), 81*, 108-116.

Faraone, S. V., Biederman, J., Mennin, D., Russell, R., & Tsuang, M. T. (1998). Familial subtypes of attention deficit hyperactivity disorder: A 4-year follow-up study of children from antisocial-ADHD families. *Journal of Child Psychology Psychiatry, 39*(7), 1045-1053.

Fargason, R. E., & Ford, C. V. (1994). Attention deficit hyperactivity disorder in adults: diagnosis, treatment, and prognosis. *Southern Medical Journal, 87*(3), 302-309.

Feagans, L. V. (1991). Preface. In L. V. Feagans, E. J. Short, & L. J. Meltzer (Eds.), *Subtypes of learning disabilities: Theoretical perspectives and research* (pp. iv-ix). Hillsdale, NJ: Earlbaum.

Feagans, L. V., & McKinney, J. D. (1991). Subtypes of learning disabilities: A review. In L. V. Feagans, E. J. Short, & L. Meltzer (Eds.), *Subtypes of learning disabilities: Theoretical perspectives and research* (pp. 3-31). New Jersey: Earlbaum & Associates.

Federal Register. (1977, Thursday, December 29). 65082-65085. Washington, DC.

Felton, R. H., Naylor, C. E., & Wood, F. B. (1990). Neuropsychological profile of adult dyslexics. *Brain and Language, 39*, 485-497.

Fibiger, H. C., & Phillips, A. G. (1988). Mesocorticolimic dopamine systems and reward. *Ann NY Academy of Science, 537*, 206-215.

Filpek, P. A., Samrud-Clikeman, M., Steingard, R. J., Renshaw, P. F., & et al. (1997). Volumetreic MRI analysis comparing subjects having attention-deficit hyperactivity disorder with normal controls. *Neurology, 48*, 589-601.

Finucci, J. M., Guthrie, J. T., Childs, A. L., Abbey, H., & Childs, B. (1976). The genetics of specific reading disability. *Annals of Human Genetics, 40*, 1-23.

Finucci, J. M., Whitehouse, C. C., Isaacs, S. D., & Childs, B. (1984). Derivation and validation of a quantitative definition of specific reading disability for adults. *Developmental Medicine and Child Neurology, 26*, 143-153.

Fisher, B. C. (1998). *Attention Deficit Disorder Misdiagnosis*. Boston, MA: CRC Press.

Fleischner, J. E., Garnett, K., & Shepherd, M. (1982). Proficiency in arithmetic basic fact computation by learning disabled and nondisabled children. *Focus on Learning Problems in Mathematics, 4*, 47-55.

Fletcher, J. M. (1985). External validation of learning disability subtypes. In B. P. Rourke (Ed.), *Neuropsychology of learning disabilities: Essentials of subtypal analysis*. New York: Guilford Press.

Fletcher, J. M. (1989). Nonverbal learning disabilities and suicide: Classification leads to prevention. *Journal of Learning Disabilities, 22*, 176, 179.

Fletcher, J. M., Foorman, B. R., Shaywitz, S. E., & Shaywitz, B. A. (in press). Conceptual and methodological issues in dyslexia research: A lesson for developmental disorders. In H. Tager-Flusberg (Ed.), *Cognitive neuroscience of developmental disorders* . Cambridge, MA: MIT Press.

Fletcher, J. M., Francis, D. J., Rourke, B. P., Shaywitz, S. E., & Shaywitz, B. A. (1992). The validity of discrepancy-based definitions of reading disabilities. *Journal of Learning Disabilities, 25*(9), 555-573.

Fletcher, J. M., Francis, D. J., Rourke, B. P., Shaywitz, S. E., & Shaywitz, B. A. (1993). Classification of learning disabilities: Relationships with other childhood disorders. In G. R. Lyon, D. B. Gray, J. F. Kavanagh, & N. A. Krasnegor (Eds.), *Better understanding learning disabilities: New views from research and their implications for education and public policies* (pp. 27-55). Baltimore, MD: Paul H. Brookes Publishing Co.

Fletcher, J. M., Shaywitz, S. E., Shankwiler, D., Katz, L., Liberman, I., Stuebing, K., Francis, D. J., Fowler, A., & Shaywitz, B. A. (1994). Cognitive profiles of reading disability: Comparisons of discrepancy and low achievement definitions. *Journal of Educational Psychology, 86*, 6-23.

Flynn, J. M., & Deering, W. M. (1989). Subtypes of dyslexia: Investigation of Boder's system using quantitative neurophysiology. *Developmental Medicine and Child Neurology, 31*, 215-223.

Foorman, B., Francis, D., Shaywitz, S., Shaywitz, B., & Fletcher, J. (1997). The case for early reading intervention. In B. Blachman (Ed.), *Foundations of reading acquisition* (pp. 243-264). Hillsdale, NJ: Earlbaum.

Foss, J. M. (1991). Nonverbal learning disabilities and remedial interventions. *Annals of Dyslexia, 41*, 128-140.

Frith, U., & Snowling, M. (1983). Reading for meaning and reading for sound in autistic and dyslexic children. *British Journal of Developmental Psychology, 1*, 329-342.

Fuchs, D., Fuchs, L. S., Mathes, P. H., & Simmons, D. C. (1997). Peer-assisted strategies: Making classrooms more responsive to diversity. *American Educational Research Journal, 34*, 174-206.

Gadbow, N. F., & DuBois, D. A. (1998). *Adult Learners with Special Needs*. Malabar, FL: Krieger Publishing.

Gainetdinov, R. R., Wetsel, W. C., Jones, S. R., & et al. (1999). Role of serotonin in the paradoxical calming effect of psychostimulants on hyperactivity. *Science, 28*(283), 397-401.

Gajar, A. (1996). Current and future research priorities. In J. R. Patton & E. A. Pollock (Eds.), *Learning disabilities: The challenge of adulthood* (pp. 185-203). Austin, TX: Pro-Ed.

Galaburda, A. M., Sherman, G. F., Rosen, G. D., Aboitz, F., & Geschwind, N. (1985). Developmental dyslexia: Four consecutive patients with cortical anomalies. *Annals of Neurology, 18,* 222-233.

Gander, M., & Shea, L. C. (1998). Rethinking the writing classroom: Meeting the needs of diverse learners. In P. L. Dwinell & J. Higbee (Eds.), *Developmental education: Meeting diverse student needs.* Morrow, GA: National Association of Developmental Education.

Gardiner, S., & Schwean, V.L. (1998). *The role of protective mechanisms in resilient adults with AD/HD.* Manuscript submitted for publication.

Garfinkel, B. D. (1986). Recent developments in attention deficit disorder. *Psychiatric Annals, 16,* 11-15.

Gaub, M., & Carlson, C. (1997). Gender differences in ADHD: A meta-analysis and critical review. *Journal of American Academy of Child & Adolescent Psychiatry, 36*(8), 1036-1044.

Geary, D. C. (1990). A componential analysis of an early learning deficit in mathematics. *Journal of Experimental Child Psychology, 49,* 363-383.

Geary, D. C. (1993). Mathematical disabilities: Cognitive, neuropsychological, and genetic components. *Psychological Bulletin, 114,* 345-362.

Geary, D. C. (2000). Mathematical disorders: An overview for educators. *Perspectives, The International Dyslexia Association, 26*(3), 6-9.

Geary, D. C., Hamson, C. O., & Hoard, M. K. (in press). Numerical and arithmetical cognition: A longitudinal study of process and concept deficits in children with learning disability. *Journal of Experimental Child Psychology.*

Gelenberg, A. J., Bassuk, E. L., & Schoonover, S. C. (1991). *The practitioner's guide to psychoactive drugs.* New York: Plenum Medical Book Company.

Gerber, P. J. (1997). Life after school: Challenges in the workplace. In P. J. Gerber & D. S. Brown (Eds.), *Learning Disabilities and Employment.* Austin, TX: Pro-Ed.

Gerber, P. J., Ginsberg, R., & Reiff, H. B. (1992). Identifying patterns in employment success for highly successful adults with learning disabilities. *Journal of Learning Disabilities, 25,* 475-487.

Gerber, P. J., & Reiff, H. (Eds.). (1993). *Learning disabilities in adults.* Stoneham, MA: Butterworth-Heinemann.

Gerber, P. J., & Reiff, H. (Eds.). (1994). *Learning disabilities in adulthood: Persisting problems and evolving issues.* Stoneham, MA: Butterworth-Heinemann.

Gerber, P. J., & Reiff, H. B. (1991). *Speaking for themselves: Ethnographic interviews with adults with learning disabilities.* Ann Arbor, MI: The University of Michigan Press.

Gerber, P. J., Reiff, H. B., & Ginsberg, R. (1996). Reframing the learning disabilities experience. *Journal of Learning Disabilities, 29*(1), 97-101.

Gersten, R. (1998). Recent advances in instructional research for students with learning disabilities: An overview. *Learning Disabilities Research and Practice, 13*(3), 162-170.

Gerstman, J. (1940). Syndrome of finger agnosia, disorientation for right and left, agraphia and acalculia. *Archives of Neurology and Psychiatry, 44,* 398-408.

Geschwind, N. (1982). Why Orton was right. *Annals of Dyslexia, 32,* 13-30.

Geschwind, N. (1985). Dyslexia in neurological perspective. In F. H. Duffy & N. Geschwind (Eds.), *Dyslexia: A Neuroscientific Approach to Clinical Evaluation.* Boston, MA: Little, Brown & Co.

Geschwind, N., & Behan, P. O. (1982). *Left-handedness: Association with immune disease, migraine, and developmental learning disorder.* Paper presented at the Proceedings of the National Academy of Sciences.

Geschwind, N., & Behan, P. O. (1984). Laterality, hormones, and immunity. In N. Geschwind & A. Galaburda (Eds.), *Cerebral Dominance: The Biological Foundations*. Cambridge, MA: Harvard University Press.

Gibbs, N. (1998,). The age of Ritalin. *Time Magazine, November,* 87-96.

Gill, M., Daley, G., Heron, S., Hawi, Z., & Fitzgerald, M. (1997). Confirmation of association between attention deficit hyperactivity disorder and a dopamine transporter polymorphism. *Mol Psychiat, 2,* 311-313.

Gillberg, C. (1983). Perceptual, motor and attentional deficits in Swedish primary school children: Some child psychiatric aspects. *Journal of Child Psychology and Psychiatry, 25,* 377-403.

Gillberg, C. (1985). Asperger's Syndrome and recurrent psychosis -- A neuropsychiatric case study. *Journal of Autism and Developmental Disorders, 15,* 389-387.

Gillberg, C., & Coleman, M. (1992). *The biology of the autistic syndromes.* (2nd ed.). London: MacKeith Press.

Gillingham, A., & Stillman, B. (1973). *Remedial Training for Children with Specific Disabilities in Reading, Spelling and Penmanship.* Cambridge, MA: Educators Publishing Service.

Gillis, J. J., Gilger, J. W., Pennington, B. F., & DeFries, J. C. (1992). Attention deficit disorder in reading-disabled twins: Evidence for a genetic etiology. *Journal of Abnormal Child Psychology, 20,* 303-315.

Gittelman, R., Mannuzza, S., Shenker, R., & Bonagura, N. (1985). Hyperactive boys almost grown up: I. Psychiatric status. *Archives of General Psychiatry, 42,* 937-947.

Gladwell, M. (1999, February). Running from Ritalin. *The New Yorker,* 80-84.

Glennon, S., & Kipp, J. (1997). *Practical strategies for teaching writing: Integrating process, form, and student metacognition.* Paper presented at the Sharing Our Gifts conference, Landmark College, Burlington, Vermont.

Goldberg, T. (1987). On hermetic reading abilities. *Journal of Autism and Developmental Disorders, 17,* 29-44.

Golden, C. J. (1978). *Stroop Color and Word Test: A Manual for Clinical and Experimental Use.* Chicago, IL: Stoelting.

Golden, C. J., Purisch, A. D., & Hammeke, T. A. (1985). *Luria-Nebraska Neuropsychological Battery: Manual.* Los Angeles, CA: Western Psychological Services.

Goldman, L. S., Genel, M., Bezman, R. J., & et al. (1998). Diagnosis and treatment of attention-deficit/hyperactivity disorder in children and adolescents. *Journal of American Medical Association, 279*(14), 1100-1107.

Goldman, S. R. (1989). Strategy instruction in mathematics. *Learning Disability Quarterly, 12,* 43-55.

Goldman-Rakic, P.S. (1987). Development of cortical circuitry and cognitive function. *Child Development, 58*(3), 601-622

Goldman-Rakic, P.S. (1994) Working memory and the mind. *Scientific American 267*(3), 110-117

Goldstein, D. E., Murray, C., & Edgar, E. (1998). Employment earnings and hours of high school graduates with learning disabilities through the first decade after graduation. *Learning Disabilities Research & Practice, 13*(1), 53-64.

Goldstein, G. (1999). The LNNB and other forms of neuropsychological assessment in prediction of functional capacity. In C. J. Golden (Ed.), *The Luria-Nebraska Neuropsychological Battery 20th anniversary handbook, Vol I: A guide to clinical interpretation and use in special settings* (pp. 187-199). Los Angeles, CA: Western Psychological Services.

Goldstein, G., Beers, S. R., Shemansky, W. J., & Longmore, S. (1998). An assistive device for persons with severe amnesia. *Journal of Rehabilitation Research and Development, 35,* 238-244.

Goldstein, G., Katz, L., Slomka, G., & Kelley, M. A. (1993). Relationships among academic, neuropsychological, and intellectual status in subtypes of adults with learning disability. *Archives of Clinical Neuropsychology, 8*, 41-53.

Goldstein, G., Katz, L., Slomka, G., & Kelly, M. A. (1993). Relationships among academic, neuropsychological, and intellectual status in subtypes of adults with learning disability. *Archives of Clinical Neuropsychology, 8*, 41-53.

Goldstein, G., Minshew, N. J., & Siegel, D. J. (1994). Age differences in academic achievement in high-functioning autistic individuals. *Journal of Clinical and Experimental Neuropsychology, 16*, 671-680.

Goldstein, G., Shelly, C., McCue, M., & Kane, R. L. (1987). Classification with the Luria-Nebraska Neuropsychological Battery: An application of luster and ipsative profile analysis. *Archives of Clinical Neuropsychology, 2*, 215-235.

Goldstein, K., & Scheerer, M. (1941). Abstract and concrete behavior: An experimental study with special tests. *Psychological Monographs, 53*(2), 1-151.

Goldstein, S. (1997). *Managing attention and learning disorders in late adolescence and adulthood.* New York: John Wiley & Sons, Inc.

Goodman, R., & Stevenson, J. (1989). A twin study of hyperactivity: I. An examination of hyperactivity scores and categories derived from Rutter teacher and parent questionnaires. *Journal of Child Psychology and Psychiatry, 30*, 671-589.

Gottardo, A., Siegel, L. S., & Stanovich, K. E. (1997). The assessment of adults with reading disabilities: What can we learn from experimental tasks? *Journal of Research in Reading, 20*, 42-54.

Gottesman, R. L. (1994). The adult with learning disabilities: An overview. *Learning Disabilities, 5*(1), 1-14.

Graham, S., Harris, K. R., MacArthur, C. A., & Schwartz, S. (1991). Writing and writing instruction for students with learning disabilities: Review of a research program. *Learning Disability Quarterly, 14*(2), 89-114.

Graham, S., Schwartz, S. S., & MacArthur, C. A. (1993). Knowledge of writing and the composing process, attitude toward writing, and self-efficacy for students with and without learning disabilities. *Journal of Learning Disabilities, 26*, 237-249.

Green, M. F., Satz, P., Ganzell, S., & Vaclav, J. F. (1992). Wisconsin Card Sorting Test performance in schizophrenia: Remediation of a stubborn deficit. *American Journal of Psychiatry, 149*, 62-67.

Greenbaum, B., Graham, S., & Scales, W. (1996). Adults with learning disabilities: Occupational and social status after college. *Journal of Learning Disabilities, 29*, 167-173.

Greene, G. (1999). Mnemonic multiplication fact instruction for students with learning disabilities. *Learning Disabilities Research and Practice, 14*, 141-148.

Greenhill, L. L., & Osman, B. B. (Eds.). (1991). *Ritalin Theory and Patient Management.* Larchmont, NY: Mary Ann Liebert.

Gregg, N. (1995). Eligibility for learning disabilities rehabilitation services: Operationalizing the definition. *Journal of Vocational Rehabilitation, 4*, 86-95.

Gregg, N., Scott, S., McPeek, D., & Ferry, B. (1999). Definitions and eligibility criteria applied to the adolescent and adult population with learning disabilities across agencies. *Learning Disability Quarterly, 22*, 213-223.

Gresham, F. M., & Elliott, S. N. (1989). Social skills deficits as a primary learning disability. *Journal of Learning Disabilities, 22*, 120-124.

Grodzinsky, G., & Diamond, R. (1992). Frontal lobe functioning in boys with attention deficit hyperactivity disorder. *Developmental Neuropsychology, 8*, 427-445.

Gronwall, D. M. A. (1977). Paced Auditory Serial Addition Task: A measure of recovery from concussion. *Perceptual and Motor Skills, 44*, 367-373.

Gross-Glenn, K., Duara, R., Barker, W. W., Loewenstein, D., Chang, J. Y., Yoshii, F., Apicella, A. M., Pascal, S., Boothe, T., Sevush, S., Jallad, B. J., Novoa, L., & Lubs, H. A. (1991). Positron emission tomographic studies during serial word-reading by normal and dyslexic adults. *Journal of Clinical and Experimental Neuropsychology, 13,* 531-544.

Gualtieri, C. T., Ondrusek, M. G., & Finley, C. (1985). Attention deficit disorders in adults. *Clinical Neuropharmacology, 8,* 343-356.

Guckenberger v. Boston University. (1997). 974 F. Suppp. 106, D. Mass.

Gur, R. C., Packer, I. K., Hungerbuhler, J. P., Reivich, M., Obrist, W. D., Amarnek, W. S., & Sackheim, H. A. (1980). Differences in the distribution in gray and white matter in human cerebral hemispheres. *Science, 207,* 1226-1228.

Hagman, J. O., Wood, F., Buschbaum, M. S., Tallal, P., Flowers, L., & Katz, W. (1992). Cerebral brain metabolism in adult dyslexic subjects assessed with positron emission tomography during performance of an auditory task. *Archives of Neurology, 49,* 734-739.

Hallahan, D. P., & Cottone, E. A. (1977). Attention deficit hyperactivity disorder. In T. E. Scruggs & M. A. Mastropieri (Eds.), *Advances in learning and behavioral disabilities* (pp. 27-67). Greenwich, CT: JAI Press, Inc.

Hallgren, B. (1950). Specific dyslexia ("congenital word-blindness"): A clinical and genetic study. *Acta Psychiatrica et Neurologica Scandinavica, 65,* 1-287.

Hallowell, E. M. (1995). Psychotherapy of adult attention deficit disorder. In K. Nadeau (Ed.), *A comprehensive guide to attention deficit disorder in adults* (pp. 146-167). New York: Brunner/Mazel.

Hallowell, E. M., & Ratey, J. J. (1994). *Driven to distraction.* New York: Pantheon Books.

Halperin, J. M., Newcorn, J. H., & Sharma, V. (1991). Ritalin: Diagnostic comorbidity and attention measures. In L. L. Greenhill & B. Osman (Eds.), *Ritalin Theory and Patient Management.* Larchmont, NY: Mary Ann Liebert.

Hammill, D. D. (1985). *DTLA-2: Detroit Tests of Learning Aptitude.* Austin, TX: Pro-Ed.

Hammill, D. D., & Larsen, S. C. (1996). *Test of Written Language (TOWL-3).* (3rd ed.). Odessa, FL: PAR.

Hanfman, E., & Kasanin, J. (1936). A method for study of concept formation. *Journal of Psychology, 3,* 521-240.

Hansen, C., Weiss, D., & Last, C. G. (1999). ADHD boys in young adulthood: Psychosocial adjustment. *Journal of American Academy of Child and Adolescent Psychiatry, 38,* 165-171.

Harnadek, M. C. S., & Rourke, B. P. (1994). Principal identifying features of the syndrome of nonverbal learning disabilities in children. *Journal of Learning Disabilities* (27), 144-154.

Harris, K. R., & Pressley, M. (1991). The nature of cognitive strategy instruction: Interactive strategy construction. *Exceptional Children, 57,* 392-404.

Hart, E. R., & Speece, D. L. (1998). Reciprocal teaching goes to college: Effects for postsecondary students at risk for academic failure. *Journal of Educational Psychology, 90*(4), 670-681.

Hartje, W. (1987). The effects of spatial disorders on arithmetic skills. In G. DeLoche & X. Seron (Eds.), *Mathematical disabilities* (pp. 121-136). Hillsdale, NJ: Lawrence Earlbaum.

Hartzell, H. E., & Compton, C. (1984). Learning disability: 10 year follow-up. *Pediatrics, 74,* 1058-1064.

Harvey, J. R., & Wells, M. (1989, February). *Diagnosis of adult learning disabilities and vocational rehabilitation: A descriptive analysis.* Paper presented at the ACLD International Conference, Miami, FL.

Hassett, I., & Gurian, A. (1984, August). *The learning disabled girl: A Profile.* Paper presented at the 92nd Annual Convention of the American Psychological Association, Toronto, Ontario.

Heaton, R. K. (1981). *A manual for the Wisconsin card sorting test.* Odessa, TX: Psychological Assessment Resources.

Heaton, R. K., Chelune, G. J., Talley, J. L., Kay, G. G., & Curtiss, G. (1993). *Wisconsin Card Sort Test Manual: Revised and Expanded*. Odessa, FL: Psychological Assessment Resources.

Hebert, B. M., & Murdock, J. Y. (1994). Comparing three computer-aided instruction output modes to teach vocabulary words to students with learning disabilities. *Learning Disabilities Research & Practice, 9*(3), 136-141.

Hecaen, H., Angelergues, R., & Houillier, S. (1961). Les varieties cliniques des acalculies au cors des lesions retrorolandiques: Approche statistique du probleme [The clinical varieties of the acalculies in retrorolandic lesions: A statistical approach to the problem]. *Revue Neurologique, 105*, 85-103.

Hechtman, L. (1989). Attention-deficit hyperactivity disorder in adolescence and adulthood: An updated follow-up. *Psychiatric Annals, 19*, 597-603.

Hechtman, L., Weiss, G., Perlman, T., & et al. (1981). Hyperactives as young adults: Various clinical outcomes. *Adolescent Psychiatry, 9*, 295-306.

Hechtman, L., Weiss, G., Perlman, T., Hopkins, J., & Wener, A. (1981). Hyperactives as young adults: Prospective ten-year follow-up. In K. D. Gadow & J. Loney (Eds.), *Psychosocial aspects of drug treatment for hyperactivity* (pp. 417-442). Boulder, CO: Westview Press, Inc.

Heilman, K. M., Voeller, K. K. S., & Nadeau, S. E. (1991). A possible pathophysiological substrate of attention deficit hyperactivity disorder. *Journal of Child Neurology, 6*(Supplement), S74-S79.

Helfgott, D. & Westhaver, M. (1997). Inspiration Software. , Portland, OR.

Henderson, C. (1999). *College Freshmen with Disabilities. A triennial statistical profile*: American Council on Education, HEATH Resource Center.

Henningfield, J. E., Clayton, R., & Pollin, W. (1990). Involvement of tobacco in alcoholism and illicit drug use. *British Journal of Addictions, 85*, 279-291.

Higgins, E. L., & Raskind, M. H. (1995). Compensatory effectiveness of speech recognition on the written composition performance of postsecondary students with learning disabilities. *Learning Disability Quarterly, 18*, 159-174.

Himelstein, J., Schulz, K. P., Newcorn, J. H., & Halperin, J. M. (2000). The neurobiology of Attention-Deficit Hyperactivity Disorder. *Frontiers in Biosciences, 5*, 461-478.

Hinchley, J., & Levy, B. A. (1988). Developmental and individual differences in reading comprehension. *Cognitive Instruction, 5*, 3-47.

Hiscock, M., & Hiscock, C. K. (1991). On the relevance of neuropsychological data to learning disabilities. In J. E. Obrzut & G. W. Hynd (Eds.), *Neuropsychological foundations of learning disabilities* (pp. 743-774). San Diego, CA: Academic Press.

Hoffman, F. J., Sheldon, K. L., Minskoff, E. H., Sautter, S. W., Steidle, E. F., Baker, D. P., Bailey, M. B., & Echols, L. D. (1987). Needs of learning disabled students. *Journal of Learning Disabilities, 20*, 43-52.

Hoffman, W. L., & Prior, M. R. (1982). Neuropsychological dimensions of autism in children: A test of the hemispheric dysfunction hypothesis. *Journal of Clinical Neuropsychology, 4*, 27-41.

Holdanack, J. A., Moberg, P. J., Arnold, S. E., & et al. (1995). Speed of processing and verbal learning deficits in adults diagnosed with attention deficit disorder. *Neuorpsychiatry Neuropsychology Behavioral Neurology, 8*, 282-292.

Holliday, G. A., Koller, J. R., & Thomas, C. D. (1999). Post-high school outcomes of high IQ adults with learning disabilities. *Journal for the Education of the Gifted, 22*, 266-281.

Hooper, S. R., Montgomery, J., Schwartz, D., Reed, M., Sandler, A., Levine, M., & Watson, T. (1994). Measurement of written language expression. In G. R. Lyon (Ed.), *Frames of reference for the assessment of learning disabilities: New views on measurement issues* (pp. 375-418). Baltimore, MD: Paul H. Brookes.

Hooper, S. R., & Olley, J. G. (1996). Psychological comorbidity in adults with learning disabilities. In N. Gregg, C. Hoy, & A. F. Gay (Eds.), *Adults with learning disabilities* (pp. 162-183). New York: Guilford Press.

Hooper, S. R., & Willis, W. G. (1989). *Learning disability subtyping: Neuropsychological foundations, conceptual models, and issues in clinical differentiation.* New York: Springer-Verlag.

Horn, J. L., O'Donnell, J. P., & Leicht, D. J. (1988). Phonetically inaccurate spelling among learning-disabled, head-injured, and nondisabled young adults. *Brain and Language, 33,* 55-69.

Horn, W. F., O'Donnell, J. P., & Vitulano, L. A. (1983). Long-term follow-up studies of learning-disabled persons. *Journal of Learning Disabilities, 16*(9), 542-555.

Horn, W. F., Wagner, A. E., & Ialongo, N. (1989). Sex differences in school-aged children with pervasive attention deficit hyperactivity disorder. *Journal of Abnormal Child Psychology, 17,* 109-125.

Hornig, M. (1998). Addressing comorbidity in adults with Attention-Deficit/Hyperactivity Disorder. *Clinical Psychiatry, 59,* 69-75.

Houck, C. K., & Billingsley, B. S. (1989). Written expression of students with and without learning disabilities: Differences across the grades. *Journal of Learning Disabilities, 22,* 561,567,572.

Hoy, C., Gregg, N., Wisenbaker, J., Manglitz, E., King, M., & Moreland, C. (1997). Depression and anxiety in two groups of adults with learning disabilities. *Learning Disability Quarterly, 20,* 280-291.

Hughes, C. (1996). Brief report: Planning problems in autism at the level of motor control. *Journal of Autism and Developmental Disorders, 26,* 99-107.

Hughes, C., & Russell, J. (1993). Autistic children's difficulty with mental disengagement from an object: Its implications for theories of autism. *Developmental Psychology, 29,* 498-519.

Hunt, R. D. (1997). Nosology, neurobiology, and clinical patterns of ADHD in adults. *Psychiatric Annals, 27,* 572-581.

Hunt, R. D., Arnsten, A. F. T., & Asbell, M. D. (1995). An open trial of Guanfacine in the treatment of attention-deficit hyperactivity disorder. *Journal of American Academy of Child and Adolescent Psychiatry, 34*(1), 50-54.

Hunt, R. D., Capper, L., & O'Connell, P. (1990). Clonidine in child and adolescent psychiatry. *Journal of Child and Adolescent Psychopharmacology, 1*(1), 87-102.

Hutt, C., Hutt, S. J., Lee, D., & Ounsted, C. (1964). Arousal and childhood autism. *Nature,* 908-909.

Hynd, G. W., Hern, K. L., Novey, E. S., Eliopolus, D., & et al. (1993). Attention-Deficit Hyperactivity Disorder (ADHD) and asymmetry of the caudate nucleus. *Journal of Child Neurology, 8,* 339-347.

Hynd, G. W., Lorys, A. R., Semrud-Clikeman, M., Nieves, N., Huettner, M. I. S., & Lahey, B. B. (1991). Attention deficit disorder without hyperactivity: A distinct behavioral and neurocognitive syndrome. *Journal of Child Neurology, 6*(Supplement), S36-S43.

Hynd, G. W., Semrud-Clikeman, M., Lorys, A. R., Novey, E. S., & Eliopulos, D. (1990). Brain morphology in developmental dyslexia and Attention Deficit Disorder/Hyperactivity. *Archives of Neurology, 47,* 916-919.

Hynd, G. W., Semrud-Clikeman, M., Lorys, A. R., Novey, E. S., Eliopulos, D., & Lyytinen, H. (1991). Corpus callosum morphology in Attention-Deficit Hyperactivity Disorder: Morphometric analysis of MRI. *Journal of Learning Disabilities, 24,* 141-155.

Ialongo, N. S., Horn, W. F., Pascoe, J. M., Greenberg, G., & et al. (1993). The effects of a multimodal intervention with attention-deficit hyperactivity disorder children: A 9-month follow-up. *Journal of the American Academy of Child and Adolescent Psychiatry, 32,* 182-189.

Individuals with Disabilities Education Act (IDEA). (1990). P.L. 101-476, 20 U.S.C. 1400 et seq.

Inge, K. J., & Tilson, G. P. (1993). Supported employment: Issues and applications for individuals with learning disabilities. In P. J. Gerber & H. B. Reiff (Eds.), *Learning disabilities in adulthood: Persisting problems and evolving issues* (pp. 179-193). Boston, MA: Andover.

Interagency Committee on Learning Disabilities. (1987). *Learning disabilities: A report to the U.S. Congress.* Washington, DC: Government Printing Office.

Jaffe, S. L. (1989). Pemoline and liver function. *Journal of the American Academy of Child and Adolescent Psychiatry, 28,* 457-458.

Jastak, J. F., & Wilkinson, G. S. (1984). *The Wide Range Achievement Test - Revised.* Wilmington, DE: Jastak Associates.

Jenkins, M., Cohe, R., Malloy, P., & et al. (1998). Neuropsychological measures which discriminate among adults with residual symptoms of attention deficit disorder and other attentional complaints. *Clinical Neuropsychology, 12,* 74-83.

Jensen, J. B., Burke, N., & Garfinkel, B. D. (1988). Depression and symptoms of attention deficit disorder with hyperactivity. *Journal of the American Academy of Child and Adolescent Psychiatry, 27,* 742-747.

Jensen, P. S., Kettle, L., Roper, M. T., & et al. (1999). Are stimulants overprescribed? *Journal of the American Academy of Child and Adolescent Psychiatry, 38,* 797-804.

Johnson, D. (1994). Clinical study of adults with severe learning disabilities. *Learning Disabilities: A Multidisciplinary Journal, 5*(1), 43-50.

Johnson, D. J., & Blalock, J. W. (1987). *Adults With Learning Disabilities: Clinical Studies.* New York: Grune & Stratton.

Johnson, D. J., & Myklebust, H. R. (1967). *Learning Disabilities: Educational Principles and Practices.* New York: Grune & Stratton.

Johnson, D. J., & Myklebust, H. R. (1971). *Learning disabilities.* New York: Grune and Stratton.

Jones, B. F. (1988). Text learning strategy instruction: Guidelines from theory and practice. In C. E. Weinstein, E. T. Goetz, & P. A. Alexander (Eds.), *Learning and study strategies, issues in assessment, instruction, and evaluation.* New York: Academic Press.

Jones, E. D., Wilson, R., & Bhojwani, S. (1997). Mathematics instruction for secondary students with learning disabilities. *Journal of Learning Disabilities, 30,* 151-163.

Jones, E. D., Wilson, R., & Bhojwani, S. (1998). Mathematics instruction for secondary students with learning disabilities. In D. P. Rivera (Ed.), *Mathematics education for students with learning disabilities* (pp. 155-176). Austin, TX: Pro-Ed.

Jordan, N. C., & Montani, T. O. (1997). Cognitive arithmetic and problem solving: A comparison of children with specific and general mathematics difficulties. *Journal of Learning Disabilities, 30,* 624-634.

Judd, T. P., & Bilsky, L. H. (1989). Comprehension and memory in the solution of verbal arithmetic problems by mentally retarded and nonretarded individuals. *Journal of Educational Psychology, 81,* 541-546.

Jueptner, M., Rijntjes, M., Weiller, C., Faiss, J. H., & et al. (1995). Localization of a cerebellar timing processing unit using PET. *Neurology, 45,* 1540-1545.

Kamps, D., Walter, D., Maher, J., & Rotholz, D. (1992). Academic and environmental effects of small group arrangements in classrooms for students with autism and other developmental disabilities. *Journal of Autism and Developmental Disorders, 22,* 277-293.

Kanner, L. (1943). Autistic disturbances of affective contact. *Nervous Child, 2,* 217-250.

Kanner, L. (1971). Follow-up study of eleven autistic children originally reported in 1943. *Journal of Autism and Childhood Schizophrenia, 1,* 119-145.

Kanner, L., Rodriguez, A., & Ashenden, B. (1972). How far can autistic children go in matters of social adaptation? *Journal of Autism and Childhood Schizophrenia, 2,* 9-33.

Katz, J. J., Wood, D. S., Goldstein, G., Auchenbach, R. C., & Geckle, M. (1998). The utility of neuropsychological tests in evaluation of Attention-Deficit/Hyperactivity Disorder (ADHD) versus depression in adults. *Assessment, 5*(1), 45-51.

Katz, L., & Goldstein, G. (1993). The Luria-Nebraska neuropsychological battery and the WAIS-R in assessment of adults with specific learning disabilities. *Rehabilitation Counseling Bulletin, 36*(4), 190-197.

Katz, L., Goldstein, G., Rudisin, S., & Bailey, D. (1993). A neuropsychological approach to the bannatyne recategorization of the Wechsler Intelligence Scales in adults with learning disabilities. *Journal of Learning Disabilities, 26*(1), 65-72.

Katz, L. J., Goldstein, G., & Geckle, M. (1998). Neuropsychological and personality differences between men and women with ADHD. *Journal of Attention Disorders, 2*(4), 239-248.

Katz, L. J., Kelly, M. A., Goldstein, G., Bartolomucci, E., & Comstock, E. J. (1992, November). *MMPI subtypes in a mixed LD sample.* Paper presented at the 12th Annual Meeting of the National Academy of Neuropsychology.

Kaufman, A. S., & Kaufman, N. L. (1985). *Kaufman Tests of Educational Achievement.* Circle Pines, MN: AGS.

Kavale, K. A., & Fornes, S. R. (1995). *The nature of learning disabilities: Critical elements of diagnosis and classification.* Mahwah, NJ: Earlbaum.

Kelly, J. (1998). Recording for the blind & dyslexic: Learning through listening for half a century. *Perspectives* (Summer), 28-30.

Kelly, K., & Ramundo, P. (1995). *You mean I'm not lazy, stupid, or crazy: A self-help book for adults with attention deficit disorder.* New York: Scribner.

Kelman, M., & Lester, G. (1997). *Jumping the Queue.* Cambridge, MA: Harvard University Press.

Kerka, S. (1998). Adults with learning disabilities. *ERIC Digest, 189.*

Kershner, J. S. (1991). Neuropsychological perspectives in special education. In J. E. Obrzut & G. W. Hynd (Eds.), *Neuropsychological foundations of learning disabilities* (pp. 711-741). San Diego, CA: Academic Press.

Kim, S. G., Ugurbil, K., & Strick, P. L. (1994). Activation of a cerebellar output nucleus during cognitive processing. *Science, 265,* 949-951.

Kinsborne, M. (1968). Developmental Gerstmann syndrome. *Pediatric Clinics of North America, 15,* 771-778.

Kinsborne, M. (1997). Nonverbal learning disability. In T. E. Feinberg & M. J. Farah (Eds.), *Behavioral neurology and neuropsychology* (pp. 789-794). New York: McGraw Hill.

Kirsch, I. A., Jungeblut, A., Jenkins, L., & Kilstad, A. (1993). *Adult literacy in America: A first look at the results of the National Adult Literacy Survey.* Washington, DC: U. S. Department of Education, Office of Educational Research and Improvement, National Center for Education Statistics.

Kite, J. L. (1984). Rehabilitation planning with learning disabled persons. *Journal of Rehabilitation,* 59-63.

Kitz, W. R., & Thorpe, H. W. (1995). A comparison of tne errecuveness of videodisc and traditional algebra instruction for college-age students with learning disabilities. *Remedial and Special Education, 16,* 295-306.

Klee, S. H., Garfinkel, B. D., & Beauchesne, H. (1986). Attention deficits in adults. *Psychiatric Annals, 16*(1), 52-56.

Klein, K., & Hecker, L. (1994). The write moves. In A. Brand (Ed.), *R. Graves.* Portsmouth, NH: Boyton/Cook Heinemann.

Klin, A., Volkmar, F. R., Sparrow, S. S., Cicchetti, D. V., & Rourke, B. P. (1995). Validity and neuropsychological characterization of Asperger syndrome: Convergence with nonverbal learning disabilities syndrome. *Journal of Child Psychology and Psychiatry, 7,* 1127-1140.

Kohaska, C. J., & Skolnik, J. (1986). Employment suggestions from LD adults. *Academic Therapy, 2,* 573-575.

Kopin, I. J. (1978). Measuring turnover of neurotransmitters in human brain. In M. A. Lipton, A. DiMaascio, & K. F. Killam (Eds.), *Psychopharmacology: A Generation of Progress* (pp. 9333-9342). New York: Raven Press.

Kornetsky, C. (1970). The psychopharmacology of the immature organism. *Psychopharmacologia, 17,* 105-136.

Kowalchuk, B., & King, J. D. (1989). Adult suicide versus coping with nonverbal learning disorder. *Journal of Learning Disabilities, 22,* 177-178.

Kronick, D. (1981). *Social development of learning disabled persons.* San Francisco, CA: Jossey-Bass.

Kurzweil 3000. (1999). Kurzweil Educational Systems, Lernout & Hauspie Speech Products N.V. Burlington, MA.

LaHoste, G. J., Swanson, J. M., Wigal, S. B., Glabe, C., Wigal, T., King, N., & Kenney, J. L. (1996). Dopamine D4 receptor gene polymorphism is associated with Attention Deficit Hyperactivity disorder. *Mol Psychiatry, 1,* 121-124.

Laine, M., & Butters, N. (1982). A preliminary study of the problem solving strategies of detoxified long-term alcoholics. *Drug and Alcohol Dependence, 10,* 235-242.

Lambert, N., & Hartsough, C. S. (1998). Prospective study of tobacco smoking and substance dependencies among samples of ADHD and non-ADHD participants. *Journal of Learning Disabilities, November,* 533-551.

Lapan, R., Koller, J., & Holliday, G. (1991). A role for counselors in school-to-work transition programs for learning disabled students. *Counseling Interviewer, 23,* 21-23.

Latham, P. H. (1995). Legal issues pertaining to the postsecondary student with ADD. *Journal of Postsecondary Education and Disability, 11,* 53-61.

Latham, P. H., & Latham, P. S. (1997). Legal rights. In S. Goldstein (Ed.), *Managing attention and learning disorders in late adolescence and adulthood. A guide for practitioners.* New York: John Wiley & Sons.

Latham, P. H., & Latham, P. S. (1998). Learning disabilities/attention deficit hyperactivity disorder and test accommodations in provisional licensing under the Americans with Disabilities Act. *Learning Disabilities, 9*(1), 17-18.

Latham, P. S., & Latham, P. H. (1993). *ADD and the law.* Washington, DC: JKL Communications.

Latham, P. S., & Latham, P. H. (Eds.). (1994). *Succeeding in the workplace.* Washington, DC: JKL Communications.

Leckman, J. F., & Cohen, D. J. (Eds.). (1999). *Tourette's Syndrome - Tics, Obsessions, Compulsions.* New York: John Wiley & Sons, Inc.

LeCouteur, A., Rutter, M., Lord, C., Rios, P., Robertson, S., Holdgrafer, M., & McLennan, J. (1989). Autism diagnostic interview: A standardized investigator-based instrument. *Journal of Autism and Developmental Disorders, 19,* 363-387.

Leicht, D. J. (1987). *Personality/social/behavior subtypes of learning disabled young adults.* , Southern Illinois University, Carbondale, IL.

Lennox, C., & Siegel, L. S. (1993). Visual and phonological spelling errors in subtypes of children with learning disabilities. *Applied Psycholinguistics, 14,* 473-488.

Leong, C. K. (1999). Phonological and morphological processing in adult students with learning/reading disabilities. *Journal of Learning Disabilities, 32*(3), 224-238.

Lerner, J. W. (1989). Educational interventions in learning disabilities. *Journal of the American Academy of Child & Adolescent Psychiatry, 28,* 326-331.

Lerner, J. W. (2000). *Learning disabilities: Theories, diagnosis and teaching strategies.* Boston, MA: Houghton Mifflin Company.

Levine, M., & Fuller, G. (1972). Sex differences on psychoeducational tests with three classified deficit reading groups. *Slow Learning Child, 19*, 165-174.

Levine, M. D. (1987). *Developmental variation and learning disorders.* Cambridge, MA: Educators Publishing Service.

Levine, M. D. (1994). *Educational care: A system for understanding and managing learning disorders.* Cambridge, MA: Educators Publishing Service.

Levine, P., & Edgar, E. (1995). An analysis by gender of long-term postschool outcomes for youth with and without disabilities. *Exceptional Children, 61*(3), 282-300.

Levine, P., & Nourse, S. W. (1998). What follow-up studies say about postschool life for young men and women with learning disabilities: A critical look at the literature. *Journal of Learning Disabilities, 31*(3), 212-233.

Levine, S. (1995). Career counseling for people with attention deficit disorder. In T. Hartman (Ed.), *ADD success stories: A guide to fulfillment for families with attention deficit disorder.* Grass Valley, CA: Underwood Books.

Lewandowski, L., & Arcangelo, K. (1994). The social adjustment and self-concept of adults with learning disabilities. *Journal of Learning Disabilities, 27*, 598-605.

Lewis, R. D., & Lorion, R. P. (1988). Discriminative effectiveness of the Luria-Nebraska Battery for LD adolescents. *Learning Disabilities Quarterly, 11*, 62-69.

Lewitter, F. I., DeFries, J. C., & Elston, R. C. (1980). Genetic models of reading disability. *Behavior Genetics, 10*, 9-30.

Leyser, Y., Vogel, S., Wyland, B., & Brulle, A. (1998). Faculty attitudes and practices regarding students with disabilities: Two decades after implementation of Section 504. *Journal of Postsecondary Education and Disability, 13*(3), 5-19.

Liberman, I. Y., Shankweiler, D., Liberman, A. M., Fowler, C., & Fischer, F. W. (1977). Phonetic segmentation and recoding in the beginning reader. In A. S. Reber & D. L. Scarborough (Eds.), *Toward a psychology of reading.* Hillsdale, NJ: Earlbaum.

Light, J. G., DeFries, J. C., & Olson, R. K. (1998). Multivariate behavioral genetic analysis of achievement and cognitive measures in reading-disabled and control twin pairs. *Human Biology, 70*, 215-237.

Lincoln, A. J., Courchesne, E., Kilman, B. A., Elasian, R., & Allen, M. (1988). A study of intellectual abilities in high-functioning people with autism. *Journal of Autism and Developmental Disorders, 18*, 505-524.

Lindamood, C., & Lindamood, P. (1975). *Lindamood Auditory Conceptualization Test.* Hingham, MA: Teaching Resources Corporation.

Livingstone, M. S., Rosen, G. D., Drislane, F. W., & Galaburda, A. M. (1991). *Physiological and anatomical evidence for a magna cellular defect in developmental dyslexia.* Paper presented at the Proceedings of the National Academy of Science, USA.

Loge, D. V., Staton, R. D., & Beatty, W. W. (1990). Performance of children with ADHD on tests sensitive to frontal lobe dysfunction. *Journal of the American Academy of Child and Adolescent Psychiatry, 29*, 540-545.

Lord, C., Rutter, M., & Goode, S. (1989). Autism diagnostic observation schedule: A standardized investigator-based instrument. *Journal of Autism and Developmental Disorders, 19*, 185-212.

Lord, C., Rutter, M., & LeCouteur, A. L. (1994). Autism diagnostic interview revised: A revised version of a diagnostic interview for caregivers of individuals with possible pervasive developmental disorders. *Journal of Autism and Developmental Disorders, 24*, 659-685.

Lou, H. C. (1996). Etiology and pathogenesis of attention-deficit hyperactivity disorder (ADHD): Significance of prematurity and perinatal hypoxic-haemodynamic encephalopathy. *Acta Paediatr, 85*, 1266-1271.

Lou, H. C., Henriksen, L., & Bruhn, P. (1984). Focal cerebral hypoperfusion in children with dysphasia and/or attention deficit disorder. *Arch Neurol, 41*, 825-829.

Lou, H. C., Henriksen, L., Bruhn, P., Borner, H., & Nielsen, J. B. (1989). Striatal dysfunction in Attention Deficit and Hyperkinetic disorder. *Archives of Neurology, 46*, 48-52.

Lovaas, O. I., Koegel, R., & Schriebman, L. (1979). Stimulus overselectivity in autism. A review of research. *Psychological Bulletin, 86*, 1236-1254.

Lovejoy, D. W., Ball, J. D., Keats, M., & et al. (1999). Neuropsychological performance of adults with attention deficit hyperactivity disorder (ADHD): Diagnostic classification estimates for measures of frontal lobe/executive functioning. *Journal Int Neuropsychology Soc, 5*, 222-233.

Lovett, M. W. (1984). A developmental perspective on reading dysfunction: Accuracy and rate criteria in the subtyping of dyslexic children. *Brain and Language, 22*, 67-91.

Lovett, M. W. (1987). A developmental approach to reading disability: Accuracy and speed criteria for normal and deficient reading skill. *Child Development, 58*, 234-260.

Ludwikowski, K., & DeValk, M. (1998). Attention-deficit hyperactivity disorder. The psychostimulants and beyond. *Advance for Nurse Practitioners, 6*, 55-60.

Lyon, G. R. (1983). Learning-disabled readers: Identification of subgroups. In H. R. Myklebust (Ed.), *Progress in learning disabilities* (Vol. 5, pp. 103-134). New York: Grune & Stratton.

Lyon, G. R. (1985). Educational validation studies of learning disability subtypes. In B. P. Rourke (Ed.), *Neuropsychology of learning disabilities*. New York: Guilford Press.

Lyon, G. R. (1985b). Identification and remediation of learning disability sub-types: Preliminary findings. *Learning Disability Focus, 1*, 21-35.

Lyon, G. R. (1995a). Research initiatives in learning disabilities: Contributions from scientists supported by the National Institute of Child Health and Human Development. *Journal of Child Neurology, 10*, 120-126.

Lyon, G. R. (1995b). Toward a definition of dyslexia. *Annals of Dyslexia, 45*, 3-26.

Lyon, G. R. (1996). The state of research. In S. C. Cramer & W. Ellis (Eds.), *Learning disabilities: Lifelong issues*. Baltimore, MD: Paul H. Brooks.

Lyon, G. R., Rietta, S., Watson, B., Porch, B., & Rhodes, J. (1981). Selected linguistic and perceptual abilities of empirically derived subgroups of learning disabled readers. *Journal of School Psychology, 19*, 152-166.

Lyon, R., Stewart, N., & Freeman, D. (1982). Neuropsychological characteristics of empirically derived subgroups of learning disabled readers. *Journal of Clinical Neuropsychology, 4*, 343-365.

Ma, X. (2000). A longitudinal assessment of antecedent course work in mathematics and subsequent mathematical attainment. *The Journal of Educational Research, 94*, 16-28.

MacArthur, C., & Graham, S. (1987). Learning disabled students' composing under three methods of text production: Handwriting, word processing, and dictation. *Journal of Special Education, 21*, 22-42.

MacArthur, C. A. (1999). Word prediction for students with severe spelling problems. *Learning Disability Quarterly, 22*, 158-172.

MacArthur, C. A., Schwartz, S., Graham, S., Molloy, D., & Harris, D. (1996). Integration of strategy instruction into whole language classroom: A case study. *Learning Disabilities Research and Practice, 11*, 168-176.

Maccini, P., & Hughes, C. A. (2000). Effects of a problem-solving strategy on the introductory algebra performance of secondary students with learning disabilities. *Learning Disabilities Research and Practice, 15*, 10-21.

Magoun, H. W. (1952). An ascending reticular activating system in the brain stem. *Archives of Neurology and Psychiatry, 67*, 145-154.

Malhotra, A. K., Virkkunen, M., Rooney, W., Eggert, M., Linolla, M., & Goldman, D. (1996). The association between the dopamine D4 receptor (D4DR) 15 amino acid repeat polymorphism and novelty seeking. *Molecular Psychiatry, 1*, 388-391.

Mann, V. A., & Brady, S. (1988). Reading disability: The role of language deficiencies. *Journal of Consulting and Clinical Psychology, 56*, 811-816.

Mannuzza, S., Klein, R. G., Bessler, A., Malloy, P., & LaPadula, M. (1993). Adult outcome of hyperactive boys: Educational achievement, occupational rank and psychiatric status. *Arc Gen Psychiatry, 50,* 565-576.

Mannuzza, S., Klein, R. G., Bessler, A., Malloy, P., & LaPadula, M. (1998). Adult psychiatric status of hyperactive boys grown up. *American Journal of Psychiatry, 155,* 493-498.

Marsh, L. G., & Cook, N. L. (1996). The effects of using manipulatives in teaching math problem solving to students with learning disabilities. *Learning Disabilities Research and Practice, 11,* 58-65.

Marshall, R. M., Hynd, G. W., Handwerk, M. J., & Hall, J. (1997). Academic underachievement in ADHD subtypes. *Journal of Learning Disabilities, 20,* 635-642.

Matochik, J. A., Leibenauer, L. L., King, C., Szymanski, H. V., Cohen, R. M., & Zametkin, A. J. (1994). Cerebral glucose metabolism in adults with attention deficit hyperactivity disorder after chronic stimulant treatment. *American Journal of Psychiatry, 151*(5), 658-664.

Matochik, J. A., Rumsey, J. M., Zametkin, A. J., & et al. (1996). Neuropsychological correlates of familial attention deficit hyperactivity disorder in adults. *Neuropsychiatry, Neuropsychology Behav. Neurol, 9,* 186-191.

Mattek, P. W., & Wierzbicki, M. (1998). Cognitive and behavioral correlates of depression in learning-disabled and nonlearning-disabled adult students. *Journal of Clinical Psychology, 54,* 831-837.

Mattes, J. A. (1980). The role of frontal lobe dysfunction in childhood hyperkinesis. *Comp Psychiatry, 21,* 358-369.

Mattes, J. A., Boswell, L., & Oliver, H. (1984). Methylphenidate effects on symptoms of Attention Deficit Disorder in adults. *Archives General Psychiatry, 41,* 1059-1063.

Mattis, S. (1978). Dyslexia syndromes: A working hypothesis that works. In A. L. Benton & D. Pearl (Eds.), *Dyslexia: An appraisal of current knowledge* (pp. 43-58). London: Oxford University Press.

McCarney, S. B., & Anderson, P. D. (1996). *Adult attention deficit disorder evaluation scale (AADDES).* Columbia, MO: Hawthorne Educational Services.

McCracken, J. T. (1991). A two-part model of stimulant action on Attention-Deficit Hyperactivity Disorder in children. *Journal Neuropsychiatry Clin Neurosci, 3,* 201-209.

McCue, M. (1984). Assessment and rehabilitation of learning-disabled adults. *Rehabilitation Counseling Bulletin*(May), 281-290.

McCue, M. (1993). Clinical and diagnostic functional assessment of adults with learning disability. In P. J. Gerber & H. B. Reiff (Eds.), *Learning disabilities in adulthood: Persisting problems and evolving issues* (pp. 55-71). Boston, MA: Andover Medical Publishers.

McCue, M. (1994). *Neuropsychological Diagnostic and Functional Interview.* Unpublished manuscript.

McCue, M., & Goldstein, G. (1991). Neuropsychological aspects of learning disability in adults. In B. Rourke (Ed.), *Neuropsychological validation of learning disability subtypes* (pp. 311-329). New York: Guilford Publications, Inc.

McCue, M., Goldstein, G., Shelly, C., & Katz, L. (1986). Cognitive profiles of some subtypes of learning disabled adults. *Archives of Clinical Neuropsychology, 1,* 13-23.

McCue, M., Katz, L., & Goldstein, G. (1985). *A Training Program in Specific Learning Disability (SLD) for Rehabilitation Psychologists.* Unpublished manuscript.

McCue, M., Shelly, C., Goldstein, G., & Katz-Garris, L. (1984). Neuropsychological aspects of learning disability in young adults. *The International Journal of Clinical Neuropsychology, 6,* 229, 233.

McDermott, P. (1996). A nationwide study of developmental and gender prevalence for psychopathology in childhood and adolescence. *Journal of Abnormal Child Psychology, 2*(1), 53-66.

McEvoy, R. E., Rogers, S. J., & Pennington, B. F. (1993). Executive function and social communication deficits in young autistic children. *Journal of Child Psychology and Psychiatry, 34,* 563-578.

McGuffin, P., Owen, M. J., O'Donovan, M. C., & et al. (1994). *Seminars in psychiatric genetics.* London: Gaskell.

McGuire, J. M., Hall, D., & Litt, A. V. (1991). A field-based study of the direct service needs of college students with learning disabilities. *Journal of College Student Development, 32,* 101-108.

McNaughton, D., Hughes, C., & Clark, K. (1997). The effect of five proofreading conditions on the spelling performance of college students with learning disabilities. *Journal of Learning Disabilities, 30*(6), 643-651.

McTighe, J., & Lyman, F. T., Jr. (1988). Cueing thinking in the classroom: The promise of theory-embedded tools. *Educational Leadership, 4,* 18-24.

Means, C. D., Stewart, S. W., & Dowler, D. L. (1997). Job accommodations that work: A follow-up study of adults with attention deficit disorder. *Journal of Applied Rehabilitation Counseling, 28,* 13-17.

Mefford, I. N., & Potter, W. Z. (1989). A neuroanatomical and biochemical basis for attention deficit disorder with hyperactivity in children: a defect in tonic adrenaline mediated inhibition of locus coeruleus stimulation. *Med Hypotheses, 29,* 33-42.

Meyer, M. S., Wood, F. B., Hart, L. A., & Felton, R. H. (1998a). Longitudinal course of rapid naming in disabled and nondisabled readers. *Annals of Dyslexia, 48,* 91-114.

Meyer, M. S., Wood, F. B., Hart, L. A., & Felton, R. H. (1998b). The selective predictive values in rapid automatized naming within poor readers. *Journal of Learning Disabilities, 31,* 106-117.

Meyers, J. E., & Meyers, K. R. (1995). *Rey comples figures test and recognition trial.* Odessa, FL: Psyhcological Assessment Resources, Inc.

Michaels, C. A., Lazar, J. W., & Risucci, D. A. (1997). A neuropsychological approach to the assessment of adults with learning disabilities in vocational rehabilitation. *Journal of Learning Disabilities, 30*(5), 544-551.

Michie, A. M., Lindsay, W. R., & Smith, A. H. W. (1998). Changes following community living skills training: A controlled study. *British Journal of Clinical Psychology, 37,* 109-111.

Middleton, F. A., & Strick, P. L. (1994). Anatomical evidence for cerebellar and basal ganglia involvement in higher cognitive function. *Science, 266,* 458-461.

Milberger, S., Biederman, J., Faraone, S. V., Murphy, J., & Tsuang, M. T. (1995). Attention deficit hyperactivity disorder and comorbid disorders: Issues of overlapping symptoms. *American Journal of Psychiatry, 152,* 1793-1799.

Miles, T. R. (1986). On the persistence of dyslexic difficulties into adulthood. In G. T. Pavlidis & D. F. Fisher (Eds.), *Dyslexia: Neuropsychology and treatment.* New York: Wiley.

Miller, S. P., & Mercer, C. D. (1998). Educational aspects of mathematics disabilities. In D. P. Rivera (Ed.), *Mathematics education for students with learning disabilities* (pp. 81-96). Austin, TX: Pro-Ed.

Millon, T., Davis, R. G., & Millon, C. (1997). *Millon clinical multiaxial inventory - III.* Minneapolis, MN: MCS, Inc.

Millon, T., Green, C. J., & Meagher, R. B. (1982). *Millon adolescent personality inventory manual.* Minneapolis, MN: Interpretive Scoring Systems.

Millon, T., Millon, C., & Davis, R. (1993). *Millon adolescent clinical inventory.* Minneapolis, MN: National Computer Systems, Inc.

Millstein, R. B., Wilens, T. E., Biederman, J., & Spencer, T. J. (1997). Presenting ADHD symptoms and subtypes in clinically referred adults with ADHD. *Journal of Attention Disorders, 2*(3), 159-166.

Minshew, N. J. (1996). Autism. In B. O. Berg (Ed.), *Principles of Child Neurology* (pp. 1713-1730). New York: McGraw-Hill.

Minshew, N. J., & Goldstein, G. (1993). Is autism and amnesic disorder? Evidence from the California Verbal Learning Test. *Neuropsychology, 7*, 209-216.

Minshew, N. J., Goldsetin, G., & Siegel, D. J. (1997). Neuropsychologic functioning in autism: Profile of a complex information processing disorder. *Journal of the International Neuropsychological Society, 3*, 303-316.

Minshew, N. J., & Goldstein, G. (1998). Autism as a disorder of complex information processing. *Mental Retardation and Developmental Disabilities Research Reviews, 4*, 129-136.

Minshew, N. J., Goldstein, G., Dombrowski, S. M., Panchalingam, K., & Pettegrew, J. W. (1993). A preliminary[31] PMRS study of autism: Evidence for undersynthesis and increased degradation of brain membranes. *Biological Psychiatry, 33*, 762-773.

Minshew, N. J., Goldstein, G., Muenz, L. R., & Payton, J. B. (1992). Neuropsychological functioning in non-mentally retarded autistic individuals. *Journal of Clinical and Experimental Neuropsychology, 14*, 740-761.

Minshew, N. J., Goldstein, G., Taylor, H. G., & Siegel, D. J. (1994). Academic achievement in high functioning autistic individuals. *Journal of Clinical and Experimental Nueropsychology, 16*, 261-270.

Minshew, N. J., Luna, B., & Sweeney, J. A. (1999). Oculomotor evidence for neocortical systems but not cerebellar dysfunction in autism. *Neurology, 23*, 917-922.

Minshew, N. J., & Payton, J. B. (1988). The clinical spectrum of infantile autism: Part I. *Current Problems in Pediatrics, 18*, 561-610.

Minshew, N. J., Siegel, D. J., Goldstein, G., & Weldy, S. (1994). Verbal problem solving in high functioning autistic individuals. *Archives of Clinical Neuropsychology, 9*, 31-40.

Minshew, N. J., Sweeney, J. A., & Bauman, M. L. (1997). Neurological aspects of autism. In D. J. Cohen & F. R. Volkmar (Eds.), *Handbook of autism and pervasive developmental disorders* (2nd ed., pp. 344-369). New York: John Wiley & Sons.

Minskoff, E. H., Hawks, R., Steidle, E. F., & Hoffmann, F. J. (1989). A homogeneous group of persons with learning disabilities: Adults with severe learning disabilities in vocational rehabilitation. *Journal of Learning Disabilities, 22*, 521-528.

Mirsky, A. F., Anthony, B. J., Duncan, C. C., & et al. (1991). Analysis of the elements of attention: A neuropsychological approach. *Neuropsychological Review, 2*, 109-145.

Moats, L. C. (1983). A comparison of the spelling errors of older dyslexics and second-grade normal children. *Annals of Dyslexia, 33*, 121-139.

Moats, L. C. (1993a). Assessment of spelling in learning disabilities research. In G. R. Lyons (Ed.), *Frames of Reference for the Assessment of Learning Disabilities: New Views of Measurement Issues*. Baltimore, MD: Paul Brookes.

Moats, L. C. (1993b). Spelling error analysis: Beyond the phonetic/dysphonic dichotomy. *Annals of Dyslexia, 43*, 174-185.

Moats, L. C. (1994). Principles of spelling instruction. In S. Brody (Ed.), *Teaching Reading: Language, Letters, and Thought*. Milford, NH: LARC Publishing.

Moats, L. C. (1995). *Spelling, Development Disability and Instruction*. Baltimore, MD: York Press.

Montague, M. (1998). Cognitive strategy instruction in mathematics for students with learning disabilities. In D. P. Rivera (Ed.), *Mathematics education for students with learning disabilities* (pp. 177-199). Austin, TX: Pro-Ed.

Moore, D. (1997,). Adult ADHD: Challenge of a lifetime. *The ADHD Challenge, September/October*.

Morris, R., Lyon, G. R., Alexander, D., Gray, D. B., Kavanagh, J., Rourke, B. P., & Swanson, H. L. (1994). Editorial: Proposed guidelines and criteria for describing samples of persons with learning disabilities. *Learning Disability Quarterly, 17,* 106-109.

Morris, R. D., Stuebing, K. K., Fletcher, J. M., Shaywitz, S. E., Lyon, R., Shankweiler, D. P., Katz, L., Francis, D. J., & Shaywitz, B. A. (1998). Subtypes of reading disability: Variability around a phonological core. *Journal of Educational Psychology, 90*(3), 347-373.

Morris, R. D., & Walter, L. W. (1991). Subtypes of arithmetic-disabled adults: Validating childhood findings. In B. Rourke (Ed.), *Neuropsychological validation of learning disability subtypes* (pp. 330-346). New York: Guilford Publications.

Morrison, J. R., & Stewart, M. A. (1973). The psychiatric status of the legal families of adopted hyperactive children. *Arch Gen Psychiatry, 28,* 888-891.

Morrison, S. R., & Siegel, L. S. (1991). Arithmetic disability: Theoretical considerations and empirical evidence for this subtype. In L. V. Feagans, E. J. Short, & L. J. Meltzer (Eds.), *Subtypes of learning disabilities* (pp. 198-208). Hillsdale, NJ: Earlbaum.

Morrison, S. R., & Siegel, L. S. (1991b). Learning disabilities: A critical review of definitional and assessment issues. In J. E. Obrzut & G. W. Hynd (Eds.), *Neuropsychological foundations of learning disabilities: A handbook of issues, methods, and practice* (pp. 79-97). San Diego, CA: Academic Press.

Morrow, L. A., & Beers, S. R. (1995). Neuropsychological assessment: When to ask for it, what to expect. *Journal of Psychological Practice, 1,* 182-190.

Moruzzi, G., & Magoun, H. W. (1949). Brain stem reticular formation and activation of the EEG. *Electroencephalography and Clinical Neuropsychology, I,* 455-473.

Mosberg, L., & Johns, D. (1994). Reading and listening comprehension in college students with developmental dyslexia. *Learning Disabilities Research & Practice, 9*(3), 130-135.

Mosher, F. A., & Hornsby, J. R. (1996). On asking questions. In J. S. Bruner, R. R. Olver, T. M. Greenfield, J. R. Hornsby, H. J. Kenney, M. Maccoby, N. Modiano, S. A. Mosher, D. R. Olson, M. C. Potter, L. C. Reich, & A. M. Sonstroem (Eds.), *Studies in cognitive growth* (pp. 86-102). New York: Wiley & Sons.

Murphy, K., & LeVert, S. (1995). *Out of the fog: Treatment options and coping strategies for adult attention deficit disorder.* New York: Skylight Press.

Mykelbust, H. R. (1975). Nonverbal learning disabilities: Assessment and intervention. In H. R. Myklebust (Ed.), *Progress in learning disabilities* (3rd ed., pp. 85-121). New York: Grune & Stratton.

Nadeau, K. (Ed.). (1995). *A comprehensive guide to attention deficit disorders in adults: Research, diagnosis, and treatment.* New York: Brunner/Mazel, Inc.

Naglieri, J. A., & Johnson, D. (2000). Effectiveness of a cognitive strategy intervention in improving arithmetic computation based on the PASS theory. *Journal of Learning Disabilities, 33,* 591-597.

National Center for Education Statistics. (1995-96). *National postsecondary student aid study.* Washington, DC: U.S. Government Printing Office.

National Center for Education Statistics. (1999). *Students with disabilities in postsecondary education: A profile of preparation, participation, and outcomes.* Washington, DC: U.S. Government Printing Office.

National Educational Goals Panel (1993). *The 1993 national educational goals panel report.* Washington, DC: U. S. Government Printing Office.

Newby, R. F., & Lyon, G. R. (1991). Neuropsychological subtypes of learning disabilities. In J. E. Obrzut & G. W. Hynd (Eds.), *Neuropsychological foundations of learning disabilities: A handbook of issues, methods, and practice* (pp. 355-385). New York: Academic Press.

Newcomer, P. L., & Barenbaum, E. M. (1991). The written composing ability of children with learning disabilities: A review of the literature from 1980 to 1990. *Journal of Learning Disabilities, 14*, 578-593.

Nichelli, P., & Venneri, A. (1995). Right hemisphere developmental learning disability: A case study. *Neurocase, 1*, 173-177.

Nichols, P. (1980). Early antecedents of hyperactivity. *Neurology, 30*, 439.

Nielson, K. H., Mrazik, M., Hiemenz, J. R., & Hynd, G. W. (1994). *Rates of birth complications and prenatal toxin exposure in children with attention deficit hyperactivity disorder* : University of Georgia.

Nightengale, D., Yudd, R., Anderson, S., & Barnow, B. (1991). *The learning disabled in employment and training programs* (Research and Evaluation Report Series 91-E). Washington, DC: Urban Institute.

NIH Consensus Statement. (1998). Diagnosis and Treatment of Attention Deficit Hyperactivity Disorder. Nov. 16-18, 16, 2: 1-37.

Nolting, P. D. (1991). *Math and the learning disabled student: A practical guide for accommodations.* Pompano Beach, FL: Academic Success Press.

Nolting, P. D. (1997). *Winning at math: Your guide to learning mathematics through successful study skills.* Bradenton, FL: Academic Success Press, Inc.

Norman, C. A., & Zigmond, N. (1980). Characteristics of children labeled and served as learning disabled in school systems affiliated with Child Service Demonstration Center. *Journal of Learning Disabilities, 13*, 542-547.

Nussbaum, N. L., Grant, M. L., Roman, M. J., Poole, J. H., & Bigler, E. D. (1990). Attention deficit disorder and the mediating effect of age on academic and behavioral variables. *Developmental and Behavioral Pediatrics, 11*, 22-26.

O'Donnell, J. P. (1991). Neuropsychological assessment of learning-disabled adolescents and young adults. In J. E. Obrzut & G. W. Hynd (Eds.), *Neuropsychological foundations of learning disabilities* (pp. 331-353). San Diego, CA: Academic Press.

O'Donnell, J. P., Romero, J. J., & Leicht, D. J. (1990). A comparison of language deficits in learning-disabled, head-injured and nondisabled young adults: Results from an abbreviated aphasia screening test. *Journal of Clinical Psychology, 46*, 310-315.

Oestreicher, J. M., & O'Donnell, J. P. (1995). Validation of the General Neuropsychological Deficit Scale with nondisabled, learning-disabled, and head-injured young adults. *Archives of Clinical Neuropsychology, 10*, 185-191.

Olson, R., Forsberg, H., Wise, B., & Rack, J. (1994). Measurement of word recognition, orthographic, and phonological skills. In G. R. Lyon (Ed.), *Frames of reference for the assessment of learning disabilities: New views on measurement issues.* Baltimore, MD: Brookes.

Ornitz, E. M. (1988). Autism: A disorder of directed attention. *Brain Dysfunction, 1*, 309-322.

Ornitz, E. M., & Ritvo, E. R. (1968). Perceptual inconstancy in early infantile autism. *Archives of General Psychiatry, 18*, 76-98.

Ornitz, E. M., Sugiyama, T., & deTraversay, J. (1993). Startle moducation studies in autism. *Journal of Autism and Developmental Disorders, 23*, 619-637.

Orton, J. L. (1966). The Orton-Gillingham approach. In J. Money (Ed.), *The disabled reader: Education of the dyslexic child* (pp. 243-277). Baltimore, MD: Brookes.

Orton, S. T. (1925). "Word-blindness" in school children. *Archives of Neurology and Psychiatry, 14*, 581-615.

Orton, S. T. (1937). *Reading, writing and speech problems in children: A presentation of certain types of disorders in the development of the language faculty.* New York: W. W. Norton.

Osterrieth, P. A. (1944). Le test de copie d'une figure complexe. *Archives de Psychologie, 30*, 206-356.

Owens, N., & Owens, B. W. (1993). *Adult attention deficit disorder behavior rating scales.*

Ozonoff, S. (1995a). Reliability and validity of the Wisconsin Card Sorting Test in studies of autism. *Neuropsychology, 9,* 491-500.

Ozonoff, S. (1995b). *Executive functions in autism.* New York: Plenum Press.

Ozonoff, S., Pennington, B. F., & Rogers, S. J. (1991). Executive function deficits in high-functioning autistic individuals: Relationship to theory of mind. *Journal of Child Psychology and Psychiatry, 32,* 1081-1105.

Ozonoff, S., Strayer, D. L., McMahon, W. M., & Filloux, F. (1994). Executive function abilities in autism and Tourette syndrome: An information processing approach. *Journal of Child Psychology and Psychiatry, 35,* 1015-1032.

Palinscar, A. S., & Brown, A. L. (1984). Reciprocal teaching of comprehension-fostering and comprehension-monitoring activities. *Cognition and Instruction, 1,* 117-175.

Pardo, J. V., Fox, P. T., & Raichie, M. E. (1991). Localization of a human system for sustained attention by positron emission tomography. *Nature, 349,* 61-64.

Pascualvaca, D. M., Fantie, B. D., Papageorgiou, M., & Mirsky, A. F. (1998). Attentional capacities in children with autism: Is there a general deficit in shifting focus. *Journal of Autism and Developmental Disabilities, 28,* 467-478.

Pasto, L., & Burack, J. A. (1995, June). *A developmental study of visual filtering: Can windows facilitate filtering efficiency?* Paper presented at the Canadian Psychological Association, Charlottetown, Canada.

Patton, J. R., & Polloway, E. A. (1992). Learning disabilities: The challenges of adulthood. *Journal of learning disabilities, 25*(7), 410-415, 447.

Pauls, D. L., Alsobrook, J. P., Gelernter, L., & Leckman, J. F. (1999). Genetic vulnerability. In J. F. Leckman & R. T. Schulz (Eds.), *Tourette's syndrome - tics, obsessions, compulsions* (pp. 194-212). New York: John Wiley & Sons, Inc.

PeBenito, R. (1987). Developmental Gerstmann Syndrome: Case report and review of the literature. *Journal of Developmental and Behavioral Pediatrics, 8,* 229-232.

PeBenito, R., Fisch, C. B., & Fisch, M. L. (1988). Developmental Gerstmann Syndrome. *Archives of Neurology, 45,* 977-982.

Pelham, W., & Swanson, J. (1999, October). *Do time-response effects vary among stimulant medications?* Symposium presented at the 46th Annual Meeting of the American Academy of Child and Adolescent Psychiatry, Chicago, Illinois.

Pennington, B. F. (1991). *Diagnosing learning disorders: A neuropsychological framework.* New York: Guilford.

Pennington, B. F., & Gilger, J. W. (1996). How is dyslexia transmitted? In C. H. Chase, G. D. Rosen, & G. F. Sherman (Eds.), *Developmental dyslexia* (pp. 41-61). Baltimore, MD: York Press.

Pennington, B. F., Rogers, S. J., Bennetto, L., Griffith, E. M., Reed, D. T., & Shyu, V. (In press). Validity tests of the executive dysfunction hypothesis of autism. In J. Russell (Ed.), *Autism as an executive disorder.* Oxford, UK: Oxford University Press.

Pennington, B. F., Van Orden, G. C., Smith, S. D., Green, P. A., & Haith, M. M. (1990). Phonological processing skills and deficits in adult dyslexics. *Child Development, 61,* 1753-1758.

Peter, B. M., & Spreen, O. (1979). Behavior rating and personal adjustment scales of neuropsychologically and learning handicapped children during adolescence and early adulthood: Results of a follow-up study. *Journal of Clinical Neuropsychology, 1,* 75-91.

Peterson, K. *Coaching interventions and strategies for adults with attention deficit disorder.*

Petrauskas, R., & Rourke, B. P. (1979). Identification of subgroups of retarded readers: A neuropsychological, multivariate approach. *Journal of Clinical Neuropsychology, 1,* 17-37.

Pierce, K., Glad, K. S., & Scheiebman, L. (1997). Social perception in children with autism: An attentional deficit? *Journal of Autism and Developmental Disorders, 27*, 265-282.

Pliszka, S. R., Carlson, C. L., & Swanson, J. M. (1999). *ADHD with comorbid disorders.* New York: Guilford Press.

Pliszka, S. R., McCracken, J. T., & Maas, J. W. (1996). Catecholamines in Attention-Deficit Hyperactivity Disorder: Current perspectives. *Journal of American Academy of Child & Adolescent Psychiatry, 35*(3), 264-272.

Policy statement for documentation of attention-deficit/hyperactivity disorder in adolescents and adults. (1998). Office of Disability Policy, Educational Testing Service, Princeton, NJ.

Pollens, R., McBratnie, B., & Burton, P. (1988). Beyond cognition: Executive functions in closed head injury. *Cognitive Rehabilitation* (September/October).

Pontius, A. A. (1973). Dysfunction patterns analogous to frontal lobe system and caudatae nucleus syndromes in some groups of minimal brain dysfunction. *Journal of American Medical Women Association, 28*, 285-292.

Posner, M. L., & Raichle, M. (1996). *Images of mind.* (Revised ed.). Washington, DC: Scientific American Books.

Poteet, J. A. (1978). Characteristics of written expression of learning disabled and non-learning disabled elementary school students. *Diagnostique, 4*, 60-74.

Pratt, A. C., & Brady, S. (1988). Relation of phonological awareness to reading disability in children and adults. *Journal of Educational Psychology, 80*(3), 319-323.

Price, L. A., Johnson, J. M., & Evelo, S. (1994). When academic assistance is not enough: Addressing the mental health issues of adolescents and adults with learning disabilities. *Journal of Learning Disabilities, 27*(2), 82-90.

Prior, M., & Hoffman, W. (1990). Neuropsychology testing of autistic children through an exploration with frontal lobe tests. *Journal of Autism and Developmental Disorders, 4*, 581-590.

Public Law 94-142. (1975, November 29). *Education for All Handicapped Children Act.* U. S. Congress.

Rack, J. (1997). Issues in the assessment of developmental dyslexia in adults: Theoretical and applied perspectives. *Journal of Research in Reading, 20*(1), 66-76.

Rack, J. P., Snowling, M. J., & Olson, R. K. (1992). The nonword reading deficit in developmental dyslexia. *Reading Research Quarterly, 27*, 28-53.

Rapin, I. (1997). Current concepts: Autism. *The New England Journal of Medicine, 337*, 97-104.

Rapoport, J. L., Donnelly, M., Zametkin, A., & Carrougher, J. (1986). Situational hyperactivity in a U.S. clinical setting. *Journal of Child Psychology & Psychiatry, 27*, 639-646.

Raskind, M. H. (1993). Assistive technology for adults with learning disabilities: A rationale for use. In P. J. Gerber & H. B. Reiff (Eds.), *Learning disabilities in adulthood: Persisting problems and evolving issues* (pp. 152-162). Boston, MA: Andover.

Raskind, M. H. (1995). Assistive technology for adults with learning disabilities. In P. J. Gerber & H. B. Reiff (Eds.), *Learning disabilities in adulthood.* Austin, TX: Pro-Ed.

Raskind, M. H., & Higgins, E. (1995). Effects of speech synthesis on the proofreading efficiency of postsecondary students with learning disabilities. *Learning Disability Quarterly, 18*, 141-158.

Raskind, M. H., & Higgins, E. L. (1998). Assistive technology for postsecondary students with learning disabilities: An overview. *Journal of Learning Disabilities, 31*(1), 27-40.

Ratey, J., Hallowell, E. M., & Leveroni, C. L. (1993). *Pharmacotherapy for ADHD in adults.* Paper presented at the 5th Annual CHADD Conference, San Diego, CA.

Ratey, J. J., Greenberg, M. S., & Lindem, K. J. (1991). Combination of treatments for attention deficit hyperactivity disorder in adults. *Journal of Nerv Ment Dis, 179*, 699-701.

Ratey, J. J., Hallowell, E., & Miller, A. (1997). Psychosocial issues and psychotherapy in adults with attention deficit disorder. *Psychiatric Annals, 27*(8), 582-587.

Ratey, N. (1997). Supporters give ADD coaching credit for low attrition rates, improved grades. *Disability Compliance for Higher Education, 3*, 5.

Rawson, M. (19968). *Developmental and Language Disability: Adult Accomplishments of Dyslexic Boys.* Baltimore, MD: Johns Hopkins Press.

Reback, M. B. (1996). Accommodating workers with learning disabilities. In S. C. Cramer & W. Ellis (Eds.), *Learning disabilities: Lifelong issues.* Baltimore, MD: Paul H. Brookes.

Rehabilitation Act of 1973. Public Law 93-112, 87 Stat. 355

Rehabilitation Services Administration. (1981, July 27). *Acceptance of specific learning disabilities as a medically recognized disability program instruction.* Program Information Memorandum RSA-PI-81-22, 1-7.

Rehabilitation Services Administration. (1985, January 24). *Program policy directive.* Washington, DC: U.S. Office of Special Education and Rehabilitation Services.

Reichler, R. J., & Schopler, E. (Eds.). (1976). *Developmental therapy: A program model for providing individual services in the community: Psychopathology and child development.* New York: Plenum Press.

Reiff, H. B., & Gerber, P. J. (1993). Social/emotional and daily living issues for adults with learning disabilities. In P. J. Gerber & H. B. Reiff (Eds.), *Learning disabilities in adulthood: Persisting problems and evolving issues* (pp. 72-81). Boston, MA: Andover.

Reiff, H. B., Gerber, P. J., & Ginsberg, R. (1997). *Exceeding expectations: Successful adults with learning disabilities.* Austin, TX: Pro-Ed.

Reitan, R. M., & Wolfson, D. (1993). *The Halstead-Reitan Neuropsychological Test Battery: Theory and clinical interpretation.* (2nd ed.). Tucson, AZ: Neuropsychology Press.

Rey, A. (1941). L'examen psychologique dans les cas d'encephalopathie traumatique. *Archives Psychology, 28*, 286-340.

Reynolds, C. R. (1985). Measuring the aptitude-achievement discrepancy in learning disability diagnosis. *Remedial and Special Education, 6*(5), 37-55.

Reynolds, W. M. (1987). *Reynolds adolescent depression scale.* Odessa, FL: Psychological Assessment Resources, Inc.

Reynolds, W. M. (1998). *Adolescent psychopathology scale.* Odessa, FL: Psychological Assessment Resources, Inc.

Riccio, C. A., & Hynd, G. W. (1996). Neurobiological research specific to the adult population with learning disabilities. In N. Gregg, C. Hoy, & A. F. Gay (Eds.), *Adults with Learning Disabilities: Theoretical & Practical Perspectives* (pp. 127-143). New York: Guilford Press.

Riccio, C. A., Hynd, G. W., & Cohen, M. J. (1997). Etiology and neurobiology of ADHD. In W. N. Bender (Ed.), *Understanding ADHD, a practical guide for teachers and parents.* New Jersey: Prentice-Hall.

Riccio, C. A., Hynd, G. W., Cohen, M. J., & Gonzalez, J. J. (1993). Neurological basis of attention deficit hyperactivity disorder. *Exceptional Children, 60*(2), 118-124.

Richard, M. M. (1995). Pathways to success for the college student with ADD accommodations and preferred practices. *Journal of Postsecondary Education and Disability, 11*, 16-30.

Richard, M. M., Finkel, M. F., & Cohen, M. D. (1998). Preparing reports documenting Attention-Deficit/Hyperactivity disorder for students in post-secondary education: What neurologists need to know. *The Neurologist, 4*, 277-283.

Rincover, A., & Ducharme, J. M. (1987). Variables influencing stimulus overselectivity and "tunnel-vision" in developmentally disabled children. *American Journal of Mental Deficiency, 91*, 422-430.

Rivera, D. P. (Ed.). (1998). *Mathematics education for students with learning disabilities.* Austin, TX: Pro-Ed.

Roberts, R., & Mather, N. (1997). Orthographic dyslexia: The neglected subtype. *Learning Disabilities Research & Practice, 12*(4), 236-250.

Robinson, F. P. (1946). *Effective Study.* New York: Harper & Brothers.

Rogan, L. L., & Hartman, L. D. (1990). Adult outcomes of learning disabled students ten years after initial follow-up. *Learning Disabilities Focus, 5*(2), 91-102.

Rogeness, G. A., Javors, M. A., & Pliska, S. R. (1992). Neurochemistry and child and adolescent psychiatry. *American Academy of Child & Adolescent Psychiatry, 3*, 765-781.

Rogers, J. C., & Holm, M. B. (1998). Geriatric rehabilitation. In G. Goldstein & S. R. Beers (Eds.), *Rehabilitation* (pp. 89-109). New York: Plenum.

Rojewski, J. W. (1999). Occupational and educational aspirations and attainment of young adults with and without LD 2 years after high school completion. *Journal of Learning Disabilities, 32*, 533-552.

Rosner, J., & Simon, D. (1971). The auditory analysis test: An initial report. *Journal of Learning Disabilities, 4*, 40-48.

Ross, J. J., & Smith, J. O. (1990). Adult basic educator's perceptions of learning disabilities. *Journal of Reading, 33*(5), 340-347.

Ross, J. M. (1987). Learning disabled adults: Who are they and what do we do with them? *Lifelong Learning, 11*(3), 4-7.

Ross, J. M. (1988). Learning and coping strategies of learning disabled ABE students. *Adult Literacy and Basic Education, 12*(2), 78-90.

Ross-Gordon, J. M. (1989). Adults with Learning Disabilities: An Overview for the Adult Educator. Columbus, OH: ERIC Clearinghouse on Adult, Career, & Vocational Education.

Ross-Gordon, J. M. (1996). Sociocultural issues affecting the identification and service delivery models for adults with learning disabilities. In N. Gregg, C. Hoy, & A. F. Gay (Eds.), *Adults with Learning Disabilities: Theoretical & Practical Perspectives.* New York: Guilford Press.

Rothstein, L. (1998, April). Guidelines emerge for accommodating students who have learning disabilities. *The Chronicle of Higher Education.*

Rourke, B. P. (1982). Central processing deficiencies in children: Toward a developmental neuropsychological model. *Journal of Clinical Neuropsychology* (4), 1-18.

Rourke, B. P. (Ed.). (1985). *Essentials of subtype analysis.* New York: Guilford.

Rourke, B. P. (1985). *Neuropsychology of Learning Disabilities: Essentials of Subtype Analysis.* New York: Guilford Press.

Rourke, B. P. (1988). The syndrome of nonverbal learning disabilities: Developmental manifestations in neurological disease, disorder, and dysfunction. *The Clinical Neuropsychologist, 2*, 293-330.

Rourke, B. P. (Ed.). (1989). *Nonverbal learning disabilities: The syndrome and the model.* New York: Guilford Press.

Rourke, B. P. (1989a). *Nonverbal learning disabilities: The syndrome and the model.* New York: Guilford.

Rourke, B. P. (1989b). Nonverbal learning disabilities, socioemotional disturbance, and suicide: A reply to Fletcher, Kowalchuk and King, and Bigler. *Journal of Learning Disabilities, 22*, 186-187.

Rourke, B. P. (1991). Validation of learning disabilities subtypes: An overview. In B. P. Rouorke (Ed.), *Neuropsychological validation of learning disability subtypes* (pp. 3-11). New York: Guilford Press.

Rourke, B. P. (1993). Arithmetic disabilities, specific and otherwise; a neuropsychological perspective. *Journal of Learning Disabilities, 26*, 214-226.

Rourke, B. P. (Ed.). (1995). *Syndrome of nonverbal learning disabilities: Neurodevelopmental manifestations.* New York: Guilford.

Rourke, B. P., Bakker, D. J., Fisk, J. L., & Strang, J. D. (1983). *Child neuropsychology: An introduction to theory, research, and practice.* New York: Guilford.

Rourke, B. P., & Conway, J. A. (1998). Disabilities of arithmetic and mathematical reasoning: Perspectives from neurology and neuropsychology. In D. P. Rivera (Ed.), *Mathematics education for students with learning disabilities* (pp. 59-79). Austin, TX: Pro-Ed.

Rourke, B. P., Del Dotto, J. E., Rourke, S. B., & Casey, J. E. (1990). Nonverbal learning disabilities: The syndrome and a case study. *Journal of School Psychology, 28*, 361-385.

Rourke, B. P., & Finlayson, M. A. (1978). Neuropsychological significance of variations in patterns of academic performance: Verbal and visual-spatial abilities. *Journal of Abnormal Child Psychology, 6*, 121-133.

Rourke, B. P., & Fisk, J. L. (1981). Socio-emotional disturbances of learning disabled children: The role of central processing deficits. *Bulletin of the Orton Society, 31*, 77-88.

Rourke, B. P., & Fisk, J. L. (1992). Adult presentations of learning disabilities. In R. F. White (Ed.), *Clinical syndromes in adult neuropsychology* (pp. 451-473). New York: Elsevier.

Rourke, B. P., Fisk, J. L., & Strang, J. D. (1986a). *Neuropsychological assessment of children: A treatment oriented approach.* New York: Guilford.

Rourke, B. P., & Fuerst, D. E. (1996). Psychosocial dimenstions of learning disability subtypes. *Assessment, 3*, 277-290.

Rourke, B. P., & Strang, J. D. (1983). Subtypes of reading and arithmetic disabilities: A neuropsychological analysis. In M. Butler (Ed.), *Developmental neuropsychiatry* (pp. 473-488). New York: Guilford Press.

Rourke, B. P., Young, G. C., & Leenaars, A. A. (1989). A childhood learning disability that predisposes those afflicted to adolescent and adult depression and suicide risk. *Journal of Learning Disabilities, 22*, 169-175.

Rourke, B. P., Young, G. C., Strang, J. D., & Russell, D. L. (1986b). Adult outcomes of central processing deficiencies in childhood. In I. Grant & K. M. Adams (Eds.), *Neuropsychological assessment in neuropsychiatric disorders: Clinicla methods and empirical findings* (pp. 244-267). New York: Oxford.

Rucklidge, J. J., & Kaplan, B. J. (1997). Psychological functioning of women identified in adulthood with attention-deficit/hyperactivity disorder. *Journal of Attention Disorders, 2*(3), 167-176.

Rumsey, J. M. (1985). Conceptual problem-solving in highly verbal, non-retarded autistic men. *Journal of Autism and Developmental Disorders, 15*, 23-35.

Rumsey, J. M., Andreason, P., Zametkin, A. J., Aquino, R., King, A. D., Hamburger, S. D., Pikus, A., Rapoport, J. L., & Cohen, R. M. (1992). Failure to activate the left temporoparietal cortex in dyslexia: An oxygen 15 positron emission tomographic study. *Archives of Neurology, 49*, 527-534.

Rumsey, J. M., & Eden, G. (1998). Functional neuroimaging of developmental dyslexia: Regional cerebral blood flow in dyslexic men. In B. D. Shapiro, P. J. Accardo, & A. J. Capute (Eds.), *Specific Reading Disability: A View of the Spectrum* . Timonium, MD: York Press.

Rumsey, J. M., & Hamburger, S. D. (1988). Neuropsychological findings in high-functioning men with infantile autism, residual state. *Journal of Clinical and Experimental Neuropsychology, 10*, 201-221.

Rumsey, J. M., & Hamburger, S. D. (1990). Neuropsychological divergence of high-level autism and severe dyslexia. *Journal of Autism and Developmental Disorders, 20*, 155-168.

Rumsey, J. M., Horwitz, B., Donohue, B. C., Nace, K., Maisog, J. M., & Andreason, P. (1997). Phonologic and orthographic components of word recognition: A PET-rCBF study. *Brain, 120*, 739-760.

Rush, C. R., Kollins, S. H., & Pazzaglia, P. J. (1998). Discriminative-stimulus and participant-rated effects of Methylphenidate, Bupropion, and Triazolam in *d*-Amphetamine-trained humans. *Experimental and Clinical Psychopharmacology, 6*(1), 32-44.

Russell, D. L., & Rourke, B. P. (1991). Concurrent and predictive validity of phonetic accuracy of misspellings in normal and disabled readers and spellers. In B. P. Rourke (Ed.), *Neuropsychological validation of learning disability subtypes* (pp. 57-72). New York: Guilford Press.

Russell, J., Jarrold, C., & Henry, L. (1996). Working memory in children with autism and with moderate learning difficulties. *Journal of Child Psychology and Psychiatry, 37*, 673-686.

Rutter, M., & Schopler, E. (1987). Autism and pervasive developmental disorders: Concepts and diagnostic issues. *Journal of Autism and Developmental Disorders, 17*, 159-186.

Ryan, A. G., & Price, L. (1992). Adults with learning disabilities in higher education in the 1990s. *Interventions in School and Clinic, 28*, 6-20.

Ryckman, D. (1981). Sex differences in a sample of learning disabled children. *Learning Disability Quarterly, 4*, 48-52.

Safer, D. J. (1973). A familial factor in minimal brain dysfunction. *Behav Genet, 3*, 175-186.

Sandler, A. D. (1995). Attention deficits and neurodevelopmental variation in older adolescents and adults. In K. Nadeau (Ed.), *A comprehensive guide to attention deficit disorder in adults* (pp. 58-73). New York: Brunner/Mazel.

Saracoglu, B., Minden, H., & Wilchesky, M. (1989). The adjustment of students with learning disabilities to university and its relationship to self-esteem and self-efficacy. *Journal of Learning Disabilities, 22*, 590-592.

Satz, P., Buka, S., Lipsitt, L., & Seidman, L. (1998). The long-term prognosis of learning disabled children. In B. K. Shapiro, P. J. Accardo, & A. J. Capute (Eds.), *Specific reading disability: A view of the spectrum*. Timonium, MD: York Press.

Schachar, R., Sandberg, S., & Rutter, M. (1986). Agreement between teacher ratings and observations of hyperactivity, inattentiveness, and defiance. *Journal of Abnormal Child Psychology, 14*, 331-335.

Schoenfeld, A. H. (1994). A discourse on methods. *Journal for Research in Mathematics Education, 25*, 697-710.

Schonhaut, S., & Satz, P. (1983). Prognosis of the learning disabled child: A review of the follow-up studies. In M. Rutter (Ed.), *Developmental neuropsychiatry*. New York: Guilford Press.

Schopler, E., Reichler, R. J., & Rochen-Renner, B. R. (1988). *The Childhood Autism Rating Scale*. Los Angeles, CA: Western Psychological Services.

Schreibman, L., Koegel, R. L., Charlop, M. H., & Egel, A. L. (1982). Infantile autism. In A. S. Bellack, M. Hersen, & A. E. Kazdin (Eds.), *International handbook of behavior modification and therapy* (2nd ed., pp. 763-789). New York: Plenum.

Schultz, W. (1997). Dopamine neurons and their role in reward mechanisma. *Curr Opin Neurobiol, 7*, 191-197.

Schultz, W., Dayan, P., & Montague, P. R. (1997). A neural substrate of prediction and reward. *Science, 275*, 1593-1599.

Schumaker, J. B., Deshler, D. D., Alley, G. R., Warner, M. M., & Denton, P. H. (1982). Multipass: A learning strategy for improving reading comprehension. *Learning Disability Quarterly, 5*, 295-304.

Schumaker, J. B., Nolan, S. M., & Deshler, D. D. (1985). *The error monitoring strategy: Learning Strategies Curriculum*. Lawrence, KS: The University of Kansas.

Schwean, V. L. (1999). Looking ahead: The adjustment of adults with disabilities. In Schwean & Saklofske (Eds.), *Handbook of psychosocial characteristics of exceptional children* (pp. 587-610). New York: Kluwer Academic/Plenum Publishers.

Schwiebert, V. L., Sealander, K. A., & Bradshaw, M. L. (1998). Preparing students with attention deficit disorders for entry into the workplace and postsecondary education. *ASCA Professional School Counseling, 2*(1), 26-32.

Section 504 of the Rehabilitation Act of 1973. 29, U.S.C. 794, 45 C.F.R. 81, 84.

Seidman, L. J., Biederman, J., Faraone, S. V., Weber, W., & Ouellette, C. (1997). Towards defining a neuropsychology of ADHD: Performance of children and adolescents from a large clinically referred sample. *Journal Consult Clin Psychol, 65,* 150-160.

Seidman, L. J., Biederman, J., Weber, W., & et al. (1998). Neuropsychological function in adults with attention deficit hyperactivity disorder. *Biol Psychiatry, 44,* 260-268.

Selz, M., & Reitan, R. M. (1979a). Rules for neuropsychological diagnosis: Classification of brain function in older children. *Journal of Consulting and Clinical Psychology, 47,* 258-264.

Selz, M., & Reitan, R. M. (1979b). Neuropsychological test performance of normal, learning-disabled, and brain-damaged children. *Journal of Nervous and Mental Disease, 167,* 298-302.

Semrud-Clikeman, M., & Hynd, G. W. (1990). Right hemisphere dysfunction in nonverbal learning disabilities: Social, academic, and adaptive functioning in adults and children. *Psychological Bulletin, 107,* 196-209.

Shaffer, D., & Greenhill, L. (1978). A critical note on the predictive validity of the "Hyperkinetic Syndrome". *Journal Child Psychol Psychiatry, 20,* 617-620.

Shafrir, U., Siegel, L. S., & Chee, M. (1990). Learning disability, inferential skills, and post-failure reflectivity. *Journal of Learning Disabilities, 23,* 506-517.

Shafrir, U., & Wiegel, L. S. (1994). Subtypes of learning disabilities in adolescents and adults. *Journal of Learning Disabilities, 27,* 123-134.

Shallice, T. (1988). *From neuropsychology to mental structure*. New York: University Press.

Share, D. L., & Stanovich, K. E. (1995). Cognitive processes in early reading development: Accommodating individual differences into a model of acquisition. *Issues in Education: Contributions from Educational Psychology, 1,* 1-57.

Shaw, R. A. (1999). The case for course substitutions as a reasonable accommodation for students with foreign language learning difficulties. *Journal of Learning Disabilities, 32*(4), 320-349.

Shaywitz, B. A., Cohen, D. J., & Bowers, M. B. (1977). CSF monomine metabolites in children with minimal brain dysfunction: Evidence of alteration of brain dopamine. *Journal Pediatrics, 90,* 67-71.

Shaywitz, B. A., Fletcher, J. M., Holahan, J. M., & Shaywitz, S. E. (1992). Discrepancy compared to low achievement definitions of reading disability: Results from the Connecticut longitudinal study. *Journal of Learning Disabilities, 25,* 639-648.

Shaywitz, B. A., Holford, T. R., Holahan, J. M., & et al. (1995). A Matthew effect for IQ but not for reading: Results from a longitudinal study. *Read Res Q, 30,* 894-906.

Shaywitz, B. A., Shaywitz, S. E., Byrne, T., Cohen, D. J., & Rothman, S. (1983). Attention Deficit Disorder: Quantitative analysis of CT. *Neurology, 33,* 1500-1503.

Shaywitz, B. A., Shaywitz, S. E., Fletcher, J. M., Pugh, K. R., Gore, J. C., Constable, R. T., Fulbright, R. K., Skudlarski, P., Liberman, A. M., Shankweiler, D. P., Katz, L., Bronen, R. A., Marchione, K. E., Holahan, J. M., Francis, D. J., Klorman, R., Aram, D. M., Blachman, B. A., Stuebing, K. K., & Lacadie, C. (1997). The Yale Center for the study of learning and attention: Longitudinal and neurobiological studies. *Learning Disabilities, 8,* 21-29.

Shaywitz, B. A., Shaywitz, S. E., Liberman, I. Y., & et al. (1991). Neurolinguistic and biologic mechanisms in dyslexia. In D. D. Duane & D. B. Gray (Eds.), *The Reading Brain* (pp. 27-52). Parkton, MD: York Press.

Shaywitz, S. E. (1998). Current concepts: Dyslexia. *New England Medical Journal, 338,* 307-312.

Shaywitz, S. E., Escobar, M. D., Shaywitz, B. A., Fletcher, J. M., & Makuch, R. (1992). Evidence that dyslexia may represent the lower tail of a normal distribution of reading ability. *New England Journal of Medicine, 326,* 145-150.

Shaywitz, S. E., Fletcher, J. M., Holahan, J. M., Schneider, A. E., Marchione, K. E., Stuebing, K. K., Francis, D. J., Pugh, K. R., & Shaywitz, B. A. (1999). Persistence of dyslexia: The Connecticut longitudinal study at adolescence. *Pediatrics, 104*(6), 1351-1359.

Shaywitz, S. E., Fletcher, J. M., & Shaywitz, B. A. (1994). Issues in the definition and classification of attention deficit disorder. *Top. Lang. Disord., 14,* 1-25.

Shaywitz, S. E., & Shaywitz, B. A. (1988). Attention deficit disorder: Current perspectives. In T. Kavanagh & T. Truss (Eds.), *Learning Disabilities.* Parkton, MD: York Press.

Shaywitz, S. E., Shaywitz, B. A., Fletcher, J. M., & Escobar, P. L. (1990). Prevalence of reading disability in boys and girls. *Journal of the American Medical Association, 264,* 998-1002.

Shaywitz, S. E. (1996,). Dyslexia. *Scientific American, November,* 98-104.

Shea, V., & Mesibov, G. B. (1985). Brief report: The relationship of learning disabilities and high-level autism. *Journal of Autism and Developmental Disorders, 15,* 425-435.

Shekim, W. O. (1989). Comprehensive evaluation of attention deficit disorder-residual type. *Comprehensive Psychiatry, 31,* 416-425.

Shekim, W. O., Asarnow, R. F., Hess, E., Zaucha, K., & Wheeler, N. A. (1990). A clinical and demographic profile of a sample of adults with attention deficit hyperactivity disorder, residual state. *Comprehensive Psychiatry, 31,* 416-425.

Shelly, C., & Goldstein, G. (1982). Intelligence, achievement and the Luria-Nebraska battery in a neuropsychiatric population: A factor analytic study. *Clinical Neuropsychology, 4,* 164-169.

Sherman, G. F. (1995). Dyslexia: Is it all in your mind? *Perspectives, The Orton Society, 21*(4), 1, 8.

Siebel, L. S., & Ryan, E. B. (1988). Development of grammatical sensitivity, phonological, and short-term memory skills in normally achieving and learning disabled children. *Developmental Psychology, 24,* 28-37.

Siegel, D. J., Goldstein, G., & Minshew, N. J. (1996). Designing instruction for the high-functioning autistic individual. *Journal of Developmental and Physical Disabilities, 8,* 1-19.

Siegel, D. J., Minshew, N. J., & Goldstein, G. (1996). Wechsler IQ profiles in diagnosis of high-functioning autism. *Journal of Autism and Developmental Disorders, 26,* 389-406.

Siegel, L. S. (1988). Evidence that IQ scores are irrelevant to the definition and analysis of reading disability. *Canadian Journal of Psychology, 42,* 201-215.

Siegel, L. S. (1989). IQ is irrelevant to the definition of learning disabilities. *Journal of Learning Disabilities, 22,* 469-478, 486.

Siegel, L. S. (1993). Alice in Iqland or why IQ is still irrelevant to learning disabilities. In R. M. Joshi & C. K. Leong (Eds.), *Reading disabilities: Diagnosis and components processes* . Dordrecht, the Netherlands: Kluwer.

Siegel, L. S. (1999). Issues in the definition and diagnosis of learning disabilities: A perspective on Guckenberger v. Boston University. *Journal of Learning Disabilities, 32,* 304-319.

Siegel, L. S., & Heaven, R. K. (1986). Categorization of learning disabilities. In S. J. Ceci (Ed.), *Handbook of cognitive, social and neuropsychological aspects of learning disabilities* (Vol. 1, pp. 94-121). Hillsdale, NJ: Earlbaum.

Siegel, L. S., & Ryan, E. B. (1989a). The development of working memory in normally achieveing and subtypes of learning disabled children. *Child Development, 60,* 973-980.

Siegel, L. S., & Ryan, E. G. (1989b). Subtypes of developmental dyslexia: The influence of definitional variables. *Reading and Writing: An Interdisciplinary Journal, 1,* 257-287.

Siegel, L. S., & Stanovich, K. E. (1997). The assessment of adults with reading disabilities: What can we learn from experimental tasks? *Journal of Research in Reading, 20*(1), 42-54.

Sitlington, P. L., & Frank, A. R. (1990). Are adolescents with learning disabilities successfully crossing the bridge into adult life? *Learning Disability Quarterly, 3,* 97-111.

Smith, A. (1982). *Symbol digit modalities test.* Los Angeles, CA: Western Psychological Services.

Smith, I. M., & Bryson, S. E. (1994). Imitation and action in autism: A critical review. *Psychological Bulletin, 116,* 259-273.

Smith, J. (1988). Social and vocational problems of adults with learning disabilities: A review of the literature. *Learning Disabilities Focus, 4,* 36-58.

Smith, J. D. (1996). Adult development theories: An overview and reflection on their relevance for learning disabilities. In J. R. Patton & E. A. Polloway (Eds.), *Learning disabilities: The challenges of adulthood* (pp. 11-23). Austin, TX: Pro-Ed.

Sohlberg, M. M., & Geyser, S. (1986). *Executive function behavioral rating scale.* Paper presented at the Whittier College Conference Series, Whittier, CA.

Southwestern Community College v. Davis. (1979). 442 U.S. 397.

Sparks, R., Phillips, L., & Ganschow, L. (1996). Students classified with learning disabled and the college foreign language requirement. In J. Liskin-Gasparro (Ed.), *The changing demographics of foreign language instruction* (pp. 123-159). Boston: Heinle & Heinle.

Speece, D. L., & Cooper, D. H. (1991). Retreat, regroup, or advance? An agenda for empirical classification research in learning disabilities. In L. V. Feagans, E. J. Short, & L. J. Meltzer (Eds.), *Subtypes of learning disabilities: Theoretical perspectives and research* (pp. 33-52). Hillsdale, NJ: Earlbaum.

Spekman, N. J., Goldberg, R. J., & Herman, K. L. (1992). Learning disabled children grow up: A search for factors related to success in the young adults years. *Learning Disabilities Research & Practice, 7,* 161-170.

Spekman, N. J., Herman, K. L., & Vogel, S. A. (1993). Risk and resilience in individuals with learning disabilities: A challenge to the field. *Learning Disabilities Research and Practice, 8*(1), 59-65.

Spellacy, F., & Peter, B. (1978). Dyscalculia and elements of the developmental Gerstmann syndrome in school children. *Cortex, 14,* 197-206.

Spencer, T., Biederman, J., Wilens, T., Harding, M., O'Donnell, D., & Griffin, S. (1996). Pharmacotherapy of attention-deficit hyperactivity disorder across the life cycle. *Journal of the American Academy of Child and Adolescent Psychiatry, 35,* 409-432.

Spencer, T., Wilens, T. E., Biederman, J., Faraone, S. V., Ablon, S., & Ras, J. F. (1995). A double blind comparison of methylphenidate and placebo in adults with attention deficit hyperactivity disorder. *Archives of General Psychiatry, 52.*

Spitzer, R. L., Williams, J. B., Gibbon, M., & First, M. B. (1992). The structured clinical interview for the DSM-III-R (SCID). *Archives of General Psychiatry, 49,* 624-629.

Spreen, O. (1982). Adult outcomes of reading disorders. In R. N. Malatesha & P. G. Aaron (Eds.), *Reading disorders, varieties and treatments* (pp. 473-498). New York: Academic Press.

Spreen, O., & Haaf, R. G. (1986). Empirically derived learning disability subtypes: A replication attempt and longitudinal patterns over 15 years. *Journal of Learning Disabilities, 19*, 170-180.

Sprich-Buckminster, S., Biederman, J., Milberger, S., Faraone, S. V., & Lehman, B. K. (1993). Are perinatal complications relevant to the manifestation of ADD? Issues of comorbidity and familiality. *Journal of the American Academy of Child and Adolescent Psychiatry, 32*, 1032-1037.

Stafford-Depass, J. M. (1998). Psychological characteristics and life experiences of highly successful learning disabled adults. *Dissertation Abstracts International: Section B: The Sciences & Engineering, 58 (9-B)*, 5142.

Stanovich, K. E. (1986). Matthew effects in reading: Some consequences of individual differences in the acquisition of literacy. *Reading Research Quarterly, 21*, 360-407.

Stanovich, K. E. (1988a). Explaining the differences between the dyslexic and the garden-variety poor reader: The phonological-core variable-difference mode. *Journal of Learning Disabilities, 21*, 590-612.

Stanovich, K. E. (1988b). The right and wrong places to look for the cognitive locus of reading disability. *Annals of Dyslexia, 38*, 154-177.

Stanovich, K. E. (1991). Conceptual and empirical problems with discrepancy definitions of reading disability. *Learning Disability Quarterly, 14*, 269-280.

Stanovich, K. E. (1991). Discrepancy definition of reading disability: Has intelligence led us astray? *Reading Research Quarterly, 26*, 7-29.

Stanovich, K. E. (1999). The sociopsychometrics of learning disabilities. *Journal of Learning Disabilities, 32*, 350-361.

Stanovich, K. E., & Siegel, L. S. (1994). The phenotypic performance profile of reading-disabled children: A regression-based test of the phonological-core variable-difference model. *Journal of Educational Psychology, 86*, 24-53.

Stanovich, K. E., Siegel, L. S., & Gottardo, A. (1997). Converging evidence for phonological and surface subtypes of reading disability. *Journal of Educational psychology, 89*, 114-127.

Steel, J. G., Gorman, R., & Flexman, J. E. (1984). Case report: Neuropsychiatric testing of an autistic mathematical idiot-savant. *Journal of the American Academy of Child Psychology, 23*, 704-707.

Stein, J., & Walsh, V. (1997). To see but not to read: The magnocellular theory of dyslexia. *Trends in Neurosciences, 20*(4), 147-152.

Stevenson, J. (1992). Evidence for a genetic etiology in hyperactivity in children. *Behavior Genetics, 22*, 337-344.

Stevenson, J., Graham, P., Fredman, G., & McLoughlin, V. (1987). A twin study of genetic influences on reading and spelling ability and disability. *Journal of Child Psychology and Psychiatry, 28*(2), 229-247.

Stevenson, J., Pennington, B. F., Gilger, J. W., DeFries, J. C., & Gillis, J. J. (1993). Hyperactivity and spelling disability: Testing for shared genetic actiology. *Journal of Child Psychology and Psychiatry and Allied Disciplines, 34*, 1137-1152.

Stewart, M. A., Cumming, C., Singer, S., & Deblois, C. S. (1981). The overlap between hyperactive and undersocialized aggressive children. *Journal Child Psychol Psychiatry, 22*, 35-45.

Still, G. F. (1902). Some abnormal psychical conditions in children. *The Lancet, I*, 1008-1012, 1077-1082.

Strauss, A. A., & Lehtinen, L. E. (1947). *The psychopathy and education of the brain-injured child.* (Vol. 1). New York: Grune & Stratton.

Stroop, J. R. (1935). Studies of interference in serial verbal reactions. *Journal of Experimental Psychology, 18*, 643-662.

Stuss, D. T., & Benson, D. F. (1986). *The Frontal Lobes.* New York: Raven Press.

Sullivan, C., & Grosser, G. S. (1996). *Dyslexia Research and Resource Guide*. Boston: Allyn and Bacon.

Sunohara, G., Barr, C., Jain, U., Schachar, R., & et al. (1997). Association of the D4 receptor gene in individuals with ADHD. *American Society of Human Genetics, Baltimore*.

Swanson, J., Castellanos, F. X., Miroas, M., Lahoste, G., & Kennedy, J. (1998). Cognitive Neuroscience of attention deficit hyperactivity disorder and hyperkinetic disorder. *Current Opinion in Neurobiology, 8*(2), 263-271.

Swanson, J. M., Sunohara, G. A., Kennedy, J. L., & et al. (1998). Association of the dopamine receptor D4 (DRD4) gene with a refined phenotype of attention deficit hyperactivity disorder (ADHD): A family-based approach. *Mol Psychiatry, 3*, 38-41.

Szatmari, P. (1992). The epidemiology of attention-deficit hyperactive disorders. In G. Weiss (Ed.), *Child and adolescent psychiatry clinics of North America: Attention deficit hyperactivity disorder*. Philadelphia, PA: Saunders.

Tager-Flusberg, H. (1985). The conceptual basis for referential word meaning in children with autism. *Child Development, 56*, 1167-1178.

Tager-Flusberg, H. (1991). Semantic processing in the free recall of autistic children: Further evidence of a cognitive deficit. *British Journal of Developmental Psychology, 9*, 417-430.

Tallal, P. (1976). Rapid auditory processing in normal and disordered language development. *Journal of Speech and Hearing, 19*, 561-571.

Tallal, P., Miller, S., & Fitch, R. H. (1996). Neurobiological basics of speech: A case for the preeminence of temporal processing. In C. H. Chase, G. D. Rosen, & G. F. Sherman (Eds.), *Developmental Dyslexia* (pp. 159-184). Baltimore, MD: York Press.

Tallal, P., & Piercy, M. (1979). Defects of auditory perception in children with developmental dysphasia. In M. A. Syke (Ed.), *Developmental Dysphasia* (pp. 63-84). Orlando, FL: Academic Press, Inc.

Tannock, R. (1998). Attention deficit hyperactivity disorder: Advances in cognitive, neurobiological, and genetic research. *Journal Child Psychol Psychiat, 39*, 65-99.

Tashman, B. (1995,). Misreading dyslexia. *Scientific American, August*, 14-16.

Taylor, E. (1994). Syndromes of attention deficit and overactivity. In M. Rutter, E. Taylor, & L. Hersov (Eds.), *Child and adolescent psychiatry: Modern approaches*. Oxford, England: Blackwell Scientific.

Taylor, E., Sandberg, S., Thorley, G., & Giles, S. (1991). *The epidemiology of childhood hyperactivity*. Oxford, UK: Oxford University Press.

Technology-Related Assistance for Individuals with Disabilities Act. (1988). P. L. 100-47, 29 U.S.C. 2001.

Thapar, A., Holmes, J., Poulton, K., & Harrington, R. (1999). Genetic basis of attention deficit and hyperactivity. *British Journal of Psychiatry, 174*, 105-111.

Tomb, D. A. (1998). *The psychiatric clinics of North America*. Philadelphia, PA: W. B. Saunders Company.

Torgesen, J. K. (1991). Subtypes as prototypes: Extended studies of rationally defined extreme groups. In L. V. Feagans, E. J. Short, & L. J. Meltzer (Eds.), *Subtypes of learning disabilities: Theoretical perspectives and research* (pp. 229-246). Hillsale, NJ: Earlbaum.

Torgesen, J. K., Wagner, R. K., & Rashotte, C. A. (1994). Longitudinal studies of phonological processing and reading. *Journal of Learning Disabilities, 27*, 286-286.

Torgeson, J. K. (1991). Learning disabilities: Historical and conceptual issues. In B. Y. L. Wong (Ed.), *Learning about learning disabilities*. San Diego, CA: Academic Press.

Torgeson, J. K. (1998). Instructional interventions for children with reading disabilities. In P. J. Accardo & A. J. Capute (Eds.), *Specific Reading Disability: A View of the Spectrum* . Timonium, MD: York Press.

Townsend, J., & Courchesne, E. (1994). Parietal damage and narrow "spotlight" spatial attention. *Journal of Cognitive Neuroscience, 6*, 220-232.

Traub, N., & Bloom, F. (1975). *Recipe for Reading.* Cambridge, MA: Educators Publishing Service.

Triolo, S. J. (1999). *Attention deficit hyperactivity disorder in adulthood.* Philadelphia: Taylor and Francis.

Triolo, S. J., & Murphy, K. R. (1996). *Attention-deficit scales for adults (ADSA) manual for scoring and interpretation.* New York: Brunner/Mazel.

Triolo, S. J., & Murphy, K. R. (1997). *Attention-deficit scales for adults (ADSA): Windows version.* New York: Brunner/Mazel.

TRLD. (2000, January 26-29). Technology, reading, and learning difficulties. *Reading Success for College Students.* San Francisco, CA.

Troller, J. N. (1999). Attention deficit hyperactivity disorder in adults: Conceptual and clinical issues. *Medical Journal of Australia, 171*, 421-425.

Tsatsanis, K. D., & Rourke, B. P. (1995). Conclusions and future directions. In B. P. Rourke (Ed.), *Syndrome of nonverbal learning disabilities* (pp. 476-508). New York: Guilford.

Tucker, D. M. (1986). Hemisphere specialization: A mechanism for unifying anterior and posterior brain regions. In D. Ottoson (Ed.), *Duality and Unity of the Brain: Unified Functioning and Specialization of the Hemispheres.* New York: Plenum Press.

Tucker, D. M., & Williamson, P. A. (1984). Asymmetric neural control in systems in human self-regulation. *Psychological Review, 91*, 185-215.

Turnock, P. (1998). Academic coping strategies in college students with symptoms of AD/HD. In P. Quinn & A. McCormick (Eds.), *Rethinking AD/HD.* Bethesda, MD: Advantage Books.

Tzelepis, A., Schubiner, H., & Warbasse, L. (1995). Differential diagnosis and psychiatric comorbidity patterns in adult ADD. In K. Nadeau (Ed.), *A comprehensive guide to attention-deficit disorder in adults.* New York: Brunner/Mazel.

U. S. Department of Education. (1977). *Definition and criteria for defining students as learning disabled.* 42 Fed. Reg. 65, 083. Washington, DC: U. S. Government Printing Office.

U. S. Department of Education. (1989). *To assure the free appropriate education of all handicapped children: Eleventh report to Congress on the implementation of the Education for the Handicapped Act.* Washington, DC: Department of Education.

U. S. Department of Education. (1991). *Memorandum to chief state school officers, subject: Clarification of policy to address the needs of children with attention deficit disorders within general and/or special education.* Washington, DC: Office of Special Education and Rehabilitative Services, Office for Civil Rights and Office of Elementary and Secondary Education.

van Bourgpndien, M. E., & Mesibov, G. B. (1987). Humor in high-functioning autistic adults. *Journal of Autism and Developmental Disorders, 17*, 417-424.

Van der Oord, E. J. C. G., Boomsma, D. I., & Verhulst, F. C. (1994). A study of problem behaviors in 10- to 15-year old biologically related and unrelated international adoptees. *Behavior Genetics, 24*, 193-205.

VerFaellie, M., & Heilman, K. M. (1987). Response preparation and response inhibition after lesions of the medial frontal lobe. *Arch Neurol, 44*, 1265-1271.

Voeller, K. K. S. (1986). Right hemisphere deficit syndrome in children. *American Journal of Psychiatry, 143*, 1004-1009.

Voeller, K. K. S. (1991). Social-emotional learning disabilities. *Psychiatric Annals, 21*, 735-741.

Voeller, K. K. S. (1991). Toward a neurobiologic nosology of Attention Deficit Hyperactivity disorder. *Journal of Clinical Neurology, 6,* S2-S8.

Voeller, K. K. S. (1997). Social and emotional learning disabilities. In T. E. Feinberg & M. J. Farah (Eds.), *Behavioral neurology and neuropsychology* (pp. 795-801). New York: McGraw-Hill.

Voeller, K. K. S., & Heilman, K. M. (1988, September). *Motor impersistence in children with attention deficit hyperactivity disorder: Evidence for right hemisphere dysfunction.* Paper presented at the 17th annual meeting of the Child Neurology Society, Halifax, Nova Scotia, Canada.

Vogel, S. A. (1990). Gender differences in intelligence, language, visual-motor abilities, and academic achievement in students with learning disabilities: A review of the literature. *Journal of Learning Disabilities, 23*(1), 44-52.

Vogel, S. A. (1996). Employment. A research review and agenda. In S. C. Cramer & W. Ellis (Eds.), *Learning Disabilities: Lifelong Issues.* Baltimore, MD: Paul H. Brookes.

Vogel, S. A., Hruby, P. J., & Adelman, P. B. (1993). Educational and psychological factors in successful and unsuccessful college students with learning disabilities. *Learning Disabilities Research & Practice, 8*(1), 34-43.

Vogel, S. A., Leyser, Y., Wyland, S., & Brulle, A. (1999). Students with learning disabilities in higher education: Faculty attitude and practices. *Learning Disabilities Research & Practice, 14*(3), 173-186.

Vogel, S. A., & Reder, S. (1998). Literacy proficiency among adults with self-reported learning disabilities. In M. C. Smith (Ed.), *Literacy for the Twenty-First Century* (pp. 159-171). Westport, CT: Praeger.

Volkmar, F. R., Hoder, E. L., & Cohe, D. J. (1985). Compliance, 'negativisim', and the effects of treatment structure in autism: A naturalistic, behavioral study. *Journal of Child Psychology and Psychiatary, 26,* 865-877.

Wachelka, D., & Katz, R. (1999). Reducing test anxiety and improving academic self-esteem in high school and college students with learning disabilities. *Journal of Behavior Therapy and Experimental Psychiatry, 30,* 191-198.

Wagner, M. M., & Blackorby, J. (1996). Transition from high school to work or college: How special education students fare. *Special Education for Students with Disabilities, 6*(1).

Wagner, R. K., & Torgesen, J. K. (1987). The nature of phonological processing and its causal role in the acquisition of reading skills. *Psychological Bulletin, 101,* 192-212.

Wagner, R. K., Torgesen, J. K., & Rashote, L. S. (1999). *Comprehensive Test of Phonological Processing (CTOPP).* Austin, TX: Pro-Ed.

Wainwright-Sharp, J. A., & Bryson, S. E. (1996). Visual-spatial orienting in autism. *Journal of Autism and Developmental Disorders, 26,* 423-438.

Wainwright-Sharp, J. W., & Bryson, S. E. (1993). Visual orienting deficits in high functioning people with autism. *Journal of Autism and Developmental Disorders, 26,* 423-438.

Walberg, H. J., & Tsai, S. (1983). Matthew effects in education. *American Educational Research Journal, 20,* 359-373.

Waldo, S. L., McIntosh, D. E., & Koller, J. R. (1999). Personality profiles of adults with verbal and nonverbal learning disabilities. *Journal of Psychoeducational Assessment, 17,* 196-206.

Walkup, J. T., Khan, S., Schuerholz, L., Pail, Y. S., Leckman, & Schultz, R. T. (1999). Phenomenology and natural history of tic-related ADHD and learning disabilities. In J. F. Leckman & R. T. Schulz (Eds.), *Tourette's syndrome - tics, obsessions, compulsions* (pp. 63-79). New York: John Wiley & Sons, Inc.

Weaver, S. (1993). *The validity of the use of extended and untimed testing for postsecondary students with learning disabilities.* Unpublished Doctoral dissertation, University of Toronto.

Wechsler, D. (1955). *Wechsler Adult Intelligence Scale manual.* San Antonio, TX: Psychological Corporation.

Wechsler, D. (1981). *WAIS-R manual.* San Antonio, TX: Psychological Corporation.

Wechsler, D. (1981). *Wechsler Adult Intelligence Scale - Revised.* San Antonio, TX: The Psychological Corporation.

Wechsler, D. (1987). *Wechsler memory scale.* (Third ed.). San Antonio, TX: Psychological Corporation.

Wechsler, D. (1992). *Wechsler Individual Achievement Test.* New York: The Psychological Corporation.

Wechsler, D. (1997). *WAIS-III administration and scoring manual.* San Antonio, TX: Psychological Corporation.

Wechsler, D. (1997). *Wechsler adult intelligence scale.* (Third ed.). San Antonio, TX: Psychological Corporation.

Weinberg, W. A., & McLean, A. (1986). A diagnostic approach to developmental specific learning disorders. *Journal of Child Neurology, 1,* 158-172.

Weintraub, S., & Mesulam, M. (1983). Developmental learning disabilities of the right hemisphere: Emotional, interpersonal, and cognitive components. *Archives of Neurology, 40,* 463-468.

Weintraub, S., & Mesulam, M. M. (1985). Mental state assessment of young and elderly adults in behavioral neurology. In M. M. Mesulam (Ed.), *Principles of Behavioral Neurology* (pp. 71-123). Philadelphia, PA: Davis.

Weiss, G., Hechtman, L., Milroy, T., & Perlman, T. (1985). Psychiatric status of hyperactives as adults: A controlled prospective 15-year follow-up of 63 hyperactive children. *Journal of the American Academy of Child Psychiatry, 24,* 211-220.

Weiss, L. (1992). *Attention deficit disorder in adults: Practical help for sufferers and their spouses.* Dallas, TX: Taylor Publishing.

Weiss, L. (1994). *The attention deficit disorder in adults workbook.* Dallas, TX: Taylor Publishing Company.

Welsh, M. C., Pennington, B. F., & Rogers, S. (1987). Word recognition and comprehension skills in hyperlexic children. *Brain and Language, 32,* 76-96.

Wender, E. H. (1995). Attention-deficit hyperactivity disorders in adolescence. *Journal of Developmental and Behavioral Pediatrics, 16,* 192-195.

Wender, P. H. (1971). *Minimal brain dysfunction in children.* New York: Wiley-Interscience Publishers, Inc.

Wender, P. H. (1998). Attention-Deficit Hyperactivity Disorder in adults. In D. A. Tomb (Ed.), *The Psychiatric clinics of North America* (pp. 761-775). Philadelphia, PA: W. B. Saunders Co.

Wender, P. H., & Reimherr, F. W. (1990). Bupropion treatment of attention-deficit hyperactivity disorder in adults. *American Journal of Psychiatry, 147*(8), 1018-1020.

Wender, P. H., Reimherr, F. W., Wood, D., & Ward, M. (1985). A controlled study of methylphenidate in the treatment of Attention Deficit Disorder, residual type, in adults. *American Journal of Psychiatry, 142*(5), 547-552.

Wender, P. H., Reimherr, F. W., & Wood, D. R. (1981). Attention Deficit Disorder ('minimal brain dysfunction') in adults. *Arch Gen Psychiatry, 38,* 449-456.

Wender, P. H., Wood, D. R., & Reimherr, F. W. (1985). Pharmacological treatment of attention deficit disorder, residual type (ADD, RT, "minimal brain dysfunction," "hyperactivity") in adults. *Psychopharmacology Bulletin, 21*(2), 222-227.

Wender, P. H., Wood, D. R., Reimherr, F. W., & Ward, M. (1983). An open trial of pargyline in the treatment of attention deficit disorder residual type. *Psychiatry Research, 9*, 329-336.

Westberry, S. J. (1994). A review of learning strategies for adults with learning disabilities preparing for the GED exam. *Journal of Learning Disabilities, 27*(4), 202-209.

Wetzel, K. (1996). Speech-recognizing computers: A written-communication tool for students with learning disabilities? *Journal of Learning Disabilities, 29*, 371-380.

White, J. L., Moffit, T. E., & Silva, P. A. (1992). Neuropsychological and socio-emotional correlates of specific-arithmetic disability. *Archives of Clinical Neuropsychology, 7*, 1-16.

Whitehouse, D., & Harris, J. C. (1984). Hyperlexia in infantile autism. *Journal of Autism and Developmental Disorders, 26*, 423-438.

Wiederholt, J. L., & Bryant, B. R. (1992). *Gray oral reading tests.* Austin, TX: Pro-Ed.

Wiig, E. H., & Secord, W. (1989). *Test of Language Competence - Expanded Edition.* San Antonio, TX: Psychological Corporation.

Wilens, T., Biederman, J., Mick, E., & et al. (1997). Attention-deficit hyperactivity disorder (ADHD) is associated with early-onset substance use disorders. *Journal Nerv Ment Dis, 185*, 475-482.

Wilens, T. E., Beiderman, J., & Mick, E. (1998). Does ADHD affect the course of substance abuse? Findings from a sample of adults with and without ADHD. *The American Journal on Addictions, 7*, 156-163.

Wilens, T. E., & Biederman, J. (1992). The stimulants. In D. Shafer (Ed.), *The psychiatric clinics of North America* (pp. 191-222). Philadelphia, PA: W. B. Saunders.

Wilens, T. E., Biederman, J., & Spencer, T. (1995b). Venlafaxine for adult ADHD (letter). *American Journal of Psychiatry.*

Wilens, T. E., Biederman, J., Spencer, T. J., & et al. (1994). Comorbidity of attention-deficit hyperactivity disorder and the psychoactive substance use disorders. *Hosp Community Psychiatry, 45*, 421-435.

Wilens, T. E., Biederman, J., Spencer, T. J., & et al. (1999). A pilot controlled clinical trial of ABT-418, a cholinergic agonist, in the treatment of adults with attention deficit hyperactivity disorder. *American Journal of Psychiatry, 156*(12), 1931-1937.

Wilens, T. E., Spencer, T. J., & Biederman, J. (1995a). Pharmacotherapy of adult ADHD. In K. G. Nadeau (Ed.), *A comprehensive guide to attention deficit disorder in adults* . New York: Brunner/Mazel, Inc.

Wilkinson, G. S. (1993). *The wide range achievement test.* Wilmington, DE: Wide Range, Inc.

Willcutt, E. G., & Pennington, B. F. (2000). Comorbidity of reading disability and attention-deficit/hyperactivity disorder: Differences by gender and subtype. *Journal of Learning Disabilities, 33*(2), 179-191.

Willcutt, E. G., Pennington, B. F., Chhabildas, N. A., Frieman, M. C., & Alexander, J. (1999). Psychiatric comorbidity associated with DSM-IV ADHD in a nonreferred sample of twins. *Journal of American Academy of Child and Adolescent Psychiatry, 38*(11), 1355-1362.

Williams, D. T., Meh., R., Yudofsky, S., Adams, D., & Roseman, B. (1982). The effect of propranolol on uncontrolled rage outbursts in children and adolescents with organic brain dysfunction. *Journal of the American Academy of Child Psychiatry, 21*(2), 129-135.

Willows, D. M., Kruk, R. S., & Corcos, E. (1993). *Visual processes in reading and reading disabilities.* Hillsdale, NJ: Earlbaum Associates, Inc.

Wilson, B. A. (1987). *Rehabilitation of memory.* New York: Guilford Press.

Wilson, B. A. (1988). *Wilson Reading System Program Overview.* Millbury, MA: Wilson Language Training.

Wing, L. (1985). Early childhood autism and Asperger's syndrome. In P. Pichot, P. Berner, R. Wolf, & K. Thau (Eds.), *Psychiatry: The state of the art* (pp. 47-52). New York: Plenum.

Winokus, G. (1974). The division of depressive illness into depression spectrum disease and pure depressive disease. *International Pharmacopsychiatry, 9*, 5-13.

Witkin, H. A., Oltman, P., Raskin, E., & Karp, S. (1971). *Manual for the children's embedded figures test.* Palo Alto, CA: Consulting Psychologists Press.

Witte, R. H., Philips, L., & Kakela, M. (1998). Job satisfaction of college graduates with learning disabilities. *Journal of Learning Disabilities, 31*(7), 259-263.

Wolf, M. (1982). The word-retrieval process and reading in children and aphasics. In K. nelson (Ed.), *Children's Language* (pp. 437-493). Hillsdale, NJ: Earlbaum.

Wolf, M. (1991). *Word-wraiths: The unique contribution of the naming speed to reading prediction and intervention in developmental dyslexia.* Paper presented at the Annual meeting of the Society for Research in Child Development, Seattle, WA.

Wolf, M. (1991a). Naming speed and reading: The contribution of the cognitive neurosciences. *Reading Research Quarterly, 26*(2), 123-141.

Wolf, M. (1996, November). *The double-deficit hypothesis for the developmental dyslexias.* Paper presented at the Orton Dyslexia Society, Boston, MA.

Wolf, M. (1997). A provisional integrative account of phonological and naming-speed deficits in dyslexia: Implications for diagnosis and intervention. In B. Blachman (Ed.), *Foundations of reading acquisition* (pp. 67-92). Hillsdale, NJ: Earlbaum.

Wolf, M., & Bowers, P. G. (1999). The double-deficit hypothesis for the developmental dyslexias. *Journal of Educational Psychology, 9*(3), 415-438.

Wolf, M., Pfeil, C., Lotz, R., & Biddle, K. (1994). Towards a more universal understanding of developmental dyslexias: The contribution of orthographic factors. In V. Gerninger (Ed.), *The varieties of orthographic knowledge* (pp. 137-172). Boston: Kluwer Academic Publishers.

Wong, B. Y. L. (1996). *The ABC's of learning disabilities.* San Diego, CA: Academic Press.

Wong, B. Y. L., Butler, D. L., Ficzere, S. A., & Kuperis, S. (1996). Teaching adolescents with learning disabilities and low achievers to plan, write, and revise opinion essays. *Journal of Learning Disabilities, 29*(2), 197-212.

Wong, B. Y. L., Butler, D. L., Ficzere, S. A., & Kuperis, S. (1997). Teaching adolescents with learning disabilities and low achievers to plan, write, and revise compare-and-contrast essays. *Learning Disabilities Research & Practice, 12*(1), 2-15.

Wong, B. Y. L., Butler, D. L., Ficzere, S. A., Kuperis, S., Corden, M., & Zelmer, J. (1994). Teaching problem learners revision skills and sensitivity to audience through two instructional modes: Student-teacher versus student-student interactive dialogues. *Learning Disabilities Research & Practice, 9*(2), 78-90.

Wong, B. Y. L., Wong, R., & Blenkinsop, J. (1989). Cognitive and metacognitive aspects of learning disabled adolescents' composing problems. *Learning Disability Quarterly, 12*(4), 300-322.

Wood, D. R., Reimherr, F. W., & Wender, P. H. (1983). The use of l-Deprenyl in the treatment of attention deficit disorder, residual type. *Psychopharmacology Bulletin, 19*(4), 627-629.

Wood, D. R., Reimherr, F. W., Wender, P. H., & Johnson, G. E. (1976). Diagnosis and treatment of minimal brain dysfunction in adults. *Arc Gen Psychiatry, 33*, 1453-1459.

Wood, F., Felton, R., Flowers, L., & Naylor, C. (1991). Neurobehavioral definition of dyslexia. In D. D. Duane & D. B. Gray (Eds.), *The Reading Brain* . Parkton, MD: York Press.

Wood, F. B., Flowers, D. L., Buchsbaum, M., & Tallal, P. (1991). Investigation of abnormal left temporal functioning in dyslexia through rCBF auditory evoked potentials, and positron emission tomography. *Reading and Writing: An Interdisciplinary Journal, 4*, 81-95.

230

Woodcock, R. W. (1987). *Woodcock Reading Mastery Tests - Revised*. Circle Pines, MN: AGS.

Woodcock, R. W. (1987). *Woodcock Reading Mastery Tests - Revised*. Circle Pines, MN: American Guidance Service.

Woodcock, R. W. (1991). *Woodcock language proficiency battery - revised*. Chicago, IL: Riverside Publishing Company.

Woodcock, R. W., & Johnson, M. B. (1989). *Woodcock-Johnson tests of achievement*. Chicago, IL: Riverside Publishing Company.

Woolston, J. L., Rosenthal, S. L., Riddle, M. A., & et al. (1989). Childhood comorbidity of anxiety/affective disorders and behavior disorders. *Journal of American Academy of Child and Adolescent Psychiatry, 28*, 707-713.

Wozniak, J., Biederman, J., Kiely, K., & et al. (1995a). Mania-like symptoms suggestive of childhood onset bipolar disorder in clinically referred children. *Journal of the American Academy of Child and Adolescent Psychiatry, 34*, 867-876.

Xin, M. (2000). A longitudinal assessment of antecedent course work in mathematics and subsequent mathematical attainment. *Journal of Education Research, 94*, 16-28.

Yakovlev, P. I., & Lecours, A. R. (1967). The myelogenic cycles of regional maturation of the brain. In A. Minkowski (Ed.), *Regional development of the brain in early life* (pp. 3-23). Oxford, UK: Blackwell.

Yellin, A. M., Hopwood, J. H., & Greenberg, L. M. (1982). Adults and adolescents with Attention Deficit Disorder: Clinical and behavioral responses to psychostimulants. *Journal of Clinical Psychopharmacology, 2*(2), 133-136.

Yirmiya, N., & Sigman, M. (1991). High functioning individuals with autism: Diagnosis, empirical findings, and theoretical issues. *Clinical Psychology Review, 11*, 669-683.

Zametkin, A., & Rapoport, J. (1986). The pathophysiology of attention deficit disorder with hyperactivity: A review. In B. B. Lahey & A. Kazdin (Eds.), *Advances in clinical child psychology* (pp. 177-216). New York: Plenum Press.

Zametkin, A. J., & Liotta, W. (1998). The neurobiology of Attention-Deficit/Hyperactivity Disorder. *Clinical Psychiatry, 59*, 17-23.

Zametkin, A. J., Nordahl, T. E., Gross, M., King, C., & et al. (1990). Cerebral glucose metabolism in adults with hyperactivity of childhood onset. *New England Journal of Medicine, 323*, 1361-1366.

Zametkin, A. J., & Rapoport, J. L. (1987). Neurobiology of attention deficit disorder with hyperactivity: Where have we come in 50 years? *Journal of American Academy of Child and Adolescent Psychiatry, 26*, 676-686.

Zentall, S. S. (1993). Research on the educational implications of attention deficit hyperactivity disorder. *Exceptional Children, 60*, 143-153.

Zentall, S. S., & Ferkis, M. A. (1993). Mathematical problem solving for youth with ADHD, with and without learning disabilities. *Learning Disability Quarterly, 16*, 6-18.

Zerbin-Rudin, E. (1967). Kongenitale wortblindheit oder spezifische dyslexie (congenital word-blindness). *Bulletin of the Orton Society, 17*, 47-54.

Zigmond, N. (1990). Rethinking secondary school programs for students with learning disabilities. *Focus on Exceptional Children, 23*(1), 1-21.

Zigmond, N., & Thornton, H. (1985). Follow-up of postsecondary age learning disabled graduates and dropouts. *Learning Disabilities Research, 1*, 50-55.

Zoccolillo, M. (1993). Gender and the development of conduct disorder. *Development and Psychopathology, 5*, 65-78.

Zubin, J. (1975). Problem of attention in schizophrenia. In M. L. Kietzman, S. Sutton, & J. Zubin (Eds.), *Experimental approaches to psychopathology* (pp. 139-166). New York: Academic Press.

INDEX